Library of Old English and Medieval Literature

THE BEGINNINGS OF POETRY

Library of Old English and Medieval Literature

THE BEGINNINGS OF POETRY

BY

FRANCIS B. GUMMERE

BOOKS FOR LIBRARIES PRESS
FREEPORT, NEW YORK

First Published 1901
Reprinted 1970

STANDARD BOOK NUMBER:
8369-5313-4

LIBRARY OF CONGRESS CATALOG CARD NUMBER:
71-114908

PRINTED IN THE UNITED STATES OF AMERICA

I ne have no text of it, as I suppose,
But I shal fynde it in a maner glose.

CANTERBURY TALES, 1919 f.

PREFACE

THE opening pages of this book contain, so one may hope, an adequate answer to the objections of those who may have been led by its title to expect a more detailed treatment of poetic origins and a closer study of such questions as the early forms of rhythm, the beginnings of national literatures, and the actual history of lyric, epic, and drama. Not these problems have been undertaken, interesting and important as they are, but rather the rise of poetry as a social institution; whether or not a definite account of this process has been obtained must be left for the reader to judge.

F. B. G.

9 SEPTEMBER, 1901.

CONTENTS

CHAPTER I

PURPOSE AND METHOD

PAGE

Object of the book. Historical and comparative treatment. Sources of help. Modern scientific aids. Limitations to their value. The evidence of poetry itself. The curve of evolution . . . 1

CHAPTER II

RHYTHM AS THE ESSENTIAL FACT OF POETRY

Definitions of poetry. The line between poetry and prose. Summary of the dispute. Rhythm fundamental and essential in poetry. Proofs from ethnology, psychology, and the history of poetry itself 30

CHAPTER III

THE TWO ELEMENTS IN POETRY

The dualism in its various forms. Poetry of nature and of art. Poetry of the people. Romantic and rationalistic theories. The real dualism 116

CHAPTER IV

THE DIFFERENCING ELEMENTS OF THE POETRY OF ART

Communal and individual. Mediæval and modern conditions. Evolution of sentimental lyric. Influence of Christianity. Reactions. Modern objective poetry. Humour 139

CHAPTER V

THE DIFFERENCING ELEMENTS OF COMMUNAL POETRY

The making of communal poetry a closed account. Elements of the European ballad. Who made it. The "I" of ballads. Style

PAGE

of ballads. Incremental repetition. Variation. Siberian songs. Bridal songs. The *vocero* and kindred songs of mourning. The refrain. Refrains and songs of labour. Harvest-home. Processions. Flytings. Festal refrains. The dance . . 163

CHAPTER VI

SCIENCE AND COMMUNAL POETRY

Science and theories of poetic origins. Invention and imitation. Comparative literature and the art of borrowing. The war against instinct. Instinct not set aside. The dualism in poetry. Greek drama. Homogeneity of savages and of primitive men . 347

CHAPTER VII

THE EARLIEST DIFFERENTIATIONS OF POETRY

The poet. Improvisation in a throng. A study of the *schnaderhüpfl*. Stanzas and poems. Differentiation of poetry. Lyric, drama, and epic. Myths. Poetic style 390

CHAPTER VIII

THE TRIUMPH OF THE ARTIST

Improvisation revived. Its fate. The two forces in poetry. Past and present 453

THE BEGINNINGS OF POETRY

THE BEGINNINGS OF POETRY

CHAPTER I

PURPOSE AND METHOD

It is the object of the following pages neither to defend poetry nor to account for it, but simply to study it as a social institution. Questions of its importance, of the place which it has held, or ought to have held, in the esteem of men, and of the part which it is yet to play, are interesting but not vital to one who is bent upon the investigation of it as an element in human life. A defence is doubtless needed now and then by way of answer to the pessimist like Peacock, or to the moralist, the founder of states ideal or real, like Plato and Mahomet. Scattered about the Koran are hints that verse-making folk, like the shepherd's turncock, are booked for an unpleasant future, although it is well known that the prophet in earlier days had been very fond of poetry; while Plato himself, if one may believe his editors, began as a poet, but took to prose because the older art was declining; with the change he turned puritan as well, and saw no room for poets in his ideal state. Attacks of this sort, however, are as old as poetry itself, which, like "the service, sir," has been going to the dogs time out of mind, and very early formed the habit of looking back to better days. For mediæval relations these remembered arguments of Plato, backed by a band of Christian writers, had put the art to its shifts; but Aristotle's fragment[1] served the renaissance as adequate

[1] Twining, *Aristotle*, 2d ed., I. 183, thinks the original treatise was written as a defence against the "cavils of prosaic philosophers" and the objections of Plato.

answer, and it is interesting to note that the champion of poetry in Aristotle long outlived the philosopher.[1] Petrarch, taking the laurel, was moved to defend poetry against her foes, and yet found, as critics find now, that she had come by some of her worst wounds at the hands of her votaries; for who, in any age, as Goethe asked and answered in his *Divan*, "Who is driving poetry off the face of the earth?—The poets." Certainly not the philosophers and men of science, though that is the common belief. Lefebvre,[2] in 1697, thought that he had given poetry its mortal blow when he attacked it in the name of morals and of science; and his onslaught is worth the notice if only to show how little Renan and others urge to-day which has not been urged at any time since Petrarch. Selden,[3] Newton, Bentham, have been among the scoffers; so, too, Pascal. As to Newton, "A friend once said to him, 'Sir Isaac, what is your opinion of poetry?' His answer was, 'I'll tell you that of Barrow; he said that poetry was a kind of ingenious nonsense.'"[4] All this is no more than disrespectful allusion to the equator, jocose moments of the learned; yet it is quoted very seriously by those who think to preach a funeral sermon over the poetic art. So that when Renan expects to see poetry swallowed up by science, and when it is said that Goethe, born a century later, would throw poetry to the winds and give full play to his scientific genius, that Voltaire would live altogether for mathematics, and that Shakspere himself, "the great psychologist," would "leave the drama of humanity for

[1] In his curious book, *La Philosophie du Bon-Sens*, 1737, p. 15, D'Argens speaks of Aristotle "dont les Ouvrages sur la Poëtique sont aussi bons, que ceux dans lesquels il traite de la Philosophie sont peu utiles."

[2] *De Futilitate Poetices auctore Tanaquillo Fabro Tanaquilli filio Verbi Divini Ministro* . . ., Amstel., 1697. It was answered by the Abbé Massieu in a *Defense de la Poésie* (in *Hist. d. l. Poës. Françoise*, Paris, 1739), a pious but heavy performance.

[3] *Table Talk*, ed. Arber, pp. 85 f.

[4] Lord Radnor in Spence's *Anecdotes*, ed. Singer, p. 368.

the drama of the world," abjure wings, and settle to the collar with psychical research folk and societies for child-study, — even then the friends of poetry need feel no great alarm; all this, allowing for conditions of the time, was said long ago, and has been repeated in the dialect of each generation. As for the past of poetry, kings have been its nursing fathers and queens its nursing mothers; and for its future, one may well be content with the words of the late M. Guyau, a man of scientific training and instincts, who has looked carefully and temperately at the whole question and concludes[1] that "poetry will continue to be the natural language of all great and lasting emotion."

Vindication apart, there is the art of poetry, the technique, the Horatian view; and with this treatment of the subject the present work has as little to do as with defence and praise. From Vida even to Boileau writers on poetry were mainly concerned to teach the art, and seemed to assume that every bright boy ought to be trained as a poet. With this idea went the conception of poetry as sum and substance of right living and embodiment of all learning, sacred and profane, — witness not only the famous lines of Milton, but a part of the epitaph which Boccaccio composed for his own tomb: *studium fuit alma poesis*. J. C. Scaliger, when that early enthusiasm of the renaissance had begun to wane, turned from art to science; his son and Casaubon and the rest took up the work of research and let the art of poetry languish. On this scientific ground, where, in spite of the overthrow of Aristotelian authority, in spite of changes in method and a new range of material, one may still learn much from these pioneers, there are now three ways by which one can come to poetry from the outside, and regard it not technically but in the spirit of research: there is the theory of poetic impulses and processes in general; there is the criticism of

[1] *Problèmes de l'Esthétique Contemporaine*, pp. 89 ff., 255.

poems and poetry as an objective study; and there are the recording, the classifying, and the comparing of the poetic product at large. The present work belongs to this third division, and in its method must keep mainly within historical and comparative bounds. It is not concerned in any way with the poetic impulse, or with the poem as object of critical study; it regards the whole poetic product as a result of human activity working in a definite field. This must be clearly understood. At the outset of an attempt to throw some light upon the beginnings of poetry, it is well to bear in mind that by poetry is meant, not the poetic impulse, but the product of that impulse, and that by beginnings are meant the earliest actual appearances of poetry as an element in the social life of man, and not the origins or ultimate causes, biologically or psychologically considered, of poetic expression. What the origin of poetry may have been, and to what causes, however remote, in the body and life of man must be attributed the earliest conceivable rhythmic utterance, are questions for a tribunal where metaphysics and psychology on the one hand, and biology on the other hand, have entered conflicting claims. As for biology, until one has found the source of life itself, it is useless to follow brain dissections in an effort to discover the ultimate origins of poetry. To be sure, psychology has a legitimate field of inquiry in discussing the source of æsthetic manifestations;[1] and going deeper into things, it would be pleasant if one could lay hold of what philosophers call "the germinal power of whatever comes to be," the *keimkraft des seienden;* but times are hardly ripe for such a feat. Even Weismann[2] concedes a "soul," a capacity not yet explainable, for appre-

[1] Ribot, *Psychology of the Emotions*, pp. 329 ff., rejects Guyau's emendation of Grant Allen, and backs Groos in his view of the play theory.

[2] "Gedanken über Musik bei Thieren und beim Menschen," 1889, in *Deutsche Rundschau*, LXI. 50 ff.

ciating music, and, by implication, poetry. It is better in the present state of things to assume poetry as an element in human life, and to come as close as possible to its primitive stages, its actual beginnings. What these beginnings of poetry were, in what form it first made a place for itself among human institutions, and over what paths it wandered during the processes of growth and differentiation even in prehistoric times, are questions belonging to the answerable part of that catechism about his own life which man has been making and unmaking and making again ever since he began to remember and to forecast. We have here no concern with the perplexing question why æsthetic activity was first evolved; it is quite another matter when we undertake to learn how æsthetic activity made itself seen and felt. In brief, to seek the origins of poetry would be to seek the cause of its existence as a phenomenon, to hunt that elusive *keimkraft des seienden;* to inquire into the beginnings of poetry is to seek conditions and not causes.

Nothing, however, is harder than to carry out this simple plan; from a work on poetry take away both theory and criticism, and what is left? It is true that since F. Schlegel, a hundred years ago, said[1] of art in general that its science is its history, historical and comparative treatment of poetry has come speedily to the fore; but that mystery which rightly enough clings to a poetic process, the traditions of sanctity which belong to genius, and the formidable literature of æsthetics, have all worked together to keep the study of poetry out of line with the study of other human institutions, and to give it an unchartered freedom from the control of facts which has done more harm than good. Consider that touch of futility which vexes the mind when it sets about discussion of a topic so far from the daily business of life; consider the great cloud of witnesses who can be summoned

[1] *Athenæum*, III. 67.

from any library to prove that of all printed silliness nothing reaches quite so silly a pitch as twaddle about the bards; add, too, that no process is so difficult to observe and analyze as the making of a poem; and it is easy to see why writers on poetry are always flying to cover in psychology and æsthetics or in criticism.[1] Facing the facts of poetry, a scholar can treat the poetic impulse and keep the facts at arm's length, or even quite out of his range. Treating the poetic product, whether genetically or historically or comparatively, tracing the evolution of poetry as a whole, for its own laws of growth and decay, or regarding its place as

[1] Criticism has been treated of late with scientific precision. See the bibliographical array in Gayley and Scott's admirable *Methods and Materials of Literary Criticism*, Boston, 1899. From the imperial critic, the "gentle reader" and patron represented by Montaigne, who gives no reasons but his own likes and dislikes, as witness that delightful essay on books, in its opening sentence, through the official critics, down to M. Brunetière, the scientific critic, faithful to the doctrine of evolution in general, and attentive to the law in the particular case, it is to be noted how criticism has been approaching the sociological domain, the study of poetry as an element of human life. Sainte-Beuve was still a critic of poets and poems, for all his "natural method"; Taine crossed the border and studied poetry, the product, under sociological and ethnological conditions. See Sainte-Beuve, *Nouveaux Lundis*, VIII. 87 f., 69 f.; IX. 70; and Taine, *Derniers Essais*, Paris, 1894, pp. 58 f. M. Brunetière, in carrying on the plan of Taine, and Hennequin, in opposing it, work on sociological and historical ground, rather than in the old æsthetics. Hennequin's *Critique* is "scientifique"; while a title like M. Brunetière's *Evolution of Species in Literature* can be conceded to criticism only by taking such liberties with the word as to leave it practically undefined. Still, these men work for criticism if not in it, and they give no reason for disputing what is said in the text about the paucity of books on poetry as an element in human society. They have the modern poet, the modern poem, in view; they wish to lay down metes and bounds and adjust the law. Hennequin will found a new science, "an immense anthropology," made up of all the vital sciences (*Crit. Sci.*, pp. 185 f.); but his place is with the critics, and not with scholars in historical and comparative literature. His *æsthopsychology* indicates devotion to the poetic impulse rather than to the product. Mr. Granger (*Worship of the Romans*, p. vii) has lately called up the word *ethology*, suggested by Stuart Mill (*Logic of the Moral Sciences*, pp. 213 ff., 218), in line with a hint that the foundations of comparative psychology must be laid in the study of the people and of their habits of thought. Something of this sort has been done by M. Le Bon in his *Psychologie des Foules*, quoted below.

an institution in human society, he must hold unbroken commerce with a bewildering mass of material. Hence the delight which animates to their task the numberless writers of "thoughts about poetry," and the dismay with which the historian looks upon his rough and unwieldy subject. Books beyond the power of any modern reader to compass have been written on the poetic impulse; while all the books which treat the poetic product as an element of public life could be carried in one's pocket,[1] — and one need be no Schaunard for the task. Yet the facts of poetry ought to precede the theory, — facts, moreover, that should be brought into true relations with the development of social man. A record of actual poetry; then a history of its beginnings and progress as an achievement of human society; then an account of it with regard to its origin and exercise as a function of the individual mind, — such is the process by which there could have been built up a clear and rational science of poetry, the true poetics. *Dis aliter visum.* There is a fairly good record of poetry, with gaps due to chance and neglect, many of which chance and energy may yet combine to fill. As an achievement of human society, poetry has had scant attention; and the present work is intended, in however modest and imperfect performance, to supply material and make an outline for such a study.

With such an object in view, and in such a spirit, what is the method by which one is to come at the beginnings of poetry, and what material is one to employ? Literature itself, and the comparative, historical method, are indicated by the very terms of the quest; but what of other aids?

1 Such are the *Comparative Literature* of Posnett, and the less didactic work of Letourneau, *L'Évolution Littéraire dans les diverses Races Humaines*, Paris, 1894. The former was mainly pioneer work, meant to open and define its subject; and in this it attained its end. This sociological method has been applied, of course, in a critical way, to many individual works, and to many periods of literature; not so, however, with the poetic product at large.

There is no doubt that science has opened mines of research unknown to a former generation of scholars in poetics; what have zoology, physiology, psychology, ethnology, anthropology, sociology, to say to the beginnings of rhythmic utterance? From the study of those animals which stand nearest to man in intelligence and social instincts there should come in course of time a better knowledge of the physical conditions under which primitive folk essayed their earliest poetry; but it is conceded that the present state of these studies, even in obvious cases like the singing of birds and the social dances and amusements of sundry animals, offers scant help to the student of poetry, and often leads him into absurdities. Darwin's suggestion that the lyric poem might in some way go back to the call of the male *homo* to the female at mating time, induced Scherer to put the origins of poetry in general upon this purely biological basis;[1] but Scherer's enthusiasm has met no hearty response and seems to fly in the face of certain important facts. The book of Groos, to which further reference will be made, gives a better series of analogies with the subject in hand, but is not to be used in any positive or conclusive way.

Help of a more substantial kind can be found in the researches of modern psychology; and indeed, when these shall have been put in available form, they will greatly increase the materials for a study of the poetic process. To what extent the study of the poetic product, however, may use such aids, is a quite different question. For example, there

[1] There is more to be said for the partial origin of poetry in choral songs of a sexual character sung after the communal feast of the horde or clan. This "sex-freedom," so revolting to modern ideas, left late traces in history; and Professor Karl Pearson quotes Tsakni's *La Russie Sectaire* to the effect that such license still prevails at fairs and periodic festivals in Russia, combined with choral dance. — Pearson, *The Chances of Death*, II. 243. There are Australian festivals of this sort; and license of May-Day, of Shrove-Tuesday, and the rest, is familiar in European survival. On the other hand, it will be found that erotic poetry of the individual and lyric sort is almost unknown among savages.

is one doctrine, which, if it were established upon an absolute and universal truth, could be applied to the problem of primitive verse with such success as to throw a bridge over the chasm between what is recorded and what is unrecorded, and so lead one cannily into the midst of the unknown. The theory was laid down by Haeckel[1] that "ontogenesis, or the development of the individual, is a short and quick repetition"—or recapitulation—"of phylogenesis, or the development of the tribe to which it belongs, determined by the laws of inheritance and adaptation." Schultze, in his excellent book on fetishism,[2] uses this law, if law it be, in determining the mental state of primitive folk; "what is true of the child is true of the wild man, whose consciousness is in the childish embryonic stage," and who has reached the fetishistic epoch of mental growth. A savage who gets a clock wants to wrap it in costly furs; so does a child. Professor Baldwin, too, accepts the principle as a guide in working out analogies between the development of the child and the development of the race, of society.[3] For example, the consciousness of the "I" in children seems analogous in point of development to the individual consciousness of primitive man; and it is evidently of value to the student of early poetry to find his conclusion that such poetry is mainly impersonal backed by testimony from those who have studied the inner life of infants and children to the effect that fear, anger, likes and dislikes, are emotions that precede perception of the subject's own personality. A. W. Schlegel used

[1] *History of Creation*, 2 vols., trans., New York, 1893, I. 355, quoting from his *General Morphology*. He adds that by "tribe" he means "the ancestors which form the chain of progenitors of the individual concerned."

[2] *Der Fetischismus*, Leipzig, 1871, pp. 61, 74 f. A pretty little parallel of savages and children in the worship of images and dolls was drawn by M. Anatole France in a review of Lemonnier's *Comédie des Jouets*. See France, *La Vie Littéraire*, II. 10 ff.

[3] *Mental Development in the Child and the Race*, New York, 1895, pp. 15, 335 ff.; *Social and Ethical Interpretations*, New York, 1897, pp. 9, 189, etc.

this analogy a hundred years ago;[1] and, before him, Gottsched, who had far keener historic sense than one would suppose, explained early epic by the curiosity which children show in their demand for tales of every sort, adding that "primitive folk were exactly like these little creatures, who have no experience and such store of curiosity."[2] In fact, as is so often the case with a new exact theory in science, the general idea has been a commonplace time out of mind. Shelley, declaring that "the savage is to ages what the child is to years," is echoing eighteenth-century thought, with its idea of humanity passing from childhood to riper growth; and Turgot and Condorcet[3] only added the notion of human perfectibility and infinite development to an analogy which was first made, so it would seem, by the Italian Vico. The parallel is everywhere; Macaulay uses it in his theory of poetic degeneration, Peacock in his *Four Ages*, and Victor Hugo in the preface to *Cromwell.* Not as an idea, but as a formula, Mr. Spencer makes the biological doctrine of recapitulation a part of his sociological system. Professor Karl Pearson appeals to the same doctrine when he wishes to say a word for the matriarchate;[4] in the life of the child, he notes, "the mother and the woman play the largest part; and so it is in the religion and social institutions of primitive man." Thus a child's world reproduces the primitive world; and the *märchen*, where witches are still powerful though hated and malignant beings, show what is really the priestess of early matriarchal cult fallen into disfavour under patriarchal conditions. Or, finally, to choose an unexceptionable case, Professor Bücher,[5] noting that long-continued and laborious activity is easily kept up provided it pass as play and not as labour, takes

[1] *Vorlesungen*, Stuttgart, 1884, I. 275.
[2] *Critische Dichtkunst*, 1737, p. 87.
[3] *Esquisse des Progrès de l'Esprit-Humain.*
[4] Essay on "Ashiepattle" in *The Chances of Death*, II. 53.
[5] *Arbeit und Rhythmus*, p. 15.

the dances of savages, and the games of a civilized child, as analogous to the efforts of earliest man. It is true, too, that savages, and presumably early man, are like the child in quick alternations of mood, in the possibility of laughter and tears at once, in many traits of the kind; so far Letourneau[1] is perfectly right in his parallel. Now all these cases, in varying degree, are meant as arguments from analogy, and, as is usual when one deals with analogy, may be regarded as more or less desirable aids to evidence that is direct. By itself, however, analogy must not be conclusive; in the matter under consideration it cannot be regarded as proof; and alone this rule of ontogenesis and phylogenesis is not enough to bridge the chasm and allow one to describe prehistoric poetry.

Such, however, is precisely the task that some bold pioneers have essayed. Letourneau, indeed, is hardly to be placed in this category, although he upholds the doctrine and puts it to use;[2] for his conclusions are invariably fortified by facts from ethnology and literature. But the author of a book on primitive poetry, Jacobowski,[3] belongs here; freed from all obligations of research, all study of actual facts, he trips jauntily into the unknown, hand in hand with this omnipotent theory as guide. True, he affects the scientific habit of mind, and once refers the reader, for further light on some difficult problem, to "my little essay on the Psychology of a Kiss"; for he is by way of being a lyric poet, and seems of the tribe of him whom Heine described as "personal enemy of Jehovah, believing only in Hegel and in Canova's Venus," save that one must here make the

[1] *L'Évolution Littéraire*, p. 81.

[2] *Ibid.*, pp. 15 f., "répétition, approximative, abrégée surtout; mais néanmoins elle est une répétition." But at once he quotes some striking facts, in order to prove his thesis (that song preceded speech), and goes back for a child analogy to the book of B. Perez, *L'Art et la Poésie chez l'Enfant*, a book which the present writer has been unable to consult.

[3] *Die Anfänge der Poesie*, Dresden and Leipzig, 1891.

easy substitution of Haeckel for Hegel. So, too, Jacobowski is a statistician, an observer, as witness that work on the kiss, evidently in no spirit of Johannes Secundus; and he gives incidental notes on the poetic process which have a very scientific ring. "I know a young poet," he says in a burst of confidence, and perhaps remembering Goethe's fifth Roman elegy, "who actually makes his best poems in the very ecstasy of wine and of love." He draws a diagram, like those convincing charts in history and political economy, to illustrate the "hunger-curve" and the "thirst-curve," and to answer the question why there is so much poetry that deals with drinking and so little that deals with eating. Here and there a savage tribe is named, a traveller is invoked; but Jacobowski's main trust is in the human infant and in his own poetic self. That the book has been taken seriously is perhaps due to the only part of it worth considering, which traces the origin of poetry to cries of joy or of pain. This, of course, in great elaboration; by the ontogenetic method one may study poetry, that is, emotional expression, in the modern infant, and then by a simple phylogenetic process "transfer the result to humanity." Rid of all friction from facts, literary and sociological, the pace of proof is breathless, and pampered jades of investigation are left far out of sight in the rear. What was the first poem? — A cry of fright. Why? — All observers agree that the first emotion noted in a child — as early, says Preyer, as the second day — is fear. Watch by the cradle, then, and note the infant's gasps, cooings, gurglings, cryings, grimaces, gestures; these will give in due succession the stages and the history of literature. In this attitude, too, Jacobowski watches for the "primitive lyric." He quotes Preyer's account of a baby which, on the day of its birth, showed pleasure at the presence of light and displeasure at relative darkness. There follow more statistics of the same sort, "lyrical sounds of delight," heard from another baby for the same reason. Now, says the author triumphantly, "precisely" — the word is to be noted — "*precisely the same effect of light and darkness must have been experienced by primitive man.*"[1] It is hardly worth while to argue against such an extreme of absurdity as this; the lyric expression of a new-born baby's pleasure in light and fear of darkness is no parallel to the lyric and poetic expression of primitive man, not only for the reason that overwhelming evidence shows all primitive poetical expression of emotion to have been collective, but because this emotion was based on very keen physical perceptions. The analogy of infant growth in expression with the development of primitive man's expression comes soon to wreck; who furnished for infant man the adult speech, gesture, manner, upon which the imitative, actual infant works in his progress through babyhood? Moreover, the infant individual of an adult race and the adult individual of an infant race still differ, *qua* infant and adult, as human beings. Think of the adult savage's activity, his sight, his hearing, his powers of inference from what he sees; put him with his fellows even into primitive conditions; and then consider the claim that such a wild man's earliest poem, a lyric, must be analogous to the first cry of pleasure or of pain uttered by the solitary infant on the first dull perception, say of light or of hunger! Even the biological analogy, pure and simple, will now and then break down. It has been asserted that the male voice was once far higher than now in point of pitch, phylogenetic inference from the ontogenetic fact of the boy's voice before it deepens; but Wallaschek[2] examines the facts in regard

[1] Work quoted, p. 96. Even old Gottsched, *Crit. Dichtkt.*, p. 68, called a child's weeping "a song of lament," and its laughter "a song of joy." "Every passion," he says, "*has its own tone with which it makes itself manifest,*" really a better hint of origins than this scientific masquerading of Jacobowski.

[2] *Primitive Music*, pp. 76, 78.

to this claim, and finds not only adverse evidence, but a constant tendency to raise the pitch as one passes from oldest times to the present. There is another law of relativity than that to which the argument of child and race appeals, — not how primitive poetry compares with modern emotional expression, but how primitive poetry was related to the faculty and environment of primitive man. Looked at in this light, it might well appear that "simple expression of joy," or what not, is a gross misrepresentation of the lyric in question, and that the relative childishness of savages, and, as one argues, of primitive men generally, is not a positive childishness with regard to the conditions of their life.[1] In fine, the analogy and the principle are in the present state of things useless for any direct inference about primitive poetry. When the sequence of emotions and of emotional expressions has been established for infant life, it will have an interest for the student of early literature, and may even give him substantial help by way of suggestion, corrective, test. But to set up a provisional account of the origins and growth of infant emotional expression, and then to transfer this scheme to primitive culture as the origins and growth of human poetry, is, on the face of it, absurd.

Closely akin to the error which makes unwarranted use of psychological theories is the abuse of ethnological facts. True, the value of ethnology to the study of primitive poetry is immense; until one hundred and fifty years ago,[2] the

[1] The best objection against this analogy in any definite use is made by O. Gruppe, *Griechische Culte und Mythen*, p. 199. The child and the savage, he points out, have each a small range of perceptions; the ways in which they enlarge this range are diametrically opposed. One does it productively; the other, receptively. See, too, a bit of sarcasm over the complacent scorn for the "childish" savages felt by civilized man, Grosse, *Anfänge der Kunst*, pp. 51 f.

[2] Dr. Brown, Adam Smith, Lord Monboddo, and others were leading Englishmen in the movement to use the savage to explain early man. Smith and Monboddo enjoyed this literary vivisection, the former once watching "a negro dance to his own song the war-dance of his own country, with such vehemence of action

vital fault of writers on poetry lay in their neglect of what John Evelyn calls "plaine and prodigious barbarisme," and even down to the present, this contempt for lower forms of poetry vitiates the work of writers in æsthetics; nevertheless, there is caution to be applied in arguments from the modern savage as in those from the modern infant. Briefly put, the notion is abroad that the lower one goes in the scale of culture among living savage tribes, the nearer one has come to actual primitive culture, to unaccommodated man, the thing itself, as it was in the very beginning of human life; but, unless great care be used, one will follow this path to the utter confusion of progress and retrogression. All would be easy work if one could accept the statement of Gumplowicz,[1] that "So long as one unitary homogeneous group is not influenced by or does not exert an influence upon another, it persists in the original primitive state. Hence, in distant quarters of the globe, shut off from the world, we find hordes in a state as primitive, probably, as that of their forefathers a million years ago." Surely not as primitive; the very terms of the phrase deny it; and even in the stagnation of culture, through wastes of dull and unmeaning ages, man, like men, grows old: *tacitisque senescimus annis.* Neither individual nor tribal life can stand still. What one may properly do with ethnological evidence is to note how certain conditions of culture are related to the expression of human emotion, and to conclude that the same conditions, for these

and expression, that the whole company, gentlemen as well as ladies, got up upon chairs and tables." See the *Essays*, Edinburgh, 1795, "Of the Imitative Arts," Parts II., III., and the fragment "Of the Affinity between Music, Dancing, and Poetry." The main credit, however, belongs to Turgot. In his "Plan du Prém. Disc. sur l'Hist. Universelle," *Œuvres*, II. 216, he uses the savages of America to illustrate the state of primitive man. He is also strong for the *milieu.* "Si Racine fût né au Canada chez les Hurons . . . !" he says, II. 264; and his other illustrations are suggestive (in the "Plan du 2. Disc."). II. 265, he notes the homogeneity of barbaric races.

[1] *Outlines of Sociology*, trans. Moore, p. 85.

are a stable quantity, would affect the emotional expression of primitive man in a similar way, allowing, however, — and here is the important concession, — for the different state of the intellectual and emotional powers in an early and vigorous tribal life as compared with the stagnant or degenerate life of a belated culture.[1] Two pitfalls lurk under the analogy. It will not do to argue directly from a sunken race back to a mounting race found at the same level; again, it will not do to argue that because the mounting race, when arrived at its prime, has not a certain quality or function, that it therefore never had such a quality or function.[2] If one will but look at the thing honestly, what a brazen assumption it is that this makeshift human creature is always learning but never forgetting, always gaining but never losing, and that man of to-day holds fast the unimpaired *x* of man's primitive powers along with all that change and growth and countless revolutions have brought him! It is a mistake of the first order to assume that a form of expression now unknown among men must have been unknown to those who made the first

[1] The outright degeneration assumed by Le Maistre need not come into the account. Human progress is now conceded to be a resultant of opposing forces of growth and decay. Mr. Talcott Williams has an interesting paper, "Was Primitive Man a Modern Savage?" in the *Report of the Smithsonian Inst.*, 1896, pp. 541 ff. His main point is, that the modern savage has deteriorated under pressure. Primitive man was in a more or less "empty earth," and was not crowded by his fellows. The god of war is always a junior member of Olympus. So, too, Professor Baldwin (*Social and Ethical Interpretations*, p. 214) argues for a reign of peace, a "sort of organic resting-place," in the child's second period, which answers to social coöperation, "the rest which man took after his release from the animal. . . . The social tide then sets in. The quest of domestic union and reciprocal service comes to comfort him, and his nomadic and agricultural habits are formed." One is reminded of Scherer's argument for an epoch of peace in early Germanic culture attested by names which bear that stamp as compared with the later and warlike Gerhards, Gertrudes, and the rest.

[2] It is hardly necessary to warn against fallacies of illustration. Even Bruchmann goes astray when he says the poem of Goethe is to the primitive song as a cherry tree in bloom is to a cherry stone just planted. To primitive man the primitive song was already a tree in bloom, and his appreciation of it was in line with modern appreciation of Goethe's poem.

trials of expression as in words and song. One often hears about the lost arts; it is quite possible that there were arts or modes of expression used by primitive man for which one can find no analogy to-day either among men of culture or in savage tribes. There are rudimentary growths in literature, and these must be taken into account just as the man of science considers the nails or the hair or even the often-discussed vermiform appendix. The pineal gland, which Descartes finally chose as the scene of that mysterious passage between soul and matter demanded by his system of philosophy, has been recently explained to be all that is left of an eye in the top of the head. This may be a true account of the pineal gland, or a false account; but no competent naturalist will assert that civilized man has all the bodily functions which he had at that remote period in question. So, too, with certain possible distorted survivals in poetry of forms of emotional expression now unknown; it is wrong to deny them, and it is perilous to assert them unless cumulative evidence of many kinds can establish the probability. Again, for the first of these two warnings, it is unfair to set up the Australian black fellow or the Andaman islander,[1] with his "primitive" tools, dress, habits, and then, by a forcing of the adjective, bid us look at our primitive ancestor. No one denies the value of ethnological evidence; Thucydides himself declared that barbarous nations gave one a good idea of what civilized nations had been; accounts of savage life have the enormous advantage of coming close to the conditions of primitive life; but they do not give us the infallible description of primitive man himself, and it is an illicit process to transfer a quality from savage to ancestor, to say

[1] Or, indeed, any one tribe of human beings. Even in the very beginning of human activity, that activity was, as now, conditioned by the environment, and there were doubtless several types of primitive existence. Evidently, then, there could have been different types of social union even at the outset of social progress.

that man at the dawn of history was like this belated specimen, and that tribes from whose loins sprang dominant races, races which fought, and spoiled, and set up civilizations now vanished from almost every kind of record, can be reconstructed, in each feature of mind and body, by a study of peoples long ago shunted upon the bypaths of progress. Mr. Spencer was one of the first to protest against this abuse of ethnology.[1] Professor Grosse,[2] on the other hand, makes a strong and candid effort to meet and minimize the objections to an assumption upon which his whole study of primitive art depends. He asserts that arguments in opposition rest on the theory of degradation, and he denies that degradation has taken place, pointing to the remarkable uniformity of culture conditions in the various tribes which he regards as primitive. But it is clear that one does not need the theory of degradation to make good the point which has just been urged. Grant that these savage tribes have not degenerated; they have certainly failed, in every important particular, to progress; they are stunted; and they compare with that primitive being who held the destinies of culture in his hand, who pressed forward, wrought and fought, and sang the while of what he did, somewhat as a dwarf idiot of forty compares with a healthy child of four. More than this. Long stagnation, while it cannot push culture to new habits, may well complicate and stiffen the old habits to such an extent that the latter state of them comes quite out of analogy with the beginnings. For example, the festal dances of the savage are often intricate to a degree, requiring real erudition in the teacher, and infinite patience and skill in the disciple. Now it needs no advance in culture, no change in the form

[1] *Principles of Sociology*, 3d (American) ed., I. 93, 96. Dr. Eugen Wolff is equally severe on the abuse, "Vorstudien zur Poetik," in the *Zst. f. Litteraturgesch.*, VI. 426.

[2] *Anfänge der Kunst*, pp. 33 ff. For falling off in civilization among Africans and others, see Tylor, *Primitive Culture*, I. 46, 48.

of production, which is Grosse's test for culture, to make this dance progress from wild rhythmic leapings in a festal throng to the rigid form it has found under the care of certain experts. The earliest dancers and the latest dancers, communal and artistic, may have lived the same tribal life and got their food by the same kind of hunting, the same rude gathering of plants. In fact, startling as the assertion may seem, and however it may run counter to this convenient law that the degree of culture depends on the form of production, and that the work of art depends on the degree of culture, it is nevertheless highly probable that a certain combination of dance and song used among the Faroe islanders about a century ago, and recorded by a Danish clergyman who saw it, is of a far more primitive type than sundry laborious dances of savage tribes who are assumed to be quite primitive in their culture.

Granted the need to use the analogy with caution, it is well to note how wary one must be in dealing with the evidence itself. The warning may be brought home by an illustration somewhat out of the beaten track of ethnological material.[1] Nearly a century ago, Dr. Samuel L. Mitchill, United States senator from New York, was "a sort of permanent chairman of the committee on Indian affairs"; and he gives an account of a song "in the Osage tongue," which was sung at his house in Washington, "translated into French by Mr. Choteau, the interpreter, and rendered into English immediately, January 1, 1806." It is well to see what came of this process in the shape of the song "On War."

> Say, warriors, why, when arms are sung,
> And dwell on every native tongue,
> Do thoughts of Death intrude?
> Why weep the common lot of all?
> Why think that you yourselves may fall,
> Pursuing or pursued?

[1] *Transactions and Collections of the American Antiquarian Society*, Worcester, Mass., 1820, I. 313 ff.

There is more in the same pensive but smooth and elegant vein; and one regrets to learn that this excellent Wanapaska, who would have pleased Chateaubriand, "died suddenly . . . a few nights after having sung this song to the translator," — who, however, unblushingly lived on. But he could be truthful on occasion, this translator, and he tells the truth about two Cherokee songs of friendship which may not have seemed capable of conversion into tender English monody. Here is silly sooth. The songs, one is told, "consist of but one sentence each with a chorus. Nothing of greater length seems to exist among" the Cherokees. "They repeat the song and chorus until they are tired. The words of both were written for me[1] by Mr. Hicks, a Cherokee of the half blood, with his own hand, both original and version. . . . *Neither among the Osages nor the Cherokees could there be found a single poetical or musical sentiment founded on the tender passion between the sexes.* Though often asked, they produced no song of love."[2] The two songs follow, — they have the same chorus and belong together, — with interlinear translation: —

Can, nal, li, èh, ne-was-tu.
A friend you resemble.
Chorus — Yai, ne, noo, way. E, noo, way, hā.

Ti, nai, tau, nā, cla, ne-was-tu.
Brothers I think we are.

And the chorus, as before. Now even the humblest student of poetry can sift all this evidence, on the face of it equally valuable throughout, and find that a part of it is worse than worthless, while another part is of real value; in many cases, however, the task is difficult, and this for two reasons. Either the missionaries, explorers, travellers, give only a partial account, or again, they give accounts of a misleading sort, if not actually untrue. For the former case, we may take Ellis

[1] In 1805. [2] See below, on the Darwinian theory of lyric.

and his description of a New Zealand dance.[1] "Several of their public dances seemed immoral in their tendency; but in general they were distinguished by the violent gestures and deafening vociferations of the performers." And that is all. It is enough for the purposes of the book, but it is not enough for the student of poetry. Worse yet is the tendency to state savage thought, savage habits, in terms of civilization, and so give a notion never true and often false. When, for example, one is told[2] that in the South Sea islands there are poets who retire at certain seasons from the world in order to live in solitude and compose their poems, one is surprised at this notion of poetical composition among races where the great mass of evidence is for improvised songs of a line or two, with eternal chorus — savage pattern everywhere — and with accompanying dance. However, here is the evidence, and it must be taken with the rest. Presently comes an actual song,[3] a pensive song, by one of these bards and akin to the Osage outburst translated by Dr. Mitchill: —

Death is easy.
To live, what boots it?
Death is peace.

Is this a Fijian Schopenhauer, or rather Leopardi; or does it mean contact with civilized thought and with Christian hymns? Before one accepts this as outcome of "primitive" poetic conditions, one must bring it into line with the poetry from such sources on which all evidence is agreed; at once the bard and his ditty fall under strong suspicion. Witty proverbial verses found in half-civilized tradition, say among the Finns,[4] get the same label of "primitive," until one appeals

[1] *Polynesian Researches*, American ed., III., Chap. XII.
[2] Waitz-Gerland, *Anthropologie der Naturvölker*, VI. 85.
[3] *Ibid.*, VI. 606 ff.
[4] See R. M. Meyer, *Altgermanische Poesie*, p. 434.

to the chronological sense of fitness, and to other kinds of evidence:—

> Praise no new horse till to-morrow,
> No wife till two years are over,
> No wife's brother till the third year,
> Praise thyself not while thou livest!

At this rate the letters of some Lord Chesterfield to his son will yet be reconstructed for the epoch of our hairy ancestors on the tree platform It is clear that the great body of ethnological evidence, unequal in its parts, and in sad need of sifting and revision, has something of that uncertain quality as an ally in argument which Tom Nash imputed to "law, logic, and the Switzers." They could be hired to fight, he said, for anybody.

Safety lies in making one kind of evidence control another kind, and in reckoning only with the carefully balanced result. What evidence is there that can control the evidence of ethnology? Philology, despite its overweening claims, is said to be unavailing; it may reveal verbal processes which belong to prehistoric times; but, as J. F. McLennan[1] remarked, "in the sciences of law and society, old means not old in chronology but in structure. . . . The preface of general history must be compiled from the materials presented by barbarism." Yet McLennan himself declares that "a really primitive people nowhere exists," and so puts a great restriction on the use of the material he has just praised. Can history be of help? "The study of the science of art," says Professor Grosse,[2] "should not turn to history or to prehistory. History knows no primitive peoples." Archæology, he thinks, is as powerless; the sole refuge is in ethnology, for it shows us "a whole series of primitive peoples in the full light of the present." But this

[1] *Studies in Ancient History*, First Series, new ed., 1886; see pp. 2, 35.
[2] *Anfänge der Kunst*, pp. 21 ff., 32 ff.

full light, now and then, has blinded even Professor Grosse; and there is a kind of history, not direct, indeed, not a matter of clear record, but still often as valuable as ethnological evidence, which has help of its own for the student of primitive institutions both by way of control and by way of suggestive facts. One of the first men who went about the reconstruction of prehistorical times by a sober application of the "known principles of human nature" to the facts offered by ethnology and sociology, sciences then unknown by name, was Adam Smith; in the highly interesting account of him written by Dugald Stewart and published as introduction to the Essays,[1] the name of "*theoretical* or *conjectural history*" is given to "this species of philosophical investigation which has no appropriated name in our language." Stewart is speaking of Smith's essay on the origin of speech,[2] and compares it with the famous pioneer work of Montesquieu and others in a related field of study, remarking on the way in which "casual observations of illiterate travellers and navigators" are combined into "a philosophical commentary on the history of law and of manners." These "casual observations" have risen of late to almost absolute power, and "known principles of human nature" are out of office. Now it is true that one must be chary in the application of such "known principles" to the facts from which one has to construct one's idea of human nature itself, a process close to the vicious circle; but there are, nevertheless, certain general controlling ideas to which appeal should be made when one has to set a value on a given bit of evidence. A controlling idea of this sort is the sense of literary evolution, an idea based on known literary facts, and quite valid as test for alleged facts which are brought forward as evidence in

[1] London, 1795, pp. xlii ff.

[2] Nearer to the present subject are Smith's excellent essay "Of the Imitative Arts" and the fragment "Of the Affinity between Music, Dancing, and Poetry."

questions of prehistoric stages of poetry. This sense of literary evolution, moreover, need be no whim or freak of one's own judgment. It is not merely that one feels the absurdity of those jingling platitudes which Dr. Mitchill fathers upon the lorn Wanapaska; it is the sense of evolution in the expression of emotion and of thought, a sense based on experience and due to a competent process of reasoning, which tells any person of information that savages do not make such a song. True, if a mass of such evidence lay before one, and it proved to be of the trustworthy sort, then the controlling idea would be driven off, and the old sense of evolution would be so modified as to conform to the new facts. But this is not the case.

The controlling idea, the sense of evolution, should be an object for the scholar in more limited fields than heretofore have been chosen for his work. It will be found wise, henceforth, to select a narrower path but a more distant goal, a smaller subject and a larger method, to run down a single clew, and to run it, if possible, to the end. Works on the History of Human Thought, on the History of Literature, of Religion, of Civilization, on Primitive Culture, were great in their day, — and probably no one book, apart from Darwin's, has had such a wide and wholesome influence as that masterpiece of Dr. E. B. Tylor; they initiated, fixed the general direction, were the doing of genius. But the day of discoveries has gone by, and colonization, a slower process, is rather an affair of hard if intelligent work. Histories, if the term will pass, are needed for the different functions of human expression and human emotion itself. The whimsical Nietzsche[1] has called for histories "of Love, of Avarice, of Envy, of Conscience, of Piety, of Cruelty"; but apart from his notions, and for sober purposes of literary study, there is need for such work as a history of sentiment, and this, of

[1] *Fröhliche Wissenschaft*, pp. 44 f. See also p. 180.

course, should be followed back on its different lines of expression. Two striking passages in Mr. Thomas Hardy's *Return of the Native* may be cited here as bearing on possibilities of investigation which need not be regarded as fantastic or absurd. In describing the face of his hero, as one that bore traces of a mental struggle, a half-formed query in regard to the value of existence, Mr. Hardy contrasts this face, so common now in every walk of life, with the countenance preserved by sculpture from an age when no such questions haunted the brain, and when, to use his phrase, man "could still revel in the general situation." Even more suggestive is the other passage, which treats the change of sentiment in regard to what are called "the beauties of nature." Much has been said and investigated of late on this attitude, ancient and modern, toward nature;[1] but there is metal more attractive in Mr. Hardy's introduction of Egdon Heath as a sort of tragic character in his story, and in his remark that with the saddening of life men have turned more and more from mere gardens and green meadows, and have sought wild, rugged scenes; in days to come, indeed, they may turn even from the barren coasts of the sea, from bleak mountains, and seek stretches of absolute desolation, forbidding, featureless, dead, to suit their mood and give them rest from the stress of life. These are hints, false or true, only hints; but if they can so stir one to look into the seeds of time for the sake of mere prediction, is there not sober gain in a reversal of this process and in a study of the conditions and expressions of sentiment as far back as one can follow them? It is said that the absence and the presence of personal sentiment respectively condition the poetry of France that precedes

[1] Compare Ribot's idea of what he calls the æsthetic conquest of nature, *Psychology of the Emotions*, p. 345, with Professor Patten's remorselessly economic theory that appreciation of these things depends on cheap and warm woollen underclothing.

Villon and the poetry that comes after him; what of the larger field, poetry itself, with regard to this important quality in emotional expression? Can one do for poetry what a recent writer[1] has done for civic life? Speaking of altruism, and noting the original absence of sentiment, he constructs a curve, or, as he calls it, a gradation, "the first word of which is selfishness and the last public sentiment." What curves, now, can be constructed in poetry which shall prove of value as showing a controlling idea and warranting a sense of evolution? Clearly, these controlling ideas in a history of literature must stand chiefly upon the facts of literature, and the sense of evolution must be based upon a study of literary changes and growth, the play and result of such elements as have just now been described. The sense of evolution in literature is akin to the genealogical point of view lately urged upon critics by M. Brunetière,[2] but it is not the same thing; with him the doctrine of evolution is applied to literature or to art as a safe guide through its chronology, as a clew to its progress and retrogressions, as a discovery of the relations which a genius bears to those who went before him and to those who follow, and as a test of the valid and the permanent in art. The application of the sense of evolution now to be considered has a far wider range and must lead in time to wider conquests. For example, if one will choose some particular characteristic of human nature and will essay, by the aid of literature and the arts, to follow back the manifestations of it to a point where all records and traces of it cease, one will have a history of this characteristic, — and one will have something more. There will be not only the actual record

[1] Pulszky, *The Theory of Law and Civil Society*, London, 1888, p. 107. "Selfishness," by the way, is not a good name for the quality he has in mind; but the method is relevant.

[2] "La doctrine évolutive et l'histoire de la littérature," *Revue des deux Mondes*, 15 Fev. 1898. See especially pp. 889, 892 ff. See also his *Évolution des Genres*, particularly the chapter on Taine.

made up from a series of observations which form a dotted line from furthest historical past to present, but the dots of this line, the line itself, will often form a curve which points either to a general gain or to a general loss of the characteristic in question. Or, if it is a case where one cannot speak with exactness of a loss or a gain in the characteristic itself, the curve will show loss or gain in any given form by which this characteristic has made itself known. Here, in other words, is a curve of relative tendencies; and the knowledge of such a curve not only gives us that sense of evolution to which reference has been made, but justifies us, after careful study and testing of these dotted facts, in a bold leap from the known to the unknown. If the characteristic in question, from the point where it comes into view at the beginning of records, shows a constant curve of increase or of decrease, one is justified in making a fairly definite statement about it in prehistoric times. Now this is not the evolutionary doctrine championed by M. Brunetière in literary research, for the reason that it is not dealing with poets and poems, but with poetry, or rather with the elements of poetry. To give a practical illustration, it is found that ethnological evidence puts in strong relief the almost exclusive and certainly overwhelming frequency of choral singing among rudest savage tribes. If, now, one takes a modern popular ballad and seeks to follow it back in such a way as to join it, as the end of a long line of survivals, to these primitive choral songs, one falls at once into confusion and halts sooner or later before insuperable barriers. Apart from the controversy about artistic or communal origin, apart from the theories of the epic, of the *cante-fable*, what not, it is out of the range of possible things to trace ballad or folksong, as such, back to a primitive form. Yet it seems to have occurred to no one that the way to treat the ballad for historic, comparative, and genetic purposes is to separate it into its elements, and to follow these elements back to the point where they vanish in the mists of unrecorded time. Such elements — and, unlike the ballad itself, they can be traced — are the fact of singing, the fact of dancing, the fact of universal improvisation, the fact of a predominant chorus or refrain. Are these elements, as far back as one can trace them, stronger, more insistent, as one approaches primitive conditions? What is the curve of evolution? Add to it the evidence of ethnology, and the conclusions of sociology, in regard to the composition and character of the early social group: here are materials which are solid enough to bear the weight of certain and definite conclusions in regard to the communal element in earliest verse. Again, there is another curve to consider. The poem of our day is mainly individual and artistic; how far back, and in what degree, waxing, waning, or stationary, can these elements be traced, and with what ethnological and sociological facts can they be confronted? The differencing characteristics of the poetry of art, and those of the poetry which is rightly or wrongly called communal, must be studied for themselves and traced back in their curves of evolution in order to ascertain what part they played in the beginnings of the art. And thus, too, the question must be answered, a question neither idle nor without wide sweep of interest, whether poetry has been one and the same element of human life from the outset, under varying circumstances, indeed, but under fixed conditions and with stable elements, or whether the conditions and the elements are now different from those which obtained at the start.

The method, then, of this attempt to study the beginnings of poetry is not to transfer outright the facts and conditions of savage life, result of ethnological investigation, to primitive song, not to take a supposed "popular" or communal poem of modern tradition and essay a somewhat similar transfer, but rather to use the evidence of ethnology in connection with the progress of poetry itself, as one can trace it in the growth or decay of its elements. The facts of ethnological research have been largely digested and can be easily used. The elements of poetry, in the sense here indicated, and combined with sociological considerations, have never been studied for the purpose of determining poetic evolution; and in this study lie both the intention of the present book and whatever modest achievement its writer can hope to attain. Before, however, this actual study is begun, two propositions must be established: the writer must prove that what he takes as poetry is poetry in fact; and, as was hinted just above, he must show a clear title for his use of the terms "communal" and "artistic."

CHAPTER II

RHYTHM AS THE ESSENTIAL FACT OF POETRY

FOR the purposes of this book, poetry is rhythmic utterance, rhythmic speech, with mainly emotional origin. One must not write a book on poetry without essaying that *iter tenebricosum* of a definition — a definition, too, that will define, and not land the reader in a mere maze of words. "Rhythmic speech" is a short journey, puts one on solid ground at the end, and brings about no doublings and evasions in the subsequent path of investigation. It says what Robert Browning says in his summary of his art: —

> "What does it all mean, poet ? — Well,
> Your brains beat into rhythm. . . ."

By rhythmic must be understood a regular recurrence which clearly sets off such speech from the speech of prose; and by speech is meant chiefly the combination of articulate words, although inarticulate sounds may often express the emotion of the moment and so pass as poetry. The proportionate intellectual control of emotion in this utterance is a matter of human development, and largely conditions the course of poetry itself. We agree, then, to call by the name of poetry that form of art which uses rhythm to attain its ends, just as we call by the name of flying that motion which certain animals attain by the use of wings; that the feelings roused by poetry can be roused by unrhythmic order of words, and that rhythmic order of words is often deplorably bad art, or "unpoetic," have as little to do with the case as the fact that a greyhound speeding over the grass gives the spectator quite the exhilaration and sense of lightness and grace which is roused by the flight of a bird, and the fact that an awkward fowl makes itself ridiculous in trying to fly, have to do with the general proposition that flying is a matter of wings. A vast amount of human utterance has been rhythmic; one undertakes to tell the story of its beginnings. With such a definition the task is plain though hard; let go this definition, and there is no firm ground under one's feet. The patron and the critic of poetry, to be sure, must make deeper and wider demands; from the critical point of view one must find the standard qualities of excellence to serve as test in any given case, one must ascertain what is representative, best, highest; poetry for the critic has its strength measured by the strongest and not by the weakest link in the chain. From the æsthetical point of view, again, poetry must be defined in terms of the purely poetic impulse. On the other hand, any comparative and sociological study must find a definition wide enough for the whole poetic product, whether of high or of low quality, whether due to this or to that emotion. It needs a simple and obvious test for the material. Now as a matter of fact, all writers on poetry take rhythm for granted until some one asks why it is necessary; whereupon considerable discussion, and the protest signed by a respectable minority, but a minority after all, that rhythm is not an essential condition of the poetic art. This discussion, as every one knows, has been lively and at times bitter; a patient and comprehensive review of it in a fairly impartial spirit has led to the conclusion, first, that no test save rhythm has been proposed which can be put to real use, even in theory, not to mention the long reaches of a historical and comparative study; secondly, that all defenders of the poem in prose are more or less contradictory and inconsistent, making confusion between theory and practice; and thirdly, that advocates of a rhythmic test, even in abstract definition, seem to have the better of the argument. Indeed, one might simply point to the actual use of the word "poetry," and be done. However the student and collector may proclaim the rights of prose to count as poetry, his history, his anthology, shows no prose at all, and he meekly follows in practice the definition against which, in theory, he was so fain to strive and cry. Of this, one example, but a very remarkable example. Baudelaire, in the preface to his *Poems in Prose*, speaks of one Bertrand[1] as his master in this art, and of a book, *Gaspard de la Nuit*, as its masterpiece. This book,[2] praised highly by Sainte-Beuve, this *fantaisie à la manière de Rembrandt et de Callot*, as its subordinate title runs, makes occasion for a very bold assertion, and apparently for a great innovation, by one of the editors of a collection of French poetry.[3] "To admit a prose writer," he says, "into a poetic anthology needs to be explained. It is certain there are poets in prose just as there are prosers in verse," — the dear old cry, the dear old half-truth! Now Bertrand is "poet not only by his sentiment, not only by the pomp and sublimity of his thought, . . . but by the very art itself" which he lavishes upon this poetic prose. True, he wrote verses also in his *Gaspard;* but his main work is an artistic marvel of prose. "Louis Bertrand prosodie la prose. . . ." Well, a fine defence for the prose-poet; and one turns to the selections for an example of the poetic prose, not only "main work," but very rare work of the writer, whose book is most difficult to obtain. And what are the selections from the prose-poet? Two poems in the most incorrigible verse! A sonnet, a *ballade:* —

[1] "Louis Bertrand, qui signait en bon romantique Aloïsius Bertrand," 1807-1841, born at Céra in Piedmont.

[2] Now very rare. It appeared, edited by M. Pavie, in 1842. See Sainte-Beuve, *Portraits Littéraires*, II. 343 ff.

[3] C. Asselineau in *Les Poètes Français*, Tom. IV., 1862, p. 697.

"O Dijon, la fille
Des glorieux ducs,
Qui portes bequille
Dans tes ans caducs,"—

a kind of refrain, and with the rime in *-ille* running through all the eight stanzas; and there is no prose at all! *Wozu der Lärm?* Why this thunder in the index? Why "admit a prose-writer into a poetic anthology," with all this ceremony, only to ignore his prose and to print his verse?[1]

It is to be noted, first of all, that in ignoring the test of rhythm, so as to admit great men of letters like Plato and Bacon to the poets' guild, the advocates of prose fail to set up any other satisfactory test. Sidney and Shelley, Arcadians both who said noble things about their calling, are reckoned as defenders of the poem in prose. As to the younger, all men must feel more deeply and more lovingly about poetry, for the reading of his essay on that art which "redeems from decay the visitations of the divinity in man," memorable words indeed; but his more exact definition declares poetry to be "the expression of the imagination." Nothing is said here of rhythm, for the good reason that while rhythm can be praised in its own place, it must not be a bar to claims which Shelley and his fellows deem important. Yet how tender and how inconsistent is his rejection of the rhythmic test! Rhythm is "created by that imperial faculty whose throne is curtained within the invisible nature of man"; and "the language of poets has ever affected a sort of uniform and harmonious recurrence of sound, *without which it were not poetry.*"[2] Well, is this not to set up rhythm

[1] Sainte-Beuve gives four specimens of Bertrand's "poems" in prose. Brunetière, *Questions de Critique*, p. 202, quotes with approval Gautier's words: "Vouloir séparer le vers de la poésie, c'est une folie moderne qui ne tend à rien moins que l'anéantissement de l'art lui-même."

[2] Italics not in Shelley's essay. — For these very sentences, so poetical in their prose, see Hegel (on the poetic sentence), *Aesthetik*, III. 248 f.

as a test? No, for Bacon, as well as Plato, is to be counted with the bards; and how shall this be done save by condemning "the distinction between poets and prose writers as a vulgar error," and by a widening of rhythm, so that it shall have no bounds, no necessary "traditional forms"? Thus Plato and Bacon come in, and all hope of a definite, working test of poetry goes out. Sidney, again, had in his day this mingled tenderness and contempt for rhythm. "Rhyming and versing" no more make a poet than a long gown maketh an advocate; but the "senate of poets *hath chosen verse as their fittest raiment*." Presently, however, the exquisite reason for prose in poetry is clear, when Sidney calls Xenophon's *Cyropædia* "an absolute heroical poem." So, too, there is a saving clause, which, by the way, nobody denies in its simple form, in Ben Jonson's well-known deliverance; a poet "expresses the life of man in fit measures, number, and harmony," yet "not he that writeth in measures only, but that feigneth and formeth a fable and writes things like the truth." Now the test of rhythm, which Ben does not really deny, will work in practice; the test of imagination will not work. Shelley, putting Plato with the poetic sheep, thrusts Cicero, disciple of Plato, among the goats of prose. Sound criticism, perhaps; but what is the formula? And when one is asking, not whom one shall regard as a poet, — that is, a great poet, — but what one shall regard as poetry, as material to include in a survey of the rise and progress of poetry at large, then the test of imagination fails utterly. Sidney was defending his art; "we are not mere rimers," so he seems to say, "the root of the matter is in us, and we are kin with the gods." J. C. Scaliger, who insisted on the test of rhythm, and was called many a pretty name for his pains, had a science of poetry in mind, a survey of it, and cast about for a test that would work on earth without reference to celestial origins. The Abbé Dubos[1] was not willing to think so nobly of verse, and laid main stress on style,[2] — always granting, to be sure, the conventional test of "genius." Only genius can unite in lofty degree within the limits of one verse that "poetry of style" and that "mechanics of poetry" which go to make up the ideal poem; however, it is this style that serves as practical test. In short, put genius, or even imagination, to the practical trial, and confusion reigns at once. Shelley and many more make a poet of Plato; Sidney brings in Xenophon. Coleridge,[3] insisting that all the parts of a poem must support "the purposes and known influences of metrical arrangement," thus making rhythm a test, promptly says it is not a test, after all, for along with Plato, both Bishop Taylor and Burnet must be counted as of the bards. Beattie[4] calls *Tom Jones* and the *Merry Wives of Windsor* "the two finest comic poems, the one epic, the other dramatical, now in the world." Emerson[5] thinks Thomas Taylor the

[1] *Reflexions*, ed. 1770, I. 508 ff. A poem in prose is like an engraving; all is here save colour, all is there save verse. The *Princesse de Cleves* and *Télémaque* are poems. Does not colour make the painting, though? Verse the poem? In the next section he prudently asserts, "qu'il est inutile de disputer si la partie du dessein et de l'expression est préferable a celle du coloris." It is a matter of taste; *trahit sua quemque voluptas.* Both in poetry and painting "genius" is the main thing, — so he had decided in earlier sections.

[2] "En lisant un poëme, nous regardons les instructions que nous y pouvons prendre comme l'accessoire. L'importante c'est le style, parceque c'est du style d'un poëme que dépend le plaisir de son lecteur." — I. 303.

[3] In the fourteenth chapter of *Biographia Literaria.* He has conceded the convenience of calling all compositions that have "this charm superadded" — rhythm and rime — by the name of poem.

[4] *Essays*, Edinburgh, 1776, p. 296. "I am of opinion," he says, pp. 294 f., *On Poetry and Music,* "that to poetry, verse is not essential. In a prose work we may have the fable, the arrangement, and a great deal of the pathos and language of poetry; and such a work is certainly a poem, though" — note the concession — "perhaps not a perfect one." Verse "is necessary to the perfection of all poetry that admits of it," — and how, pray, is that limitation to be adjusted? "Verse is to poetry what colours are to painting;" and, quoting Aristotle, "versification is to poetry what bloom is to the human countenance." Here are pribbles and prabbles enough.

[5] *Poetry and Imagination.*

Platonist "a better poet, or, perhaps I should say, a better feeder to a poet, than any man between Milton and Wordsworth,"—excellent second thought. Sir Thomas Browne he regards as a poet. Brought face to face with rhythm, Emerson hedges; as, indeed, all these good folk do. Goldsmith,[1] for example, in an unacknowledged essay, calls versification "one of the criteria that distinguish poetry from prose, yet it is not the sole means of distinction." The Psalms of David, and certain Celtic fragments in prose, "lay claim to the title of poetry." Hazlitt,[2] speaking of "poetry in general," seems favourable to rhythm as a test. Poetry "combines the ordinary use of language with musical expression"; and "there is a near connection between music and deep-rooted passion. Mad people sing." Then the fear of simplicity gets hold upon him, of postman's rimes and the posy in a ring; "all is not poetry that passes for such," verse is not absolutely the test; and he stops short of the inconsistency by saying there are three works "which *come as near to poetry as possible without absolutely being so;* namely, the *Pilgrim's Progress, Robinson Crusoe,*[3] and the *Tales of Boccaccio.*" Such works are "poetry in kind, and *generally fit to become so in name by being 'married to immortal verse.'*" Bagehot[4] is quite as cautious; "the exact line," he says, "which separates grave novels in verse like *Aylmer's Field* or *Enoch Arden* from grave novels not in verse like *Silas Marner* and *Adam Bede*, we own we cannot draw with any

[1] *Works*, ed. 1854, III. 309.

[2] As preface to his *Lectures on the English Poets.*

[3] M. E. M. de Vogüé has other views. To him *Robinson Crusoe* is "un bon traité de psychologie historique sur un peuple,"—an historic psychology of the English race.—*Histoire et Poésie*, p. 194.

[4] *Works*, Hartford, 1889, I. 213 f. Essay on Wordsworth, etc. Bruchmann, in his excellent *Poetik*, Berlin, 1898, gives up the attempt to mark off poetry from prose, speaks of a "neutral ground," and then defines poetry as "Steigerung durch Form und Inhalt; *die Form ist Gesang, Rhythmus, Reim*" (p. 53). What more could the defender of rhythm ask as working test?

confidence." This is to be deplored, perhaps, from Bagehot's point of view; but *Adam Bede* remains prose, and *Enoch Arden* is commonly set down as poetry, and there an end. Why, too, should Boccaccio's Tales, or the *Pilgrim's Progress*, be married to immortal verse? Jeremy Taylor's beautiful bit of prose about the lark is as satisfying in its own way as Shelley's verses are; they are different ways, and one wishes as little to turn one into verse as to turn the other into prose. Dr. Johnson, who recognizes no poet till "he has . . . distinguished all the delicacies of phrase and all the colours of words and has learned to adjust their different sounds to all the varieties of metrical modulation," yet concedes that "perhaps of poetry as a mental operation metre or music is no necessary adjunct," brings out, with his sturdy common sense, the clash of theory and practice. *As a mental operation*, that is, as the poetic impulse and as a matter of theory, poetry is not tested by rhythm; "it is, however, by the music of metre," he goes on to say, "that poetry has been discriminated in all languages," — in other words, metre will serve as a practical test. Now this hedging, this confusion of ideas, this facing one way in theory and another way in practice, is due partly to a shame and partly to a tradition. Where is the dignity of the art, if any Bavius can pin this facile badge of rhythm to his coat and strut about a bard in good standing? Ronsard had this scruple on his mind; so had Sidney, so even comfortable Opitz, so, in spite of his own definition, the elder Casaubon. Tradition of the humanists, of days when poetry held in fee all science, all the gorgeous east of wisdom itself, rules to this day, and keeps men groping for a subtle and esoteric definition. Hence, too, a series of futilities and contradictions in dealing with rhythm as a component part of poetry.

So one comes to the second argument for rhythm as the test of poetry. Not only does the test of imagination fail to work, but all the defenders of prose poems fall into contradiction and confusion so soon as they abandon the other test, so soon as they undertake to put their ideas into any but a protestant and academic form; moreover, this protest nearly always rises from the wish to count as poetry some masterpiece of prose. Take a few typical writers on the theme. Baumgarten, the founder of æsthetics, wrote[1] an essay in which he undertook an exact definition of poetry, and finally summed it up as *oratio sensitiva perfecta*, speech that is both concrete, — calling up in the mind a distinct picture, — and perfect. A few years later, in his *Aletheophilus*, he returns to the quest, and asks what a poem really is. A poem, he answers, is speech so charged with energy that it demands metrical expression. Yet the more he ponders over the quality of rhythm, which in the actual definition seemed imperative, the less he feels inclined to insist upon such a test; at last comes the inevitable concession of theory, and a piece of prose — here it is *Télémaque* — is suffered to pass as a poem. After all this conjuring and throwing about of Latin, one looks for results and finds instead confusion. But Baumgarten was a dull pedant; set genius to work; call up Friedrich Schlegel, who is said to have been the first critic to study the "poem in prose" as it deserved, and whose own performances in *Lucinde* made more than one of the judicious grieve. Poetry, he says in one place,[2] demands rhythm; for only that uniformity which lies in the corresponding succession of tones can express the uniformity needed in all true art; yet again,[3] wishing to put Tacitus as well as Plato among the poets, he makes his wise Lothario say that "*any art or science*" which uses speech as its expression, works for its own sake, and is

[1] When only one-and-twenty. *Meditationes Philosophicae de Nonnullis ad Poema Pertinentibus*, 1735.

[2] *Jugendschriften F. Schl.*, ed. Minor, I. 99; a study of Greek poetry.

[3] *Athenæum*, III. 87 f., in Talks about Poetry.

at its best, must be counted as poetry. But let this, too, pass as eccentricity of genius; call upon some one who has both genius and method, — say Schleiermacher, who lectured on æsthetics in 1819,[1] and undertook to reduce to system and clarity this matter of poetry in prose. To help matters, the subject is halved; drama and epic are "plastic," and can dispense with rhythm, while lyric is "musical" from the start. How came rhythm, then, into drama and epic? Chorus explains the drama, but epic rhythm cannot rest on any such original union of music and words; there must be an "inward" reason. Why does "free" productivity in speech seek after musical form? So one comes back to the difference between poetry and prose, explained by the nature of human speech; one draws a long breath and sets upon another exhilarating run round the circle. Two extremes of speech are possible, — when no syllable is accented at all, and when all syllables are accented alike; this, of course, will not differentiate poetry from prose. But speech alternates accent and no-accent, arsis and thesis; done for logical reasons this alternation makes prose, for musical reasons, verse. In languages like the classical, where rhythmical accent utterly neglects logical accent, there can be little interference of prose with poetry; while in tongues like the Germanic, where verse-accent and word-accent tend to agree, it is easy for poetry to pass into prose. Doubtless this is keen thinking; it explains in some degree why imaginative prose is absent from the classics as compared with modern drama and romance. But it will not do for a definition, and Schleiermacher begins a subtle but ineffectual analysis of poetry old and new. In a Greek drama there was mingling of measures, now more and now less musical; in modern drama this difference appears as a mingling of verse and prose. But if one thinks of the greater musical element in

[1] *Aesthetik*, Berlin, 1842.

classical verse, then the modern difference between poetry and prose[1] "*is not much greater than the difference in classical poetry between epic and dramatic measures.*" Now what has Schleiermacher really done for the matter in hand? For comparative literature he has done a distinctly brilliant piece of work; but, even apart from the fact that no really clear idea of poetry in itself has been gained, the difference between poetry and prose, and the function of rhythm, have not been elucidated. It has not been shown, after all, whether rhythm is or is not a necessary part of poetry. So one turns to the modern scholar, to the student of poetry as an element in human life, to one who studies it in the light of psychology; but here is the same contradiction. Guyau, who thinks this distinction of poetry and prose a problem of high importance, is in one place[2] quite confident that "poets" like Michelet, like Flaubert,[3] — he who first of Frenchmen[4] tried to give to his words an echo of the sensations described, a vague onomatopœia, and the wider hint of a general situation, — and like Renan, "have been able to dispense with rhythm." But verse, he thinks, is permanent; it will be "the natural language of all great and lasting emotions"; while in another book,[5] this excellent and lamented writer not only assigns to rhythm an *importance capitale*, but calls it "the very mainstay of poetic speech." And here again is intolerable confusion.

Into this pit of contradiction have fallen even sane and capable critics like A. W. Schlegel, and sober philologists

[1] See p. 663.

[2] *Problèmes de l'Esthétique Contemporaine*, p. 172.

[3] *Ibid.*, p. 150, — "ce poëte sans le rhythme."

[4] Gautier, too, thought that Flaubert had "invented a new rhythm" in prose, and described it; see the report of this, *Journal des Goncourt*, 1862, January 1. But later, in the same journal (1876, February 24), Goncourt refers all this sort of thing to Chateaubriand: "sa belle prose poétique, *mère et nourrice de toutes les proses colorées de l'heure actuelle. . . .*"

[5] *L'Art au Point de Vue Sociologique*, p. 312.

like Wilhelm von Humboldt.[1] Nobody could be more distinctly an advocate of the test of rhythm than the elder Schlegel was in certain Letters, widely read in their day, on Poetry, Metre, and Speech;[2] if it be objected, he says, that outpourings of a full heart ought not to be hemmed by rule, it is answer enough to say that they always have been under this control, and that, whatever the possibilities of the case, poetry is and has been governed by rhythm. Rhythm is born with poetry, and "whether by Ontario or by the Ganges," where poetry is, there too is rhythm. As for "the so-called poetic prose," Schlegel is very bitter; it "springs from poetic impotence," and it "tries to unite the prerogatives of prose and poetry, missing the perfection of both." Elsewhere,[3] in an amusing little dialogue, he sets Grammar and Poetry talking after this wise: "You speak so simply!" says Grammar. "I must," answers Poetry, "in order to distinguish myself from Poetic Prose!" And again,[4] he likens prose-poetry to the ostrich, which has a gait half flying, half running, and wholly awkward. Even the dialogue of the drama needs rhythm; for, thinks Schlegel, its style demands measured and regular movement of verse. Master of translation, like Herder before him, he is against the translation of verse save by verse itself; and the context shows that he is looking upon verse as an indispensable condition of poetry.

When, however, in the lectures at Berlin Schlegel begins to define poetry and to theorize about it, holding as he does a brief for the romantic school, for those doctrines of freedom which could not away with any sovereignty of measured speech over the play of fancy and would have no set paths

[1] See Humboldt, *Werke*, VI. 230 ff.

[2] "Briefe über Poesie, Sylbenmaas und Sprache," first in Schiller's *Horen*, reprinted in the *Charakteristiken und Critiken*, I. 318 ff.; *Werke*, ed. Böcking, VII. 98 ff.

[3] *Wettstreit der Sprachen*, Böcking, VII. 199.

[4] *Etwas über William Shakspere*, Böcking, VII. 55.

through the "moon-flooded night of enchantment," he turns squarely upon the test of rhythm.[1] It is a crude notion of the philistine, he declares, *eine bürgerliche meynung*, that whatever is in verses is a poem. Nor is much mended by saying only that can be called poetry which ought to be and has to be composed in verse; of late a kind of poetry has come to the fore which rejects verse entirely, — the romance, the novel. And where is yesterday's scorn for the poem in prose?[2]

This study of contradictions could be carried into many another field; but it is time to consider a third point, — that in actual argument defenders of the test of rhythm seem really to come off better than their foes. These opponents start in a fog, and fog besets them all their way. The main authority to which they appeal is Aristotle; but over certain passages[3] in the *Poetics*, their point of departure, hangs a haze of uncertainty if not of contradiction. It is doubtful whether Aristotle really meant to say what champions of poetry in prose declare him to have said; moreover, these brave texts must be taken along with a brief but pregnant passage in which he looks at origins and beginnings of poetry, a passage which lends itself less readily to the purposes of those who would sweep rhythm from the field. Indeed, sundry say that this is not Aristotle's meaning in the brave text itself. "Language without metre," observes Whately,[4] is a bad translation; it should be "metre without

[1] See below, p. 134, for a still more noteworthy and yet quite unnoticed change of front made by Schlegel in the article of folksong.

[2] It must be said for Schlegel that he is here — so, at least, it seems — merely clearing the way for his historical and "genetic" study of the art, and so is bound to have no hampering dogma, no *parti pris* in the case.

[3] Notably that division of *epopœia*, "which imitates by words alone or by verse." The question is whether Aristotle meant in the first case "words without metre" or "words without music." See Twining's fourth note. — It has been pointed out that nowhere in the fragment does Aristotle essay a formal definition of poetry.

[4] *Rhetoric*, III. iii. 3.

music." Twining,[1] one of the best commentators, refers to that other passage, where one is told that "imitation being natural to us, and . . . melody and rhythm being also natural, . . . those persons in whom, originally, these propensities were the strongest, were naturally led to rude and extemporaneous attempts, which, gradually improved, gave birth to poetry." Twining makes a judicious comment. "In this deduction of the art from the mimetic and musical instincts, Aristotle *includes verse in his idea of poetry*, which he at least *considered as imperfect without it.* All that he drops, elsewhere, to the disparagement of metre, must be understood only comparatively: it goes no further than to say that imitation, that is, fiction and invention, deserves the title of poetry, or making, better than verse without imitation." Elsewhere, too, as Twining shows, Aristotle puts verse among the requisites of poetry.[2] A good Aristotelian, J. C. Scaliger, a greater man, by the way, than modern criticism concedes, who first

[1] *Aristotle's Treatise on Poetry*, 2d ed., I. 289. This view of Twining is upheld in some highly sensible remarks by Mr. A. O. Prickard in a lecture, *Aristotle and the Art of Poetry*, London, 1891. What Aristotle clearly meant to say is that "metre is not the most essential characteristic of poetry, *yet it would be a misuse of language to call anything a poem which is not metrical in form*." (Italics not in original, p. 60.) Mr. Prickard agrees with Whately, Twining, and many others, that the words of the passage in question, and the instances given, do not make against this view; and "elsewhere, Plato and Aristotle invariably assume that only what is metrical is to be called poetry; nay, that metrical writing and poetry are, for the common purpose of language, convertible terms. 'In metre, as a poet,' says Plato, 'or without metre as a layman.' 'A good sentence,' says Aristotle, 'should have rhythm but not metre; if it have metre, it will be a poem.'" See the *Phædrus*, 258, D., and Aristotle's *Rhetoric*, III. 8.

[2] A clear summary of the case as argued in Italy may be found in Quadrio, *Della Storia e della Ragione d'ogni Poesia*, I. Bologna, 1739; II.–VII. Milan, 1741–1752. See I. 2 ff. Quadrio is outright for the test of verse and for a generous rendering of Aristotle. He gives the names of forgotten pleaders on both sides, and thinks the noes have it against a traditional Aristotelian view; not to quarrel forever, "Basta, che nacque la Poesia col Verso e col Canto: né, propagata fra le nazioni, fu altrimenti mai lavorato che in Verso." — Spingarn, *Literary Criticism in the Renaissance*, New York, 1899, pp. 9 ff., points out that Mantuan was for the verse-test, Savonarola, Minturno, Daniello, against it.

in his time undertook a science of poetry and not a mere guide to the art, who broke new ground, and who had at least the instincts of historical and comparative method, is squarely for the test of verse.[1] Poetry is imitation in verse. In the opening sections of his work[2] he calls the poet not so much a maker of fiction as of verses,[3] defends rhythm almost in Hamann's phrase as the mother-tongue of man, derives poetry from singing, and, with a touch of psychological method, makes appeal to the child who must go to sleep with song.[4] In the later sections,[5] he vigorously attacks the idea of poetry in prose. He is followed by another pioneer of the historic treatment of dogma, G. J. Vossius, who, tossing to the winds any notion that verse itself makes the poet, declares that verse is nevertheless condition of the poetic work.[6] For poetry was meant to be sung — the genetic consideration has a strong and wholesome influence upon these men — and how can that be sung which has no rhythm? Or take the rhythm from the Iliads; they turn to mere "fabulous stories." Briefly, while metres without the aid of diction and genius can make no poem, fiction — Aristotelian imitation — is powerless without the help of verse. To the same purpose and earlier, Isaac Casaubon; the test of poetry is rhythm,

[1] "Censet hoc ipsum . . . Caesar Scaliger, qui, *quod raro facit, hac parte ab Aristotele recedit*," says Vossius, *de art. poet.*, § 7.

[2] Iulii Caesaris Scaligeri . . . *Poetices Libri Septem* . . . 1561, the first edition, published three years after the author's death.

[3] See p. 3[b]: "Poetae igitur nomen non a fingendo . . . sed initio a faciendo versu ductum est. Simul enim cum ipsa natura humana extitit vis haec numerosa, quibus versus clauditur."

[4] *Ibid.*, "Infans quoque prius canit quam loquitur, videmus enim plerosque haud aliter somnum captare."

[5] See p. 347[a].

[6] Gerardi Joannis Vossii *de artis poeticae natura ac constitutione* . . . Amstelodami, 1647. § 4, "Atque ut multi ex solo metro male colligunt aliquem esse poetam: ita contrà aberrant alii, qui existimant, ne quidem requiri metrum, ut poeta aliquis dicatur. Haec tamen sententia à nonnullis ipsi tribuitur Aristoteli . . . § 5. At alii censent Aristotelem numquam agnovisse ullum poema ἄμετρον . . ."

and any utterance which comes under metrical laws is so far a poem.[1] Scaliger, Vossius, and Casaubon are "good"; and their credit comes down to them from their betters. Petrarch, with Latin so at his heart, could never confuse poetry and prose. Dante's definition[2] is cold comfort for the heretic about a rhythmic test. Of the smaller fry, Ronsard certainly cleaves to this test of rhythm in poetry.[3] Gascoigne, as the title of his little treatise shows, assumes with his teacher Ronsard that verse is the condition if not the essence of the art; and Puttenham, Webbe, Campion, Daniel, Harvey, even Spenser,[4] lean the same way. Sidney, it was shown above, is no real opponent. Bacon himself, quoted so often to sustain the cause of poetry in prose, should be read more carefully;[5] he really tosses to the winds all question of form, and turns to poetry as "one of the principal portions of learning."

So the great age thought of poetry; and so the balance inclines as one comes nearer to our own days. Isaac

[1] Isaaci Casauboni *de Satyrica Graecorum Poesi & Romanorum Satira Libri duo*, Parisiis, MDCV, pp. 352 f. "Certum heic discrimen statuitur inter eam orationem quae poema dici potest, & quae non potest. discrimen illud est metrum. . . . *Omnem metro astrictam orationem & posse & debere poema dici.*" The rest is instructive. Borinski, to be sure, *Poetik d. Renaissance*, p. 66, says that Casaubon wished to call Herodotus a poet; but a detached phrase of this sort — compare Scaliger's epic in prose — goes for little when it fails to force the barrier and break down the writer's definition. Dryden, on the other hand, making "invention" the sole test of poetry, clashes badly with his opinion (*Essay on Satire*) that "versification and numbers are the greatest pleasures of poetry."

[2] As Howell translates the not too clear Latin "fictio rhetorica in musicaque posita," poetry is "a rhetorical composition set to music." See also an article in the *Quarterly Review*, with reference to the *Convivio*, April, 1899, p. 303.

[3] See his works, ed. Blanchemain, VII. 320.

[4] The whole dispute about rime shows this "importance capitale" of verse itself.

[5] *Advancement of Learning*, ed. Wright, II. iii. 4 (pp. 101 ff.). Clearer in the Latin version, his antithesis, "nam et vera narratio carmine, et ficta oratione soluta conscribi potest," is not identical with the proposition that poetry is independent of rhythm. He says it "is in measure of words for the most part restrained."

Vossius, in a curious work[1] published without his name, holds to his father's view of the case. Shaftesbury[2] is peremptory for "metred prose," but, as both a lord and a wit, disdains to give his reasons; while another person of quality, Sir William Temple[3] indeed, regards metred prose as a monstrosity. Trapp, in his Oxford lectures,[4] is squarely for the rhythmic test, and will hold it in the teeth of all Aristotelians; so will another professor of poetry, Polycarp Leyser,[5] of Helmstadt, a rationalist in his day, who thinks it high time to have a modern system of poetics not drawn altogether from the ancients.

Across the channel, meanwhile, relations of poetry and prose had been discussed, now as an eddy in the maelstrom of argument about ancients or moderns, now as a question for itself. The *Télémaque* of Fénelon was defended as a great poem in prose; to the objection that it was not written in verse, came answers in abundance. One of them, for example, calls upon the ancients;[6] Aristotle, Dionysius, Strabo, said that verse is not essential to epic poetry. "One may write it in prose, as one writes tragedies without rime." And the old saw — "one can make verses without poetry, and be quite poetic without making verse" — is followed

[1] *De Poematum Cantu et Viribus Rythmi*, Oxon., 1673. The reference to origins is interesting: "illud quidem certum omnem poësin olim cantatum fuisse. . . . Unde sequitur, quicquid non canitur aut cantari nequeat, non esse poema."

[2] *Characteristics*, 5th ed., Birmingham, 1763, I. 254, note, and III. 264.

[3] *Essays*, "Of Poetry."

[4] *Praelectiones Poeticae*, 4th ed., London, 1760; see I. 24.

[5] *Programma de Vera Indole Poeseos Praelectionibus Praemissum*, Helmst., 1719. See also his programme of 1720 introducing lectures on the *Ars Poetica* of Horace.

[6] *Œuvres Complètes de M. de Fénélon*, Tome V., "Discours sur le poeme épique," pp. 34 ff. There are many discourses on this theme of prose-poetry in the *Mémoires* of the Academy of Inscriptions and Belles Lettres. The Abbé Fraguier is dull but weighty for the test; Burette, a real scholar, is sensible on the same side (*Mém.* X. 212 f., in 1730). The younger Racine is very feeble; after reading his contradictory and vapid papers, one has Chaucer on one's lips — "No more of this, for goddes dignité!"

by a definition of the whole matter; what constitutes a poem is "the lively plot, the bold figures, the beauty and variety of the images; it is the fire, the enthusiasm, the impetuosity, the force, a *je ne sais quoi* in the words and in the thoughts which only nature can give." So run a dozen other elaborate pleas for prose in poetry; but the arguments usually end in contradiction, and nothing is brought forward that really sets aside the feeling long ago expressed by Tom Dekker[1] in his sputtering, pamphleteer style, that "poetrie, like honestie and olde souldiers, goes upon lame feete unlesse there be musicke in her," and that both poets and musicians are children of Phœbus: "the one creates the ditty and gives it the life or number, the other lends it voyce and makes it speake musicke."

Even those great changes which the second half of the eighteenth century brought about in the making and in the judging of poetry, left this matter of prose and verse in its old estate. Whenever the critic has a writer to set up, a writer to pull down, this test of verse will be thrust aside; and it is no surprise to find men who belong to the same literary creed — say Warton and Lowth — failing to see eye to eye in this one article of faith. Joseph Warton,[2] in his guarded attack upon Pope, is working slowly to the inference that it is not genius, but a vast talent, shiftiness of phrase and smoothness of verse, that must explain Pope's overwhelming success. Hence Warton, in a reaction from this polished and accurate rhythm,[3] is sure that real poetry does not depend

[1] *A Knight's Conjuring*, Percy Soc., 1842, pp. 25, 75.

[2] *Essay on the Writings and Genius of Pope*, anon., London, 1756. The book is dedicated to Young, and in the dedication Warton gives these general views of poetry.

[3] Pope said, "There are three distinct *tours* in poetry; the design, the language, and the versification . . ." Spence, *Anecd.*, p. 23. As to prose poems, he could read *Telemachus* with pleasure, "though I don't like that poetic kind of prose." Its good sense was so great, "nothing else could make me forget my prejudices against the style." *Ibid.*, pp. 141 f.

on verse. The sublime and the pathetic "are the two chief nerves of genuine poetry." Lowth,[1] on the other hand, though quite in line with the new critical movement, setting about his great work, and undertaking to make his audience feel and know the Hebrew scriptures to be poetry, puts metrical questions in the forefront of his study and will prove that these poems are in verse. He would fain shun this path, thorny as it is and full of snares; but it is a necessary part of his journey, for he is sure that poetry is not to be considered apart from metrical form, and it ceases to be poetry when it is reduced to prose.[2] Here Lowth and Warton clash not only on the main point, but on this subsidiary matter of translation. Warton said that by no "process of critical chymistry," such as dropping the measure and transposing the words, can one disguise the *Iliad*, say, or the *Paradise Lost*, and "reduce them to the tameness of prose." Reduced to prose, says Lowth, poetry does cease to be poetry. It is strange to see how both sides of the controversy in this matter of verse and prose appeal to translation, and it is mournful to note the unstable character of what ought to be firm and fundamental facts. A. W. Schlegel, one remembers, stood for translations in verse. So Whately, following Lowth's opinion, appeals to translation for proof that to break the verse is to shatter the poem;[3] Racine,[4] on the other hand, appealed to a translation of Isaiah to fortify exactly the opposite opinion.

[1] *Praelectiones*, Pars Prima, Praelect. Tertia: "Poesin Hebraeam metricam esse."

[2] "Sed cum omni poesi haec sit veluti propria quedam lex et necessaria conditio constituta, a qua si discedat, non solum praecipuam elegantiam desiderabit et suavitatem, sed ne nomen suum obtinebit." It should be added that Calmet, *de Poesi vet. Hebrae.*, p. 15, is against this verse test, "Essentiale Poeseos quaerimus in certo quodam sermone vivido, animato, pathetico, figurisque hyperbolicis audacius ornato. Nec solam versificationem Poetas facere, nec a pedum mensura Poesin dici persuademur." Then Plato.

[3] *Rhetoric*, III. iii. 3.

[4] The younger, of course.

Or will it be said that Goethe has settled this question in favour of Warton's view? Every critic knows the oracle from Weimar which declared the best part of a poem to be whatever remains when it is translated into prose; every critic, however, is not at pains to quote the entire passage, with its important concession to verse and its reason for the statement as a whole. "I honour," says Goethe,[1] "rhythm as well as rime, *by which poetry really comes to be poetry;*[2] but the thorough and permanent effect, what develops one and helps one on one's way, is that which is left of the poet when he is translated into prose. Here is nothing but the contents pure and simple, — otherwise often concealed, or, if absent, replaced by a fine exterior form. *For this reason I think prose translations better than poetical in the early stages of education.*" He goes on to recommend a prose version of Homer, to praise Luther's Bible; but it is clear that the whole extract is no argument against the test of rhythm. Not to insist on Goethe's concession that it is rhythm which makes poetry to be poetry, one may note how little prose translation does for a lyric, which, after all, is the poet's poem. What would be left in prose, any prose, of Goethe's own *Ueber allen Gipfeln ist Ruh'?* The heart of poetry is another matter, its spirit, its informing life;[3] the historian meets it in terms of its bodily appearance, and must have a concrete test. There is no valid test for the historian save

[1] *Dichtung und Wahrheit*, Book XI.; Hempel ed., III. 45.

[2] "Wodurch Poesie erst zur Poesie wird," — the *erst* will bear a stronger translation. Schiller, too, said that one must put into verse whatever rises above the commonplace; and Goethe agreed with him: all poetry "should be treated rhythmically." Victor Hugo, in his Preface to *Cromwell*, pp. 33 f., defends verse for the drama; prose has not adequate resources.

[3] Milton is thinking, too, of this in his well-known passage in the treatise on Education. "I mean not here the prosody of a verse . . ." boys learn that in their grammars; but in time they must be taught the great things, — "that sublime Art which in Aristotle's *Poetics* . . . teaches what the laws are of a true Epic poem, what of a Dramatic, what of a Lyric, what Decorum is, which is the grand masterpiece to observe."

this test of rhythm. Particularly as sociological and historical responsibility begins to weigh upon the critic, he finds that such a test is demanded by his work. Adam Smith[1] — Blair[2] is almost with him, but slips in a plea for Ossian — is distinctly on the side of verse. So is Monboddo,[3] a pioneer in anthropology, keen, observant, who did his thinking for himself, and condemned "all that has been written of late in the rhapsody style, or measured prose," declaring that "poetry is nothing more than measured rhythm." Sensible things, too, were said on this matter by men who have left no traces in criticism; one of these sayings seems to be a pretty conclusion and summary of the whole debate. Dr. Thomas Barnes, a Unitarian clergyman now forgotten, but one of the founders of the Literary and Philosophical Society of Manchester, an interesting group of men, read, in December, 1781, a paper[4] "On the Nature and Essential Character of Poetry as Distinguished from Prose." He turns to origins, and refers to "the common remark that the original language of mankind was poetical"; he turns to ethnological hints, and, following Dr. John Brown, speaks of "Indian orators at this day"; then, summing up the case, he charges for rhythm. "To finished and perfect poetry, or rather to the highest order of poetic compositions, are necessary, elevation of sentiment, fire of imagination, and regularity of metre. This is the summit of Parnassus. But from this sublimest point there are gradual declinations till you come to the reign of prose. *The last line of separation is that of regular metre.*" Dr. Thomas Barnes is forgotten; but his statement of the case is memorable above a host of admired and often quoted deliverances on poetic art.

As one steps into the modern world, one finds the con-

[1] *Essay on the Imitative Arts.*

[2] No. XXXV. of the *Lectures.*

[3] *Of the Origin and Progress of Language,* II. 50; IV. 41.

[4] See the *Transactions* of the Society, Vol. I. Warrington, 1785, pp. 54 ff.

troversy in its old estate, getting no help from new methods and ridiculous enough, by this expense of motion without progress, in contrast with the gain made by sciences of every other sort. Does Coleridge,[1] master of rhythm, reject rhythm as a test, Poe[2] comes forward to declare it an essential condition, and to announce "the certainty that music, in its various modes of metre, rhythm, and rime, is of so vast a moment in poetry as never to be wisely rejected." Carlyle himself, reckoned by sundry critics as a poet in prose, names the "vulgar" definition of verse only to approve it. Germans, he says,[3] have spoken of "infinitude" as differencing true poetry from true speech not poetical; "if well meditated, some meaning will gradually be found in it. For my own part, I find considerable meaning in the old vulgar distinction of poetry being metrical, having music in it, being a song." And he really adopts the test, — of course, with characteristic riders. "Observe," he says, "how all passionate language does of itself become musical . . . all deep things are song. . . . Poetry, therefore, we will call *musical thought*." So, again, the vague and passionate protests of Stuart Mill beat in vain against such a temperate statement as Whately made in his *Rhetoric*.[4] "Any composition in verse (and none that is not) is always called, whether good or bad, a Poem, by all who have no favourite hypothesis to maintain. . . . The title of Poetry does not necessarily imply the requisite beauties of Poetry." Such a test, cried Mill,[5] is vulgarest of all definitions, and "one with which no person possessed of the faculties to which

[1] *Biographia Literaria*, Chap. XIV. — "Poetry of the highest kind may exist without metre, and even without the contradistinguishing objects of a poem."

[2] *The Poetic Principle.*

[3] *On Heroes*, "The Hero as Poet."

[4] III. iii. 3; another part of the passage is quoted above, p. 42.

[5] *Dissertations and Discussions*, I. 89 ff., "Thoughts on Poetry and its Varieties." The article first appeared in 1833.

poetry addresses itself can ever have been satisfied." This "wretched mockery of a definition" is more than inadequate; for poetry may exist in prose as well as in verse, may even do without words, and can speak through musical sounds, through sculpture, painting, and architecture. It is strange to hear Mill making a serious formula out of phrases to which one is indulgent enough when they come in half playful guise.[1] Apart from the uselessness of such a formula, — fancy the historian of poetry opening a new chapter with "We will now consider the Parthenon!"— it has no theoretical value, as is easy to see when Mill begins to run his division lines. Two definitions of poetry please him, one, by Ebenezer Elliott, that it is "impassioned truth," the other, by a writer in *Blackwood*, that it is "man's thought tinged by his feelings." But these "fail to distinguish poetry from eloquence," and Mill goes on to say that eloquence is "something heard," while poetry is "something overheard." Something overheard? I mean, he explains, that "all poetry is in the nature of a soliloquy," is "the natural fruit of solitude and meditation." Now this is sheer nonsense, although more than one critic has hailed it as an oracle; of that which comes down to us as poetry, a good part is anything but soliloquy or the fruit of solitude. "Read Homer," cried out Herder, perhaps at the other extreme, but certainly with better reason than Mill, "as if he were singing in the streets!" It will be shown how vast a proportion of poetry, too, that belongs to the higher class, was made and sung in throngs of men. Poetry is a social fact. Mill's own

[1] It would be more to the purpose if one went to the sources of poetry and religion and studied the survivals of primitive rite. At seed-time in Brandenburg, the women still go out to the fields and unbind their hair in sign that the flax may grow as long as their tresses. With such a ritual act goes nearly always a song, a repeated shout, a cry to the powers of growth; and this, if one please, is poetry in its making, while it is easy to think that the symbol would sooner or later force itself into the words — "make our flax like this hair."

words defeat him. "Whosoever writes out truly any human feeling, writes poetry"; and "what is poetry but the thoughts and words *in which emotion spontaneously embodies itself?*" A few pages before, it was "the fruit of solitude and meditation," a test that would make poetry of Kant's categorical imperative, refusing the title to Luther's outburst at the diet, although this at once becomes poetry if one accepts the later definition in terms of emotional spontaneity. And that wrath at the "vulgarity" of a rhythmic test is nothing more than the old mistake; because, forsooth, colours and lines fail to account in themselves for the grandeur of painting, one jumps to the assertion that paintings need not have colours and lines. Let us cling to vulgarity, if leaving it means to assert that the Parthenon is a poem, and, by implication, that a sigh is a statue.

One of the most consistent expositions of poetry is that given by Hegel.[1] Here is a careful abstract of propositions as carefully formulated and proved. He has ruled out the "poetic sentence." Specimens of the sublime, like that *Let there be light, and there was light* which Longinus[2] admired, are not poetry. History, too, is excluded, Herodotus, Tacitus, and the rest,[3] as well as eloquence, and not as Shelley rejects Cicero, on personal grounds, but because of the law in the case. Yet this summary is still inadequate as a practical test, and with it the historian is in a plight no better than when with Sidney or Coleridge he was including whatever piece of writing seemed certainly though indefinitely poetic. In the latter case he steered by a compass which was at the mercy of unnumbered hidden magnets; in the former case the

[1] *Aesthetik, Werke*, ed. 1838, X. III.; summary, pp. 269 f.—"So ist denn jedes wahrhaft poetisches Kunstwerk ein in sich unendlicher Organismus," etc.

[2] IX. 9. See the translation by Roberts, p. 65.

[3] Hegel, work quoted, p. 257.

signs on the card are blurred.[1] But Hegel does not leave the matter here; purposely or not, he gives a clear test for the historian when, twenty pages later, he comes to speak of versification. Professors Gayley and Scott[2] point out that the present writer has made too much of this concession; instead of saying that verse is "the only condition absolutely demanded by poetry," one should say that Hegel makes verse indispensable. But this is quite enough for the purpose. The passage in question runs thus: "To be sure, prose put into verse is not poetry, but simply verse, just as mere poetic expression in what is otherwise prosaic treatment results only in a poetic prose; *but nevertheless, metre or rime, being the one and only sensuous aroma,*[3] *is absolutely demanded for poetry, and indeed is even more necessary than store of imagery, the so-called beautiful diction.*" And now for Hegel's reason, which quite agrees with the historian's demand for an available test. He goes on to say that the fact of verse in any piece of literature shows at once, as poetry indeed demands there should be shown, that one is in another realm from the realm of prose, of daily life; this constraint, if one likes to call it constraint, forces the poet outside the bounds of common speech into a province wholly submitted to the laws of art. That poetry has to be something more than this, that there are other canons, nobody denies; but the first step for a poet is into this realm of verse where he must prove in sterner tests and by other achievements whether he is citizen or trespasser.

[1] E. S. Dallas, *Poetics*, p. 8, is sound in idea, but less happy in illustration, when he says that a poem without verse can be no more than the movement of a watch without its dial-plate.

[2] *Literary Criticism*, p. 134.

[3] "Als der erste und einzige sinnliche Duft." The passages to which Gayley and Scott refer — *e.g.* Hegel, p. 227 — do not change this statement in the present application. Nobody pretends that rhythm is the soul of poetry; it is a necessary form, a necessary condition.

Hegel, it might be said, is in the clouds; he is out of touch with science, and with that logic of facts which rules investigations of the present day. But the same way of thinking holds with a practical Englishman like Mr. Edmund Gurney,[1] whose feet are planted very firmly on solid ground, who is distinctly hostile to the poem in prose, that "pestilent heresy," as Professor Saintsbury has called it, and whose idea of art, which always includes an appeal to the sense of form, demands in poetry a definite metre or rhythm. And the same way of thinking holds with a student of modern psychology, M. Souriau,[2] who undertakes to define poetry in terms of science. Poetry itself derives from music and prose, — presumably he means by prose the speech of daily life, and not what Walter Pater means in his essay on Style when he makes "music and prose literature . . . the opposite terms of art"; poetry might therefore be called musical speech.[3] To show how much depends on the music, M. Souriau turns to translations from foreign poetry into prose vernacular. "The more poetical this original text, the more it loses in the change. . . . This depreciation is due to the change of process, and not to the change of tongue, for the translation of a piece of prose would not show these faults." On the other hand, now, take an irreproachable piece of verse, with this superiority just shown to be due to its rhythm, and look at it with regard to logical worth. How unsatisfying, how "thin," is the thought in it! Change again the point of view, and study poetry for its music; one will be no better pleased than when one hunted for its

[1] *The Power of Sound*, London, 1880. Chap. III. is on the elements of a work of art. On p. 51, again on p. 423 f., Mr. Gurney rejects poetry in prose.

[2] *Théorie de l'Invention*, thèse pour le doctorat ès Lettres, Paris, 1881, p. 142.

[3] It is perhaps superfluous to point out that imagination is utterly ignored in this analysis, and to recall Mr. Swinburne's phrase that "the two primary and essential qualities of poetry are imagination and harmony."

thought. The rhythm would be intolerably monotonous in a piece of music. The sonorous words, taken as sound, are not really pleasing to the ear. Rime, if one will look at it this way, is a *procédé enfantin.* In sum, poetry is logically inferior to prose, and musically inferior to pure melody,— and what, then, is its own charm? It pleases us, not by either one of these elements, but by their combination; it is harmony, but in a peculiar sense. "It is not the harmony of thought, logical system, and order, not the harmony of sounds or musical system, but the harmony between sounds and thoughts. *One loves to feel the idea bending and adjusting itself to the rules of verse, and the verse yielding to the demands of the idea.*" [1]

It is time to close the poll. For poetry in prose no one has spoken in such a temperate and yet forcible fashion as Mr. Frederic Harrison,[2] though his arguments are by no means new. Nothing but "poetry," he asserts, can serve as the word to express what one finds in Malory's *Death of Arthur*, in chapters of Job and Isaiah. But arguments such as he makes with energy and eloquence lose their force when confronted with the cool reasoning of Mr. Bosanquet,[3] who shows clearly that poetry, whatever else it may be, must be rhythmic utterance. Even in the clash of opinion between these modern writers, one finds what is to be found throughout the entire controversy, down from the days of the early renaissance, that the advocates of a rhythmic test for poetry have the better of the argument. It has been shown that there is no other test for the historian of poetry as a social institution; and whenever another test has been set up, its own advocates have not only abandoned it in practice,

[1] A curious passage which follows (pp. 149 f.), treats poetry as a supply of coal, rapidly used and close to exhaustion, so far as originality and freshness are concerned.

[2] *Choice of Books*, pp. 81 f., 126.

[3] *History of Æsthetics*, pp. 461 f.

but even in theory have obscured it with a mass of contradictions.[1]

There remains, of course, the *ambulando* argument; the champion of poetry in prose points to the work which passes under this name. A book could be written on the long series of concessions in matter of territory which verse has made to prose; but no sensible critic will allow these transfers to prove that poetry has ceased to be rhythmic utterance. The most obvious transfer, of course, is translation; is not the English Bible as noble poetry, one asks, as can be found in any time or clime? Mr. Theodore Watts[2] is sure of the rhythmic test until he faces the claims of this noblest prose. Yet surely what appeals to us here is not poetry, but the genius of the English tongue at its greatest and best,[3] flinging its full strength upon a task which at the time lay close to the heart of the English people. The Bible is not the masterpiece of our poetry, but of our prose; it beats not only with the divine pulse of its original, but also with that immense vitality and energy of English religious life in days when to many Englishmen life and religion were identical. That does not make it poetry. One must not open the gates of poetry to this or that passage of prose, and shut them, through whim or shame, upon a thousand other pas-

[1] Professor Masson in the *North British Review*, 1853, reviewed the *Poetics* of Dallas, printing the review later as fifth essay in *Wordsworth, Shelley, and Keats*, London, 1874; the sixth essay "On Prose and Verse," repeats a discussion of De Quincey's prose in the journal just named for 1854. Poets are led, Masson says, by the "flag" of imagery and the "flute" of verse; and while he inclines to the test of rhythm, he comes to no conclusion. Bain (*On Teaching English*, 1887; see Chap. VII. and pp. 249 ff.) also inclines to the test, but hedges after the manner of his brethren.

[2] *Encycl. Brit.*, article "Poetry," which defines its subject as "the concrete and artistic expression of the human mind in emotional and rhythmical language. . . . In discussing poetry, questions of versification touch . . . the very root of the subject."

[3] In the sense, of course, that it absorbed the best labour of two centuries.

sages.[1] Let in that great chapter of Job, and anon *Werther* is there, *Silas Marner*, *Tom Jones*, — we have marshalled this rout already. No, if the Bible be poetry, it is because it is rhythmic utterance, not because it is sublime. That tremendous reach of emotion borne on the cadence of a style majestic and clear, the voice of a solitary desolation crying to the desolation of all mankind, the wail of an eternal and unanswered question —

> Wherefore is light given to him that is in misery,
> And life unto the bitter in soul?

— is not this a poem? It is almost certainly a poem in the original; it might be a poem in English, provided the rhythm of the lines, printed as they now are, with parallelism and cadence properly brought out, seemed to the reader to have a recurrent regularity which could take it into the sphere of rhythmic law; otherwise it is prose, the prose of great literature, indeed, but prose. It must be granted, too, that the latter view is preferable. As great literature, the book of Job belongs with Dante, and Milton, and with a few passages, where Goethe touches the higher levels, in *Faust;* but it is not poetry in the sense that Dante and Milton and Goethe impress upon one when one reads their great passages. Longinus writes on the sublime in literature, and he is within his rights when he puts Thucydides and Homer and Moses upon one plane; but it is the plane of sublimity in thought and phrase, and it is not the plane of poetry. Poetry has no monopoly of the emotions; a line that stirs the heart is poetry when it belongs in a rhythmic whole, and is prose when it does not. *Tendentesque manus ripae ulterioris amore* is Vergil's verse; "the future balances and the hieroglyphic meanings of human suffering" is De Quincey's prose.

[1] The same argument, of course, applies to Plato, as in the "hymns" to Eros, noble prose indeed; and in less degree to such passages as De Quincey on the Ladies of Sorrow.

Carlyle says of his murdered Princess de Lamballe, "She was beautiful; she was good; she had known no happiness," — anvil-strokes as strong as the strongest in English speech. Webster, over his murdered Duchess of Malfi, makes the brother cry out, "Cover her face; mine eyes dazzle; she died young." What have phrases like "poetic prose" to do with great literature of this sort, and how will one distinguish between these two isolated passages, both throbbing with an intensity of expression which breaks out in the three short clauses? Well, the rhythm of one comes to its rights in the full poetic period where Webster, rough as his verses are, infused a noble harmony; while the cadence of the other falls naturally into the sweep of Carlyle's prose. Dryden, indeed, with his wonted critical felicity, gives the key of the whole matter. "Thoughts," he says in his preface to the *Fables*, "thoughts come crowding in so fast upon me, that my only difficulty is to choose or to reject, to run them into verse, *or to give them the other harmony of prose*."

Since Turgot[1] told France and the world that a new kind of poetry had come in the guise of Gessner's prose idylls the poem in prose has made many claims for Parnassian recognition. At Bertrand we have glanced already; his scholar Baudelaire[2] made as bold essay; and so, in quite recent times, the Swede Ola Hansson;[3] all these are Werther with a difference, and in the last case with a dash of Nietzsche. He, too, wrote a dithyrambic prose for his hysterical but noteworthy Zarathustra; yet who does not feel the passage, as into another realm of art, when one suddenly comes upon that powerful lyric in verse,[4] *O Mensch, gieb Acht?* Nietzsche, to be sure, had something to say; but with the little men these

[1] *Œuvres*, Paris, 1810, IX. 227 ff., "De la Prose Mesurée." See also pp. 185 ff.

[2] See his *Petits Poëmes en Prose*, in *Œuvres Complètes*, Paris, 1869, IV. p. 2, — an interesting preface.

[3] *Young Ofeg's Ditties*, trans. Egerton, London, 1895.

[4] *Also Sprach Zaruthustra*, III. "Das Andere Tanzlied."

dithyrambic phrases threaten to turn into mere raving, and often carry out the threat. What saves a poet from this danger, and the great poets know it, is the dignity, the self-restraint, and the communal human sympathy of rhythm, which binds one, as in that old consent of voice and step, to one's fellows, and checks all individual centrifugal follies; there are no bounds, no laws, there is no decorum, in such whirling words, until they whirl in ordered motion and until cosmos is where chaos was. "Slaves by their own compulsion," these sensual and dark things rebel in vain against the laws of poetic form; pastels and whatever else, they have not even the dignity of truly great prose. They are out of their sphere; to adapt a line from the *Dunciad*, prose on stilts is several degrees worse than poetry fallen lame.

Poetry, then, is still rhythmic utterance, though it has lost great stretches of territory to prose. Prose, to be sure, makes a tempting proposition to her impoverished friend. "Let us call ourselves by one name," she says, "unite all our power, and so make front against science." Such a union has long appealed to the French. Fénelon, one knows, sought thus to revive the epic; and many pens were set scratching for or against the *Télémacomanie*. Chateaubriand [1] tried a cadenced prose in his *Martyrs*, by way of putting new life into sacred poetry. Flaubert [2] and sundry of his school, above all, the Italian D'Annunzio, annex poetry to the prose romance, and not poetry as an informing spirit simply, but the cadences, the colour, the very refrain.[3] Maeterlinck uses the poetic

[1] His defence is very fine and languid and aristocratic, — "inutile dispute *de mots*," he protests at last: *Œuvres Complètes*, Paris, 1852, V. 84, 295 ("Examen des Martyrs").

[2] A foreigner is no judge in these things; but he may say how much more the lucidity of Mérimée, of M. Anatole France, appeals to him than the poetic prose of Flaubert's *Salammbô*.

[3] Has any one noted in the opening chapter of the *Trionfo della Morte* a prose refrain, "Gocce di pioggia, rare, cadevano," repeated with considerable effect?

device of repetition — say in the *Princesse Maleine* — to the verge of regular rhythm. Rime itself is not excluded; witness this from D'Annunzio's novel:[1] "rideva, gemeva, pregava, cantava, accarezzava, singhiozzava, miniaciava; ilare, flebile, umile, ironica, lusinghevole, disperata, crudele."[2] Is poetry, then, fallen by the wayside, and has prose spoiled her of her raiment, so as to stand hereafter in her stead? No. Whatever Walter Pater may have done for English or these men for Italian and French, they have at best set up a new euphemism[3] of no real promise and permanence. When the final balance is struck, these writers will perhaps take a place in prose analogous, even if in a contrary spirit, to the place of Swift in verse. Swift's "unpoetic verse" is remorselessly clear, remorselessly direct; one must read his poetry, and in great measure admire, even like it, for its compelling energy and lucidity of style. Yet, after all, one feels that these are alien virtues, imported from the realm of prose; and one reads Swift's poems much as one listens to a foreigner conversing correctly, admirably, in one's own tongue. And as with Swift's prose excellence in poetry, so with this poetic excellence in prose; in the long account, *laudatur et alget.* It makes the vain attempt to move landmarks set up, not by men, but by man, by human nature itself.

So much for the theories; but it must now be proved be-

[1] *Ibid.*, p. 396. The structure is strophic and very artistic in its complication.

[2] See D'Annunzio's dedication of this romance, and his artistic creed, quite an echo of the preface to Baudelaire's poems in prose.

[3] There is often in these prose-poems, so much praised now, a startling reminder of the golden style of certain despised folk who wrote cadenced and coloured prose in their romances three centuries ago. And not only in romances; Tom Nash tried rimed prose, both with alliteration and with actual rime, by way of helping the antithetical clause. See the "Anatomy of Absurdity," in Nash's *Works*, ed. Grosart, I. 6 ff., 24: inferre: averre; praise: daies; nose: rose; and the lilt of "to play with her dogge, than to pray to her God." The *Arcadia* is not so much a rimed or rhythmical prose, as swelling and sonorous. For mediæval rimed prose, see Wackernagel, *Gesch. d. deutsch. Lit.*, 2d ed., I. 107 ff., and Sievers, *Altger. Metrik*, p. 49, — the latter for Germanic relations.

yond question that rhythm is the vital and essential quality in the beginnings of poetic art. Where to draw the line between prose and verse, between the recurrence which is regular and which is called for our purposes rhythm, and the recurrence that is not regular, is hard indeed; but perhaps a satisfactory rule may be given in the words of Professor Budde, a distinguished student of that Hebrew poetry to which so many advocates of the prose poem have made appeal. "The fundamental law of form in all poetry," he says,[1] "by which in every race and at all times verse is distinguished from prose, is that while in prose the unchecked current of speech flows consistently as far as the thought carries it, the range of thought and the length of the sentence changing often and in many ways, verse, on the other hand, divides its store of thought into relatively short lines which appeal to the ear as distinct not only by this shortness, but also by relations determined by laws definite, indeed, but varying with different races and languages. Whenever the formal factors of poetry are enriched, these smallest units, the verses or lines, tend to join, by a new bond, in a higher unit of form."[2] This formal factor may be now alliteration, now rime; with the Hebrews, says Budde, it was the thought, which made a higher unit of the short and separated units of line or verse. Lowth's *parallelismus membrorum* does not quite cover the rhythmical structure of Hebrew verse; no matter if a fixed metre has not yet been found, the rhythm is evident, and its law is essentially equal length of the verses within the group.[3] For a test, one must fall back upon that original

[1] "Das Volkslied Israels im Munde der Propheten," in the *Preussische Jahrbücher*, LXXIII. (1893), 460 ff. See p. 465.

[2] Driver, *Introd. Lit. Old Test.*, p. 361, says that rhythm, *the restrained flow of expression*, separates poetry from prose.

[3] Professor Sievers has announced "a discovery of the principles of Hebrew metre," and his exposition will be welcome. See *Sitzungsberichte der sächsischen Akademie der Wissenschaften*, 5 February, 1899.

organ of poetry, the human voice. Slave to the eye, one often reads as prose what one could read, or what could be read to one, as poetry.[1] In any case, there will be debatable ground, perhaps neutral ground; but it is safe to say from theory, from the practical trial, from arguments of the learned, that so far the effort to obliterate verse or rhythm as the real boundary line of poetic territory, has proved a failure, and is likely to prove a failure as often as it shall be tried. The case must be taken to the court of human history and human progress; brought hither, all the arguments for poems in prose lose their power. If, as Bücher says, one is unwilling nowadays to let rhythmic speech pass, merely in so far as it is rhythmic speech, for poetry, that is because ages of culture, with increasing æsthetic demands, have quite naturally added new conditions; but the beginning of poetry as an æsthetic fact was in the sense of rhythm. The poem now laboriously wrought at the desk goes back to the rhythm of work or play or dance in the life of primitive man, and the element of rhythm is the one tie that binds beginning and end; if poetry denies rhythm, it denies itself.

This statement itself, however, certain of the learned now vehemently oppose, and bring reasons for their attitude quite different from such arguments as we have been considering for the prose poem. Rhythm itself, they maintain, is the outcome of prose. It is the child, says one bold German, of grammatical inflections and the stress of oratory. Here is fine revolution, indeed, if they have the trick to show

[1] Professional "readers" nearly always kill a poem by reading it as prose. Tennyson read his own verses almost in a chant. De Vigny, *Journal d'un Poete*, p. 70, says, "tout homme qui dit bien ses vers les chante, en quelque sorte." Ronsard, *Œuvres*, ed. Blanchemain, III. 12 f., asks the reader of his *Franciade* one thing: "Be good enough to pronounce my verses well, and suit your voice to their emotion, not reading it, after the way of certain folk, as a letter, . . . but as a poem, with good emphasis." So Quintilian; but the elocutionist has no bowels of mercy.

it. Strabo, in a classic sentence,[1] laid down the law which writer after writer has taken without question as undisputed and indisputable authority; poetry came before prose. "Flowery prose," he said, "is nothing but an imitation of poetry," which is the "origin of all rhetorical language," and was at first always sung; "the very term *prose*," he concludes, "which is applied to language not clothed in metre, seems to indicate . . . its descent from an elevation, or chariot, to the ground." Hence the *sermo pedestris* of Latin writers. Against this, now, come sundry scattered hints and at least two elaborate arguments. Vigfusson and Powell,[2] after a consideration of old Scandinavian poetry, are fain to think that Germanic rhythm was at the start simply "excited and emphatic prose," and make rhythm in general not an essential so much as an accomplishment and aftergrowth of poetry. Finding no metre in this same Norse poetry, none in Hebrew, Gottsched,[3] while he allowed that songs were the earliest poetic form, thought them to have been simple unmetrical chants, as if a child should sing the Lord's prayer. Many ballads, even English and Scottish, seem to show with other supposed primitive traits a rough and faulty structure of verse, so that certain critics, in their haste, make the lack of smooth metres a test of age, — an idea which long prevailed in regard to Chaucer's versification. It is said[4] that until the beginning of the seventeenth century Hungarian poetry was "quite without system, without rhythm, full of bad rimes, and mainly made up of verses joined in long, monotonous rows"; this, however, as in India, may have been the case not with lyric, but only with epic. Comparetti thinks that the *Kalevala* was founded upon earlier poetic or

[1] *Geography*, Introd., I. ii. 7, translation of Hamilton.

[2] *Corpus Poeticum Boreale*, I. 434.

[3] *Critische Dichtkunst*, pp. 70 f.

[4] Bruchmann, *Poetik*, pp. 161, 124, 22.

roughly rhythmic prose, — again a matter of epic; and earliest Japanese poetry, so far as it has been preserved, "is not far removed from prose."[1] Now and then, but not often, one is told that savage songs have no regular rhythm and no settled order in the verse. If it be true that mere counting of syllables was the earliest form of common Aryan versification, it is at first sight not so unreasonable to assume some sort of excited prose as a common basis for this system as well as for the systems of quantitative and of accentual rhythm. Moreover, as will be shown in later pages, there is a feeling abroad which runs counter to any notion of spontaneity, and insists upon a process of invention and imitation; this, too, would make against a natural rhythm,[2] would throw out rhythm as an essential and primitive part of poetry.[3] So much for scattered hints and observations; there are more elaborate attacks.

In a treatise by Norden[4] on ancient artistic prose, one has under one's hand all the evidence which can be gathered from the classics, particularly the Greek, for this view of the relations between prose and verse; here, too, are ranged certain arguments against that old notion of the precedence of poetry.[5] Musical sense, rhythm, was given to man with

[1] Aston, *Japanese Literature*, p. 13.

[2] The younger Racine is startling with his assertion that "poetry is the daughter of nature, while verse is the work of art." *Mém. Acad. Inscr.*, XV. 307 ff., "De la poesie Artificielle. . . ."

[3] Curiously enough, J. Grimm, though not too clear in his statement, is with the rationalists, in spite of his "divine origin" for poetry and the "mystery" of self-made song, which he advocates elsewhere; for in his *Ursprung der Sprache* (reprint, 7th ed., 1879, p. 54) he says poetry and music had their origin in the reason, emotion, and imagination of a poet, and gives a genetic process not unlike that set forth by Mr. Spencer: "denn aus betonter, gemessener recitation der Worte entsprangen gesang und lied, aus dem lied die andere dichtkunst, aus dem gesang durch gesteigerte abstraction alle übrige musik."

[4] *Die antike Kunstprosa*, 2 vols., Leipzig, 1898. Mr. Spencer's theory, analogous in some respects to Norden's, is considered below.

[5] This notion itself — see the extract above from Strabo — Norden, I. 35, refers to a desire to glorify the golden age, and to set its poetry over against the prose of degenerate modern days.

the spoken word itself, as in historical times to the Hellenic folk, whose melodious sentence is as inaudible as the music of the spheres to an ear dependent upon modern speech. Now before poetry was developed, Norden assumes, there was a rhythmic prose distinguished by some kind of emphasis from the speech of daily life; thence sprang on one hand the rhythm of regular poetry, and on the other hand a rhythm of impassioned, oratorical prose. The oratory of Greece was a kind of chanting, and the gestures that went with it were a species of dance; but these in no way could be called identical with the singing or recitation of poetry. Then came confusion. Gorgias began a new era when he imported certain elements of poetry into his prose; even the rimed prose of the Middle Ages Norden[1] calls "the result of a thousand years of development from the time of Gorgias." The early results, however, were destructive. Tragedy, thinks our author, was ruined in Hellas because all barriers were broken down between poetry and prose, and rhetoric overwhelmed the drama; great epos yielded to great history; gnomic poetry vanished; epigram supplanted elegy; dithyramb made room for lofty prose at large.[2] But this is nothing more than a process in civilized Greece analogous to the process in our own day described a few pages above. Even the tradition of the classical writers pointed back to an age of poetry which preceded prose; for while Strabo, in the passage already considered, and Varro,[3] speak of actual literature which they had in hand, Plutarch, writing on the Pythian oracle, made poetry the product of primitive times and prose the outcome of prehistorical decadence. Against this tradition, which he makes a mere glorification of the

[1] II. 762.

[2] *Ibid.*, I. 78.

[3] *Tam apud Graecos quam apud Latinos longe antiquiorem curam fuisse carminum quam prosae*, etc. Varro in Isiodor. *Orig.*, I. 38, 2, quoted and discussed by Norden, I. 32 f.

golden age, Norden argues with learning and acuteness, and from material furnished by Greek literature itself. But Greek literature is surely no criterion for primitive song; persistent as this prejudice is,[1] Norden sees that ethnology has better points of view, and in one or two places he calls upon it for aid.[2] The distinction between poetry and prose is, for him, "secondary, not essential," for the reason that he cannot find this distinction in the earliest expression of formal or solemn language known to the various races of man, whether on highest or lowest planes of culture. His summary may be quoted, temperate and reasonable as it is; it appeals to ethnological arguments, which would be close upon convincement if they did not utterly neglect, as nearly all writers on poetry have neglected, the communal basis of the art, and the fundamental consideration that earliest poetry is more a social than an individual expression. Norden's eye is fixed upon the priest, the poet, the medicine man, the lawgiver; he forgets the throng, and he forgets that the throng was mainly active and rarely passive in the primitive stages of poetry. But let his own summary be heard.[3] The line now drawn between poetry and prose, he maintains, was unknown to primitive races. Forms of magic, the language of the laws, ceremonial religious rites, were everywhere made in prose; not, however, in the prose of daily conversation, but in a prose removed from common conditions by two factors: first, it was spoken in measured, solemn tones, and so became rhythmical, — not the regular rhythm

[1] "I suppose, of course," said a writer of considerable reputation, to whom the project of the present work was mentioned, "you will begin with Homer."

[2] Indeed, the very arguments from Greek oratory hardly seem convincing. Let any one read the section of Aristotle's *Rhetoric* (III. viii.), where he speaks of prose rhythm. What is this rhythm without metre but the quality, far more musically developed in Greek, which one also recognizes in the harmony of any modern artistic prose?

[3] Work quoted, I. 30 f. See also I. 37, note; I. 156 ff.; II. 813 f.

of song, but a sort of chant or recitation,[1] so that one may figure the early priest like his modern brother, the snowy-banded, delicate-handed one, at his intoning; and, secondly, it was furnished, for emphasis and for the help of memory, with certain vocal expedients, such as alliteration and rime, which are inborn alike in the most civilized and in the wildest races. This kind of prose existed before there was any artistic poetry. Norden would like to see more work done in the field of early legal and religious forms; old Latin prayers, old Germanic laws, for example, have been coaxed or bullied into some metrical scheme, and made to pass as poetry. Elsewhere he takes the case of that prayer to Mars which Westphal and Allen called Saturnian verse; by Norden's reckoning, this is mainly alliterative, rhythmic prose; only the second half can be called metrical; and he is convinced that Saturnian verse itself is nothing but the later metrical equipment of what was once rhythmic prose solemnly spoken with two sections to the line. *Carmen*, he goes on to say, is originally any solemn formula whether spoken or sung, whether rhythmic prose, even simple prose, or verse;[2] that is "settled." It is a clever suggestion, too, that rhythmic prose belongs with what one now calls the loose sentence, while artistic prose, contemporary with artistic and metrical poetry, came into prominence with the

[1] See, however, E. Schröder, "Ueber das Spell," *Zst. f. deutsches Alterthum*, XXXVII. 241 ff. *Spell* and *lied*, he says, are related in terms of epic and lyric charms or incantations, and form the basis of the common antithesis of "say" and "sing" (p. 258). The epic part of a charm, he thinks, was recited, while the lyric part was sung. Unfortunately, Schröder comes to no very definite results; and, like most writers on early verse, he neglects the communal and choral conditions of primitive poetry.

[2] Düntzer, *Zeitschr. deutsch. Gymnasialwesen*, 1857, pp. 1 ff., the unwearied commentator, who has had so much experience in the practical reduction of poetry to prose, decided for this view, and doubtless with some show of right. A *carmen*, he said, was anything, — oath, formula, law, incantation, — spoken in loud and solemn tones. So Livy, I. 26, on that *lex horrendi carminis*. This may be true for the medicine man, but it is not true for the throng.

periodic structure;[1] so the tale, like Grimm's familiar "There was once a king's son, and he was very beautiful . . . ," in its uninvolved, consecutive phrases, would give one an idea of the early rhythmic prose.

All this is useful and suggestive; but it by no means does away with the fact of regular rhythmic utterance for primitive times. Who, for example, is going to believe that rime and alliteration were developed before regular rhythm,— regular rhythm, as will presently be shown, standing out as the one fact about savage poetry to which nearly all evidence of ethnology gives assent? Who will deny that quite as early as any priest recited his prayer or buzzed his magic in solemn prose, there was a throng of folk dancing and singing with a rhythm as exact as may be? Did the priests, even, recite in "irregular rhythmic prose" that repeated *enos Lases juvate* of the Arval rites, sung as they beat the ground in concerted measure of the dance? "So long," says Usener[2] in his book on old Greek verse, "so long as human societies turned in solemn and festal manner to the divinities, so long they made petition, thanks, laud, in measured and rhythmic verse, and the words were inseparable from singing and the steps of the march." For purposes of this kind, and such purposes are the very soul of primitive social life, chanted prose is out of the question. An excellent authority in musical matters, Dr. Jacobsthal,[3] points out that the rhythm, if one may so call it, of the chant stands to real rhythm as prose stands to verse, and that the song to which a throng must dance, as in primitive times, *can "in no case" lack the regular rhythm.* Who,

[1] The *λέξις ειρομένη* and the *λέξις καταστραμμένη*; down to Herodotus the Greeks, it is said, spoke and wrote in the former style: Norden, I. 37, note. He appeals to specimens gathered from folklore.

[2] *Altgriechischer Versbau*, p. 55.

[3] "Musikalische Bildung der Meistersänger," in Haupt's *Zeitsch. f. deutsches Alterthum*, XX. 80 f.

moreover, that has read Bücher's essay can overlook the fact that primitive labour must have begotten an exact rhythm, and very early must have given meaning to this rhythm by more or less connected words? The proof, offered not only by Norden but in those scattered hints already noted, breaks down when confronted with hard facts. Ballad metres are often rough in the copies which have come down to us, but a hundred considerations show this to have been the fault of the copy itself, not of the makers and singers,[1] and to have been due to the transfer from oral to written conditions. There seems to be no reason why a letter should not be quoted which the late Professor Child wrote in 1885 to the author of the present book; "any *volkslied*," he said, "shows as good an ear as any Pindaric ode by Gray or whomever else." It is the sense of complicated metres which is due to culture and intellectual development, and not the sense of exact and simple rhythm. As regards that protoplasmic prose of the popular tale, which Norden calls "the essential test of primitive speech," how can he prove that it is the essential test of primitive song? How different Bruchmann, who admits early prose narrative, but says distinctly that early poetry, lyric outpouring of emotion, was song; "the earliest of all poetry" for him is communal song, *gesang in gemeinschaft*, golden words indeed! Grosse is to the same effect. Who denies the tale, the loose prose style in short sentences verging on rhythmic effects? Of course the entertainer told his tale betimes; but earlier than this tale, the dance of the throng, as well as the labour of daily life, had from the very beginning mated sounds and words with rhythm, precise rhythm, as a festal and consenting act. A mass of evidence, soon to be considered, is overwhelm-

[1] The reason why a folksong often fails to have a musical effect, says Böckel in the introduction to his collection of Hessian ballads, p. civ., is because it is taken down from a single singer, whereas all these songs are essentially choral, and need the voices of a throng. This hint is valuable in many directions; for example, see below on social singing at labour.

ingly for this state of things. Norden appeals for the form of the tale to Radloff, a great authority; let us do the same for the form of the song. In an article on poetic forms among the Altaic Tartars,[1] Radloff remarks that in these isolated tribes popular literature, without even the faintest influence from the lettered world, has been developed in a quite natural way. Especially worthy of note, he says, is the strictness of metrical form in their poetry. He notes, moreover, the inseparable character, under such conditions, of poetry and song. The specimens which he gives are anything but rhythmic prose, and the rhythmic law is anything but loose. The tales on the other hand are quite different; "these are not sung," he says, "but recited," although now and then the reciter sings a verse or so. Which came first, the entertainer and his audience, or the festal, singing throng? Evidence of ethnology and conclusions of sociology certainly put the singing, dancing throng as a primary social fact, and the relation of audience to entertainer as a secondary social fact. Mr. Joseph Jacobs[2] has hailed the *cante-fable* as protoplasm alike of the metrical ballad and of the prose tale, one omitting prose, the other omitting verse; and while this does not really help Norden's claim, it is worth the while to note how it assumes a development which is counter to all the facts. Even on its chosen ground of Celtic tales, this theory meets indications that the verse is original and the prose of later date.[3] The *cante-fable*

[1] *Zeitschrift f. Völkerpsychol. u. Sprachwissensch.* IV. 85 ff. Comparetti is also unfortunate in his use of this essay to prove that poetic prose came before verse. See his *Kalewala*, p. 37.

[2] *English Fairy Tales*, 1898, p. 247. Ferdinand Wolf, a man not given to hazy and romantic views, dismisses the *cante-fable* as "jedesfalls . . . eine Entartung," a degenerate state of the communal ballad. *Proben port. u. catal. Volksromanzen*, Wien, 1856, p. 20, note 2.

[3] Alfred Nutt, *Voyage of Bran*, I. 135, citing Kuno Meyer, and saying that certain prose is "younger in appearance," need not assume it to have "suffered from change," but may take a simpler view. The verse may well be of older date.

seems like a late form, a device of the entertainer; the scraps of verse are survivals, just as the chorus in a Greek drama is the survival of a drama in which all took part, with no division into actors and spectators. In the Chinese drama[1] an Occidental ear is offended by a remarkable confusion of speaking and singing; even a single sentence in the dialogue is so divided that part is spoken and part is sung. This is no primitive and protoplasmic state; it is rather the confusion of contraries, than the germ of related and naturally developed forms of art. Poetry and prose in historic times have been approaching each other, not diverging, and the curve of evolution would indicate a wide distinction at the start. Mixture of prose, as Professor Sievers sees it, is a sign of decay in the *Muspilli*, in the Hildebrand Lay.[2] On the other hand, in vigorous poetry like the Roumanian ballad there is no mixture of prose, while the Roumanian popular tale is sprinkled with verses; yet here is precisely where the protoplasmic state ought to be found for both arts, since the poetical style is "simple as possible," has often no relative clauses for whole pages, and is full of repetition.[3] Under simple conditions, poetry often breaks up into prose, but prose is not found in its transition to poetry; for proof it is enough to quote a recent writer on German ballads.[4] "More and more," he says, "the ballads disintegrate into prose, a process which

[1] This account is taken from Bruchmann's *Poetik*, p. 217, and Letourneau, *L'Évolution Littéraire*, pp. 198 f., who gives other details. J. F. Campbell, *Popular Tales*, etc., 2d ed., IV. 84, mentions cases of dual performance in the Highlands, where a bard sang to his harp heroic passages, and a narrator "filled up the pauses by telling prose history."

[2] *Altgermanische Metrik*, pp. 165, 168.

[3] Rudow, *Verslehre und Stil der rumänischen Volkslieder*, Halle, 1886, pp. 5, 28 f., 31.

[4] Böckel, *Deutsche Volkslieder aus Oberhessen . . . mit kulturhistorisch-ethnographischer Einleitung* (the latter a valuable collection of material), Marburg, 1885, pp. clxxxiii. f.

has been noted for Spain, Sweden, Scotland, Portugal, and is also known in Germany."[1] He gives quotations and references to support his assertion, going on to name several well-known ballads which began as such and then, in the guise of prose tales, won as wide and as great a vogue as the originals had enjoyed before. Perhaps in the case of poetic composition at a time when intellect has mastered emotion, prose may be the basis of poetry, but this case has no bearing on primitive conditions. Whether a poet nowadays conceives his work in prose, as Goethe did in the *Iphigenie*, or begins with the "brains beat into rhythm," is an individual matter. "When Gautier wished to do a good piece of work, he always began in verse," say the Goncourts.[2] Tradition makes Vergil write out his *Æneid* in prose and then turn it into verse; Vida[3] commends this method for the prentice in poetry. There is a curious passage in Goethe's letter to Schiller of 5 March, 1798, about renewed work on *Faust*. "Some tragic scenes were done in prose; by reason of their naturalness and strength they are quite intolerable in relation to the other scenes. I am, therefore, now trying to put them into rime, for there the idea is seen as if under a veil, and the immediate effect of this tremendous material is softened." This, however, has nothing to do with primitive conditions of poetry; the simplicity of modern prose is an effort of art, and belongs with the intellectual empire, while rhythm, particularly in its early form of repetition, is the immediate and spontaneous expression of emotion, and likely

[1] Mingled verse and prose has always a late, artificial manner; for example, the *Satura Menippea*, imitated in Latin by Varro and Petronius (Teuffel and Schwabe, *Hist. Roman Literature*, trans. Warr, I. 255), and claimed for the half-rhythmical portion of Swift's *Battle of the Books*, by Feyerabend, *Englische Studien*, XI. 487 ff. Some of Feyerabend's scanning, by the way, is highly adventurous.

[2] *Journal*, 12 Mai, 1857.

[3] *De Arte Poet.*, I. 75.

to be more pronounced and dominant the nearer one is to the primitive state of things.

What Norden really does is to scour away accretions of silliness, romantic and sentimental phrases, which are too often held as part and parcel of a sensible belief about poetry in its early stage. Granted, as it is to be hoped the reader will ultimately grant, that singing and dancing wax in importance as one traces back the path of the arts, granted that verse and song covered a far greater field of activity in the beginning than they cover now, the notion that men with language in a fluent state, and on intellectual topics, sang instead of talking, that primitive life was like an Italian opera-stage, that the better part of man's utterance was given over to lyrical wonder at the sunset and the stars, — these ideas, even when hallowed by great names, must be tossed to oblivion. But such a jettison by no means involves the sinking of the ship itself; to change the figure, gentlemen who have overthrown a minor idol or so must not loudly proclaim that they have razed the temple and rooted out the faith. For example, Grimm of old and Kögel of late[1] were too fond of poetic laws; the former confounded quaintness with beauty, and the latter discovered too much rhythm. The Frisian code, Kögel seems to have thought, was composed and recited as poetry, as alliterative verse. Well, this is perhaps Frisiomania of a dangerous kind, and Dr. Siebs[2] is within his rights in preaching another sermon on the old but dubious text of *Frisia non cantat.* The laws, he says, were indeed alliterative; but they were neither rhythmic nor poetical. So far, so good; the advantage seems to be on the side of Siebs; the idol totters and possibly falls. But now to pull down the temple! Whence came this

[1] In Grimm's charming article on "Poetry in Law," and in Kögel's *Geschichte der deutschen Litt.* I.

[2] *Zeitschrift f. deutsche Philologie,* XXIX. 405 ff.

alliteration? Like rime, it is a product of prose, declares the iconoclast, "having, in the first place, nothing to do with poetry," and probably rising in answer to a demand of the language of trade, which needed to lay stress on the emphatic parts of one's plea for a good bargain. That is, the mainstay of all Germanic rhythm is a "drummer's" device, and begins in the shifty phrases of the early Germanic *hausierer*. This is a world of broken hopes. Norden for rime,[1] and Siebs for alliteration, which is only rime of another sort, have entered a terrific *caveat* against the historian of primitive song. Is rime, then, the fine flower and outgrowth of a stump-speech, and is alliteration, poor changeling, unmasked in these latter days as an intruder and an alien in poetic halls, a by-blow of the primitive bagman? No, the temple is not pulled down. The rhythmical or unrhythmical character of Frisian laws is one thing; the origin of rime, the functions and progress of it, cannot be even guessed on the basis of such studies.

Two attempts, however, to prove the priority of prose, not by the classics, not by folklore alone, not by alliterative laws, but by ethnological facts and by comparative methods, may now be considered. Poetry as a whole, says Professor Biedermann,[2] and regarded in the genetic way, was not originally bound up with song, not even with rhythm. Song, he says, does not make poetry, but breaks it, disturbs and corrupts it. Maori and Malay, he points out, simply recite their legends and poems; in the old Persian, as in the old Japanese poetry, there is no rhythm to be found; and he

[1] See Norden's *Anhang* on Rime, II. 810 ff. It may be noted here that the fact of which Norden makes so much, riming of inflectional endings, was pointed out by Masing, *Ursprung des Reims*, Dorpat, 1866, pp. 15 f.

[2] In a review of Bücher's *Arbeit und Rhythmus;* see *Zeitschr. f. vergl. Litteraturgesch.*, N. F. II. (1897) 369 ff. This is another darling heresy, — to break up the old tradition of evolution, and to deny that dance, song, poetry, began as a single art. Yet ethnology, as it will be seen, supports this tradition; so does a study of popular poetry. Compare, too, *Iliad*, XVIII. 569 ff., and other commonplaces, for the classic traditions, and Aristotle's famous passage on Origins, for older science in the case.

assures his reader "that attempts to prove the original unity of poetry, music, and rhythm have come to wrack," — a statement which needs great store of assurance when one considers it after reading the book under review. Biedermann's own theory is offered in a nutshell. Poetry began as mere repetition, without music or rhythm, a parlous and naked state indeed; the taste for music is simply a chastened love of noise;[1] while rhythm is the result of concerted labour. That in after ages the three wanderers now and then met and passed the time of day, Biedermann is generous enough not to deny.

More weighty objections are to be found in an article by R. de la Grasserie.[2] Spoken words, he says, fall into prose as expression of thought, and into poetry as expression of sentiment; prose is fundamental, while poetry gets its material from prose, and follows it in point of time, although it is conceded that the full development of poetry precedes the full development of prose. At first it would seem that the author regarded verse as essential to poetry; the poet and the verse-maker, he says, must be united as a single productive power. But at once he goes on to ask whether verse be the sole poetic expression, and answers in the negative. Poetry is creation, "subjective discovery" of any sort, as opposed to the objective discoveries of science, where nothing is created. Didactic, mnemonic verse is not poetry, for it is merely the verse that is mnemonic; and the reason why poetry has come to be confounded with versification is simply that verse was needed for the recording or memorizing of poetry.[3] This teleological explanation of rhythm is a

[1] "Dass . . . Musik aus dem Gefallen an selbst hervorgerufenen Lärm sich entwickelt hat. . . ."

[2] "Essai de Rythmique Comparée," in *Le Museon*, X. 299 ff., 419 ff., 589 ff.

[3] Used to explain the actual origin of rhythm by Müller and Schumann, *Zeitschr. f. Psychol. u. Physiol. d. Sinnesorgane*, VI. 282 f., quoted by Meumann, *Untersuchungen*, etc., pp. 10 f.

very weak joint in De la Grasserie's armour; it shows how easily common sense can make itself ridiculous in its excess, a tendency commonly ascribed to sentimental and enthusiastic ideas alone. Facing the splendours of rhythm, knowing how it has held itself abreast of the lordliest doings of poetry, one laughs at the notion that its only credentials on Olympus should be its mnemonic convenience; and De la Grasserie thrusts his explanation handily away among the mists of primitive song. Then he turns to his theory of poetic growth. Poetry passed through three stages of expression, — first, prose; next, rhythmic prose; last, verse. How did poetry begin in prose? Well, it was "prose à courte haleine,"[1] prose with thought-pauses as frequent as rhythmic pauses, so that there was no distinction between prose and verse, — and no good reason, the reader is tempted to add, why this same prose should not be called verse outright. Exactly what thought-pauses have to do with a period when poetry consisted in the indefinite repetition of a very short phrase or even of a single word, and when, by all evidence, the pause is rhythmic entirely, the author does not say; he is dealing with a theory and not with facts, and so he assumes a majestic periodic prose as primitive utterance. Next after "prose" came "rhythmic prose," and then verse; but the evolutionary process goes on, and from verse, as in these latter days, one turns back to prose in rhythm, and yet again to prose outright. If one asks for a bill of particulars, if one asks how verse came out of rhythmic prose, one is told that two propositions may have had the same number of words, just as in Arabic, just as in the *Avesta*,[2] — that the "two propositions" were once mere repetition, and sung in perfect time is, of course, not noted, — so that the psychic

[1] See Hoffmann's similar theory, quoted below.

[2] The old mistake of confounding literal chronology with evolution. As if the *Avesta* were primitive!

pause grows to be one with the rhythmic pause. But, accepting the impossible terms of the case, what proof is offered that word-counting and syllable-counting are of higher date than actual rhythm? Granting this, to be sure, the next step is easy; interior symmetry now comes into play, the measure of feet, the perfect rhythm of Greek and Latin verse. What cause, then, was at work thus to develop verse out of prose? Music and singing, answers the ingenious essayist; but the ingenious essayist has calmly shut out all facts save such as suit his case, and one is curious to know what he would do with ethnological evidence in regard to the priority and primacy of dance and song. Did man come to this fine mastery of metres and this subtle sense of quantities before he had begun to dance to his own singing?

If M. de la Grasserie were right, if Professor Norden were right, in this plea for prose as the parent of verse, a work on the beginnings of poetry could have nothing to do with verse, and only a little to do with rhythmic prose. Barring the way to their conclusions stand two facts. Rhythm is the prime characteristic, the essential condition, of the dance, and oldest poetry is by common consent found in close alliance with dance and song. Secondly, as the brilliant essay of Bücher has made more than probable, backed as it is by evidence of a really primitive character, and not by theories based upon a highly developed literature, poetry in some of its oldest forms, older indeed than that supposed period of earliest prose which M. de la Grasserie assumes for the start, was not only the companion but the offspring of labour. In postponing rhythmic utterance to the third great period of the development of poetry, the champion of prose origins is running counter to tradition, counter to the consent of science, counter to a formidable array of facts. It is quite wrong, too, to say[1]

[1] So M. de la Grasserie asserts in an ingenious account of the retrograde process by which in modern times poetry has retraced its old evolution, passing

that rhythm nowadays depends upon music to keep it sound and alive; the rhythm of Tennyson's *Bugle Song*, of Kipling's *Recessional*, of any haunting and subtle lyric, may stir the composer to set it to music, but in no way depends upon music for its charm. It is quite as wrong to say that rhythm is less effective now than it has been; a century that knew Goethe, Heine, Shelley, Tennyson, not to leave Germanic bounds, has no concessions to make in this respect. Moreover, the account which the essayist gives of Arabic verse, as developed from prose, is good until another account turns up, — say that of M. Hartmann,[1] where rhythm is beginning and end of the matter; and it happens that this account is by an Arabic scholar of repute.

Considered in all fairness, these attacks have not shaken the belief in rhythm as something that lies at the heart of poetry. They may well brush aside some absurdity of romantic origin, but they fail to make probable or even possible a theory which would overthrow a settled literary tradition touching all quarters of the globe. It cannot be said that Norden has proved the growth of poetry out of prose even in the rhetorical clauses of oratory. From Longinus[2] one learns that an oration among the Greeks had rhythm, although it was not metrical, and in its delivery stopped just short of singing; so that one may concede that the speech of an orator carried to an extreme would give song, while his harmonious gestures, an art now as good as lost, needed but little more action and detail to become what the Greeks knew as a dance. But does any one pretend to say that singing and dancing spring from individual oratory? Orators now

from verse back through rhythmic prose to prose outright. The only use which he now concedes to verse is in . . . the opera. In all other fields, — epic, drama, lyric, — he thinks it is dead as King Pandion.

[1] *Die Entstehung der arabischen Versmasse*, Giessen, 1896.

[2] A remarkable passage. See the translation of Roberts, p. 149.

and then still sing or chant in their speeches. One would like to know more about the sermons which Dr. Fell preached "in blank verse";[1] and one is in doubt whether this phrase, along with Selden's sneer[2] at those who "preach in verse," meant a distinct metrical order of words or only a sing-song of the voice — literally "cant," as in the Puritan sermons and in the chant common not long ago with preachers of the Society of Friends. Any one who has heard this "singing" of hortatory speech knows that the rhythms of regular verse, of song and dance, could not possibly be derived from it. Each form of development must be studied for itself under the control of ethnological and sociological facts; and the written oration, with its cadences, goes back to the orator and his listening crowd, just as the written poem goes back to the improvising poet, and through him to the dancing communal throng. The attempt to derive exact rhythms of poetry from loose rhythms of oratorical speech has failed; it remains to show how these exact rhythms spring from primitive song, dance, and labour, mainly under communal conditions, and that exact rhythm lies at the heart of poetry. There are two social situations to be taken for granted. It is natural for one person to speak or even to sing, and for ninety-nine persons to listen. It is also natural for a hundred persons,

[1] Evelyn's *Diary*, 24 February, 1664–1665: "Dr. Fell, Canon of Christ Church, preached before the king . . . a very formal discourse, and in blank verse, according to his manner."

[2] The whole passage is interesting with its fling at poetry, not, however, to be taken as a serious indictment: *Table Talk*, ed. Arber, p. 85: "'Tis a fine thing for children to learn to make verse; but when they come to be men, they must speak like other men, or else they will be laugh't at. 'Tis ridiculous to speak, or write, or preach in verse." Again, "'Tis ridiculous for a Lord to print verses, 'tis well enough to make them to please himself, but to make them publick is foolish. If a man in his private chamber twirls his bandstrings, or plays with a rush to please himself, 'tis well enough; but if he should go into Fleet Street," — and so on. He thinks there is no reason why plays should be in verse; but he rescues the old poets who were forced to write verse "because their verse was sung to music."

under strong emotion, to shout, sing, dance, in concert and as a throng, not as a matter of active and passive, of give and take, but in common consent of expression. The second situation, still familiar now and then, is discouraged by civilized conditions, although, as foundation of social consent, it must have preceded the other situation and must have been of far greater frequency and importance in the beginnings of social life. It is this state of things which writers like Norden fail to take into account; and it is this state of things, with its communal consent resting on the vital and unifying fact of rhythm, which is now to be positively proved by the evidence of ethnology, the conclusions of sociology, and the controlling sense of evolution in poetical as in social progress.

In treating the positive side of such a subject, one turns instinctively to the latest word of science; and it would seem that the method which combines physical facts with psychological processes ought to be an adequate court of appeal. Dr. Ernst Meumann has undertaken a study of this sort with regard to rhythm;[1] but his investigations do little for the historical and genetic side of the case. From his essay, to be sure, one learns much that is of value, and one is made to see that certain views of rhythm heretofore in vogue must be considerably modified; for the main question of primitive rhythm, however, and for historical purposes at large, one can here learn nothing, since Meumann uses in his research only that declamatory style of reciting poetry by which the rhythm is always disguised and usually suppressed.[2] He denies Paul's assertion that rhythmic measures in a verse are of equal duration, — a traditional statement, — because Brücke's famous experiments, to which Paul appeals, were made upon

[1] *Untersuchungen zur Psychologie und Aesthetik des Rhythmus*, Leipzig, 1894; reprinted from Vol. X. of Wundt's *Philosophische Studien*.

[2] See p. 77, where he chooses "die Freiheit des declamirten Rhythmus gegenüber dem allgemeinen rhythmischen Princip der Regelmässigkeit." See also pp. 82, 87, 101, and especially 91.

folk who "scanned" their verses and did not recite them. But, for the purposes just named, it is begging the question when Meumann rejects the scanning of verse as something "counter to the nature of poetic material." What is the nature of poetic material, — essentially rhythmic, or essentially free from rhythm? All reports of primitive singing, that is, of singing among races on a low plane of culture, make rhythm a wholly insistent element of the verse; and when a logical explanation which fits modern facts is at odds with the chronological course of things, then the danger signal is up for any wary student. It is easy to see that Meumann could make experiments on nothing but a modern reading of poetry, and it was natural that he should choose the sort of reciting most in vogue; his results in such a case, however, can be valid only for modern conditions. Poetry, for purposes of public entertainment, is mainly read in the free, declamatory style. This, to be sure, is not the way in which Tennyson, a master of poetic form, recited his verses; it is not the way in which one reads, or ought to read, lyric poems generally, where even the most ruthless and resolute Herod of "elocution" finds it impossible to slay all the measures of three syllables and under; and, by overwhelming evidence, it is not the way of quite savage folk, who dance and sing their verses. It is not even the way of races in more advanced stages of culture,[1] who recited their verses with strong rhythmical accents, using a harp, or some instrument of the sort, for additional emphasis. Rhythm is obscured or hidden by declamation only in times when the eye has usurped the functions of the ear, and when a highly developed prose makes the accented rhythm of poetry seem

[1] For example, classical rendering of verse, and even modern recitation, as among the Italians. "La plupart des Italiens ont, en lisant les vers, une sorte de chant monotone, appelé *cantilene*, qui détruit toute émotion," says Mme. de Staël, *Corinne*, Chap. III.; but the "elocutionary" emotion is usually an impertinence in simple and cadenced lyric.

either old-fashioned or a sign of childhood. Not that one wishes to restore a sing-song reading, but rather a recognition of metrical structure, of those subtle effects in rhythm which mean so much in the poet's art; verse, in a word, particularly lyric verse, must not be read as if it were prose. Dramatic verse is a difficult problem. French and German actors mainly ignore the rhythm; on the Parisian stage, competent critics say, whole pages of comedy or tragedy may be recited with exquisite feeling, and yet without letting one know whether it is verse or prose that one hears. For in drama one wishes nowadays to hear not rhythm, but the thought, the story, the point; imagine Sheridan's comedies in verse! Even in tragedy dull emotions are now to be roused, not keen emotions soothed; or rather it is thought, penetrated by emotion, to be sure, but thought, and not the cadence which once soothed and carried off the emotion,— thought, indeed, as the comment and gloss on emotion,—in which a modern world wishes to find its consolations and its æsthetic pleasure. As thought recedes, as one comes nearer to those primitive emotions which were untroubled by thought, they get expression more and more in cadenced tones. And, again, this cadenced emotional expression, as it grows stronger, grows wider; the barriers of irony and reserve which keep a modern theatre tearless in the face of Lear's most pathetic utterance, break down; first, as one recedes from modern conditions, comes the sympathetic emotion of the spectators expressed in sighs and tears,—one thinks of those performances in Germany a century and a half ago, and the prodigious weeping that went on,—so that the emotional expression is echoed; then comes the partial activity of the spectators by their deputed chorus; and at last the throng of primitive times, common emotion in common expression, with no spectators, no audience, no reserve or comment of thought,—for thought is absorbed in the perception and action of communal consent;[1] and here, by all evidence, rhythm rules supreme. Go back to these conditions, and what have the tricks of individual accent, the emphasis of logic, the artistic contrasts, the complicated process of interpretation, to do with social or gregarious poetry, with primitive song, with the rhythmic consent of that swaying, dancing multitude uttering a common emotion as much by the cadence of step and cry as by articulate words? Ethnology will be heard in abundance; a word or two may be in place from comparative literature and philology, and a controlling idea, a curve of evolution, may be found in this way if one takes a long stretch of poetic development in some race just forging to the front of civilized life. Song, one may assert, passes naturally into a sort of chant, especially as the epic form of poetry takes shape, into a saying rather than a singing, and then into an even easier movement. There seems to be little doubt that the recitation of classical poetry was a matter of scanning, an utterance which brought out the metre of the verse; even advocates of prose as the forerunner of poetry grant that the ancient writers made a careful distinction between the two, and always recited metre as metre. Emphasis, moreover, due to the regular steps of the original dance, is still heard in that popular verse of four measures which long held its place in Greek, Latin, Germanic, and other languages; once it accompanied the dancing throng, and by Westphal's reckoning[2] consisted of eight steps forward and as many backward, so

[1] Compare Lessing's different but analogous antithesis in the *Laokoon*, XI.: "Bei dem Artisten dünkt uns die Ausführung schwerer als die Erfindung; bei dem Dichter, hingegen, ist es umgekehrt."

[2] See his article in Kuhn's *Zeitschr. f. vergl. Sprach.*, IX. 437 ff.; and the second volume of his *Metrik der Griechen*. For the four-accent verse as popular measure, see H. Usener, *Altgriechischer Versbau*, Bonn, 1887, a suggestive book. For the same verse in Russian, see Bistrom in the *Zeitsch. f. Völkerpsychol.*, V. 185.

that the companion sounds of the voice made two verses with four pairs of syllables in each verse, right and left in step, with one syllable bearing the emphasis. Bergk in 1854 assumed that the hexameter is a combination of two such verses; Usener, correcting Bergk's details, added the Nibelungen verse as made in the same way from two "popular" verses, that is, from the common Aryan metre, and called this a "mark of the oldest European verse"[1] wherever found, still lingering in the folksongs of many peoples. Bruchmann, noting its occurrence with Malays, Esthonians, Tartars, concludes that the verse is thus prevalent because of its convenience for the breath; it is neither too short nor too long. If, now, the curve of evolution in Aryan verse begins with an absolutely strict rhythm and alternate emphasis of syllables, often, as in Iranian,[2] to the neglect of logical considerations; if the course of poetry is to admit logical considerations more and more, forcing in at least one case the abandoning of movable accent and the agreement of verse-emphasis with syllabic emphasis, an undisputed fact; if poetry, too, first shakes off the steps of dancing, then the notes of song, finally the strict scanning of the verse, until now recited poetry is triumphantly logical, with rhythm as a subconscious element; if, finally, this process exactly agrees with the gradual increase of thought over emotion, with the analogous increase of solitary poetry over gregarious poetry, — then, surely, one has but to trace back this curve of evolution, and to project it into prehistoric conditions, in order to infer with something very close to certitude that rhythm is the primal fact in the beginnings of the poetic art. Such a

[1] Wilmanns thinks the case for this "original" verse has not been made out in any convincing way.

[2] F. D. Allen, in Kuhn's *Zeitsch. f. vergl. Sprach.*, XXIV. 558 ff., showed that this Iranian syllable-counting verse, one of the oldest of metres, is not merely counting, but a rhythmic affair, and that the rhythm lay in successive equal intervals marked by verse accent.

curve is assumed as true by two Germanic scholars who differ absolutely with regard to certain questions of chronology. When did the rhythmic, measured chant of Germanic poetry pass into free recited verse? Before the date of such oldest Germanic poetry as is preserved, answers Professor Sievers; not until later, answers Professor Möller. Sievers, it is well known, declares the Germanic alliterative verse, as it lies before us, to have been spoken and not chanted; Möller insists on strophes and a rhythmical chant. To maintain his view, Möller[1] brings forward certain facts. Germanic poetry was at first mainly choral and communal song, poetry of masses of men, the *concentus*, mentioned by Tacitus, of warriors moving into battle, or of a tribe dancing at their religious rites. A *concentus* of warriors in chorus of battle, he notes quite happily, is meant not so much to terrify the foe as to strengthen and order their own emotions, precisely, one may add, as the communal songs which led to the Hellenic chorus, and so to tragedy, were at first a matter of social expression altogether, and not an artistic effort made by a few active persons for the entertainment of a great passive throng. So, too, Möller goes on to remark, song in mass is song in movement; and here a regular cadence or rhythm must be the first, the absolute condition. "To say that primitive Aryans had neither poetry nor song — and nobody says it — would be like saying that they had no speech; to say that their poetry — and poetry is poetry only when marked by regular rhythm — had no regular rhythm, is almost as much as to say that their speech did not go, even unconsciously, by grammatical rules." So far Möller.

What has Sievers to say against this? Does he prove his *sprechvortrag*, the declamatory recitation of verse, by assum-

[1] *Zur althochdeutchen Alliterationspoesie*, 1888, pp. 109 ff., particularly 146 ff., "über den Takt."

ing with Wilmanns[1] that Germanic verse is not developed from any common Aryan rhythm, but rather springs, as Norden asserted that all verse springs, from the corresponding parts of balanced sentences in prose? By no means. Wilmanns argues that this "common Aryan inheritance," the verse of four accents, has not been proved as a fact, and has been simply set up as a theory; moreover, if it is proved, then one must assume that the Germanic lost it, "for the four accents appear only in later development." Because the alliterative verse follows forms and tones of ordinary speech, Wilmanns makes it a modification of that speech, an outgrowth of prose. But that such a development is unnatural and contrary to facts as well as to common sense, that song of the masses is the earliest song, that it must be strictly rhythmic, that it passes later into rhythmic recitation, and then into free, declamatory recitation, — all this is so clear to Sievers, however it may seem to work against his own theory, as in Möller's argument, that he casts about for a true explanation of alliterative verse with two accents as the outcome of that assumed Aryan verse of four accents. On a hint from Saran,[2] Sievers assumes that Germanic poetry had already made the step from strophes, which were chanted or sung in half-verses with four accents, and with a regular rhythm, to continuous or stichic verses with halves of two accents, and with free rhythmic structure fitted for saying rather than for singing. So it might well have gone with the hexameter; two verses with four accents each became one verse of six accents, and this had the swing and freedom of spoken poetry. Now whether Sievers is right or wrong in all this is apart from the question in hand; it is simply a matter of evolution on the lines already indicated, and of the

[1] *Beiträge zur Geschichte der älteren deutschen Litteratur*, III., "Der altdeutsche Reimvers," Bonn, 1887, pp. 141 f.

[2] Sievers, *Altgermanische Metrik*, 1893, pp. 172 ff.

stage in that evolution to which Germanic verse had come. On the priority of strictly rhythmic verse[1] sung by masses of men, both Sievers and Möller are agreed.

Modern individual recitation, then, by this evidence of philology and by the sense of evolution in poetic form, can be no criterion for primitive poetry; hence the inadequate character of such investigations into the nature of poetic rhythm as neglect the facts offered by ethnology and by comparative literature. One must not neglect choral and communal conditions when one deals with primitive verse. For a study of modern epic and dramatic verse as it is read aloud or declaimed, for a study even of verse on the Shaksperian stage, Meumann's essay is useful in many respects; it is useless for the study of rhythm in that larger sweep of poetic origins and growth.

We must turn, then, to scientific material which deals with primitive stages of human life. A very primitive, perhaps a pre-primitive stage of human life is involved in Darwin's theory, stated in his *Descent of Man*, reaffirmed briefly in his book on the expression of emotions, and adopted by Scherer for the explanation of poetic origins, that a study of sexual calls from male to female among animals might unlock the secret of primitive rhythm. This, as has been said, will lead to no good. Love songs, the supposed development of such calls, actually diminish and disappear as one retraces the path of verse and comes to low stages of human progress, to savage poetry at large;[2] the curve of evolution is against recourse to facts such as Darwin would find convincing; and those "long past ages when . . . our early progenitors courted each other by the aid of vocal tones," are less help-

[1] That strophic hymns were known in earliest Germanic poetry is shown, Sievers points out, by the fact that Middle High German *liet* is the same as Old Norse *ljóð*, "strophe." For the old choral poetry, he says, "wird ein im gleichen Takte fortschreitender Sangesvortrag ohne weiteres zuzugeben sein," *Ibid.*, p. 20.

[2] Above, p. 8, and Grosse, *Anfänge*, p. 233.

ful to the understanding of rhythm and poetry, when restored in such furtive and amiable moments, than when they present the primitive horde in festal dance and song, finding by increased ease of movement and economy of force, by keener sense of kind, by delight of repetition, the possibilities of that social consent which is born of rhythmic motion. Scherer, indeed, saw how much more this social consent and this festal excitement have to do with the matter, and undertook to fix the origin of poetry in an erotic and pantomimic choral, such as one still finds in certain obscene Australian dances;[1] but the erotic impulse is not social, save in some questionable exceptions; and social consent, as Donovan has shown, began rather on public and frankly social occasions, like the dance of a horde after victory in war.[2]

Sociological considerations, again, have weight with Mr. Herbert Spencer[3] when he finds, like Norden, but for different reasons, that rhythm, as used in poetry and in music, is developed out of highly emotional and passionate speech. This doctrine of Mr. Spencer has been denied on musical grounds, and must be denied still more strongly on ethnological grounds. The objections on musical grounds brought forward by Mr. Gurney,[4] are difficult to answer, and one is bound to admit that Mr. Spencer has not answered them convincingly in the essay of 1890; moreover, in making recitative a step between speech and song, he is not only ignoring communal singing, but is reversing the facts of an evolutionary process. To develop song out of an impassioned

[1] See above, p. 8, note.

[2] Other motions than that of the communal dance may induce rhythm. The movement of labour will be considered in detail; but it may be noted here that swinging, a solitary performance, tempts the savage of Borneo to sing a monotonous song and ask the spirits for a good crop (Bruchmann, *Poetik*, p. 18).

[3] See "The Origin and Function of Music," *Essays*, 1857; "The Origin of Music," in *Mind*, XV. (1890) 449 ff.; and a note on certain criticisms of this article, *Mind*, XVI. 535 ff.

[4] *The Power of Sound*, London, 1880, pp. 476 ff.

speech is plausible enough until one fronts this primitive horde dancing, singing, shouting in cadence, with a rhythm which the analogy of ethnological evidence and the facts of comparative literature prove to have been exact.[1] In Mr. Spencer's essay of 1857, the "connate" character of dancing, poetry, and music is emphasized; but the choral, communal element is unnoticed. Precisely such social conditions, however, controlled the beginning of poetry, and the main factor in them seems to have been the exact rhythm of communal consent. Against the evidence for communal rhythm little can be urged; and the few cases brought forward for this purpose by Biedermann not only rest on imperfect observation but often prove to be contradictory in the form of the statement. So, too, with other evidence. Burchell, for example, said that the Bushmen in singing and dancing showed an exact sense of rhythm; while Daumas said that they never danced except after heavy meals, and then in wild, disordered fashion, with no rhythm at all. Grosse[2] throws out this negative evidence as counter to overwhelming evidence on the other side. Again, one often finds a statement which denies rhythm to savage poetry, nevertheless affirming most exact rhythm in the songs or cries to which the savages dance. Here is evidently a confusion of the communal "poem" or song, and the individual tale or what not chanted in a kind of recitative. It may be concluded from a careful study of ethnological evidence that all savage tribes have the communal song, and most of them have the recitative. Silent folk who do nothing of the sort, tribes that neither sing nor dance, must not be brought into the argument; if they do occur, and the negative fact is always hard to establish, they are clearly too abnormal to count. Human intelligence is not measured by the idiot. These are decadent

[1] This is the basis of Wallaschek's convincing argument against Mr. Spencer's theory: *Primitive Music*, London, 1893, pp. 251 ff.

[2] *Anfänge der Kunst*, p. 206, note.

groups, extreme degenerates, links severed from the chain; and no one will summon as witnesses for the primitive stage of poetry those Charruas of Uruguay, who are said to have no dance, no song, no social amusements, who speak only in a whisper, "are covered with vermin," and know neither religion nor laws,—in a word, no social existence, and almost no humanity. So one comes back to the normal folk. East Africans[1] are reported to have "no metrical songs," and they sing in recitative; but at once it is added that they dance in crowds to the rhythm of their own voices, as well as to the drum, moving in cadence with the songs which they sing: and here can be no recitative.[2] Moreover, when cleaning rice, they work to the rhythm of songs, to foot-stamping and hand-clapping of the bystanders,—in other words, choral dance, choral song, exact time, rhythm absolute; although, by culling a bit here and there, the theorist could have presented fine evidence from Bushmen and East Africans that savages in low levels of culture have no rhythm in their songs, and dance without consent or time. True, there is the recitative, and that, as a thing interesting to Europeans, is pushed into the foreground of the traveller's account. Yet this recitative of the singer who does a turn for the missionary or other visitor is not the main fact in the case, although it is often the only fact of the sort that is set down. It may be cheerfully conceded that the recitative occurs among savage tribes throughout the world; but the manner of its occurrence must be considered. Along with choral singing, in intervals of the dance, some person chants a sentence or two in a fashion usually described as recitative. One would like to know more of this chanting; but sometimes it is without exact rhythm or measure, and will not "scan" in any regular way. So, too, with music itself; most of the ruder tribes, as Wallaschek points

[1] Wallaschek, *Primitive Music*, p. 11.

[2] See the positive statement of Dr. Jacobsthal, quoted above, p. 69.

out,[1] know both systems of music, the rhythmic and the "free." On the Friendly Islands natives have two kinds of song, "those similar to our recitative, and others in regular measure." African singers tell a tale of their wanderings "in an emphatic recitative"; but the choral songs are always sung in exact rhythm to the dance. Not only, too, with savages; hasty generalizations and inexact statements due to this double character of singing have robbed more advanced peoples of the rhythmical sense. A Swedish writer[2] telling about the Lapps and what seemed to him their lack of any idea of melody, quotes one Blom, who "denies that the Lapps have any sense for rhythm." Why? They cannot keep harmony; of six or eight, no two agree, and each is a bit above or below the rest, — not a question of rhythm, then, and alien to the case. Scarcely any savages have the sense of melody and harmony, although their sense of exact rhythm is universal and profound.

It is not hard to follow so plain a hint as one finds in the ethnological evidence; and it is clear that recitative is a matter of the individual singer, while to choral singing it is unknown and from the nature of the case impossible. As the savage laureate slips from the singing, dancing crowd, which turns audience for the nonce, and gives his short improvisation, only to yield to the refrain of the chorus, so the actual habit of individual composition and performance has sprung from the choral composition and performance. The improvisations and the recitative are short deviations from the main road, beginnings of artistry, which will one day become journeys of the solitary singer over pathless hills of song, those "wanderings of thought" which Sophocles has

[1] Work quoted, pp. 31, 42, 68, 180 f. 184, 186, 252. The evidence collected in this interesting book is so varied, so extensive, and so impartially set forth, that the conclusions drawn by Wallaschek ought to be convincing.

[2] Gustaf von Düben, *Om Lappland och Lapparne*, . . . Stockholm, 1873 (colophon), p. 319.

noted; and the curve of evolution in the artist's course can show how rapidly and how far this progress has been made. But the relation must not be reversed; and if any fact seems established for primitive life, it is the precedence of choral song and dance. An entertainer and an audience, an artist and a public, take for granted preceding social conditions; and it is generally admitted that social conditions begin with the festal dance as well as with communal labour. Indeed, as Professor Grosse points out, rhythm was the chief factor in social "unification"; but this was never the rhythm of Norden's rhythmical prose, or the irregular measures of a recitative. Where and when the individual recitative became a thing of prominence, as it undoubtedly did, is a matter to be studied in the individual and centrifugal impulse, in the progress of the poet; here it is enough to show that rhythmic verse came directly from the choral song, and that neither the choral song, nor any regular song, could have come from the recitative. The latter, as Jacobsthal assures us, will not go with dancing; and earliest singing, as is still the case in Africa,[1] must not be sundered from the dance. Baker,[2] who made a careful study of music among our Indians, sums up the matter by saying that "the characteristic feature of primitive song was the collectiveness of amusement," and that "recitatives have a flow of words and a clearness of expression which are both incompatible with primitive song." They need, that is, a developed stage of speech when the logical sentence has shaken itself free, to some extent, of mere emotional cadence and of almost meaningless repetitions. Here, indeed, begin the orator, the teller of tales, the artistic poet; but dance, song, and poetry itself begin with a communal consent, which is expressed by the most exact rhythm. Emotional speech is an ambiguous phrase. In one sense it is an

[1] As impossible, says one authority, quoted by Wallaschek, *Primitive Music*, p. 187, "as to separate the colour from the skin."

[2] *Ibid.*, p. 186.

individual, broken, irregularly regular sequence of phrases and words; oratory and oratorical cadences came out of such a chaos, but never the ordered rhythm of dancing throngs. The emotional speech in which exact rhythm began was the loud and repeated crying of a throng, regulated and brought into consent by movements of the body, and getting significance from the significance of the festal occasion.[1]

Evidence is everywhere for the asking in this matter of communal consent and choral rhythm; but instead of taking detached and random facts from many different sources, it will be well to select three groups of facts which can offer in each case compact and consistent testimony. For the present purpose one may look at the case of the Botocudos of South America, a tribe very low in the social scale, as studied by Dr. Ehrenreich; at the case of the Eskimos as studied by Dr. Boas; and finally at the case of African negroes in this country, studied by Colonel Higginson thirty-five years ago, under most favourable circumstances, and with particular reference to their communal singing. With all respect for the zeal and truthfulness of missionaries, one will thus do well to leave them out of the account, and to take evidence which comes in two cases from a professed ethnologist and in the third case from an impartial observer.

[1] It is the neglect of choral conditions and communal consent which takes away the value for general purposes from Dr. Otto Hoffman's otherwise praiseworthy study of the *Reimformeln im Westgermanischen* (Leipzig, 1886, pp. 9 ff.). Man, he says, naturally speaks in breath-lengths, in periods which tend to be of equal duration. "Whoever could give to these periods, with their tendency to equal quantities, the most symmetrical and equal portions of actual speech, passed for an artist." To this symmetry in duration was added similarity of sound; so came the short riming phrases, as well as the verse-lengths themselves. But poetry did not wait until clever artists furbished up into verse-lengths and attractive harmonies these breath-lengths of a spoken sentence. Language itself, as one will presently see, had more a festal than an individual origin; and long before the artist was practising his breath-lengths for a connected story, the rhythm of verse was fixed by the muscular rhythm of steps in a communal dance accompanied by words, often by one sound, repeated indefinitely, but in exact cadence with the steps.

The Botocudos[1] are little better than a leaderless horde, and pay scant heed to their chieftain; they live only for their immediate bodily needs, and take small thought for the morrow, still less thought for the past. No traditions, no legends, are abroad to tell them of their forbears. They still use gestures to express feeling and ideas; while the number of words which imitate a given sound "is extraordinarily great." An action or an object is named by imitating the sound peculiar to it; and sounds are doubled to express greater intensity or a repetition. To speak is *aŏ;* to speak loudly, or to sing, is *aŏ-aŏ.* And now for their æsthetic life, their song, dance, poetry, as described by this accurate observer. "On festal occasions the whole horde meets by night round the camp fire for a dance. Men and women alternating . . . form a circle; each dancer lays his arms about the necks of his two neighbours, and the entire ring begins to turn to the right or to the left, while all the dancers stamp strongly and in rhythm the foot that is advanced, and drag after it the other foot. Now with drooping heads they press closer and closer together; now they widen the circle. Throughout the dance resounds a monotonous song to the time of which they stamp their feet. Often one can hear nothing but a continually repeated *kalauī ahā!* . . . again, however, short improvised songs in which are told the doings of the day, the reasons for rejoicing, what not, as 'Good hunting,' or 'Now we have something to eat,' or 'Brandy is good.'[2] Now and then, too, an individual begins a song, and is answered by the rest in chorus. . . . *They never sing*

[1] Dr. Paul Ehrenreich, "über die Botocuden," in the *Zeitschr. f. Ethnologie*, XIX. 30 ff.

[2] The gnomic verses preserved in Anglo-Saxon, especially the shorter sentences in the Exeter Ms. (see Grein-Wülker, *Biblioth.*, I. 345 f.) are a curious instance of the survival of *quasi*-Botocudan maxims on a higher plane of culture. As to the æsthetic value of the South American utterance, how far is it inferior to the sonorous commonplaces of our own verse, — say *The Psalm of Life?*

without dancing, never dance without singing, and have but one word to express both song and dance."

As the unprejudiced reader sees, this clear and admirable account confirms the doctrine of early days, revived with fresh ethnological evidence in the writings of Dr. Brown and of Adam Smith, that dance, poetry, and song were once a single and inseparable function; and is in itself fatal to the idea of rhythmic prose, of solitary recitation, as foundation of poetry. The circle, the close clasp, the rhythmic consent of steps and voices; here are the social foundation and the communal beginnings of the art. Then comes the improvised song, springing, however, from these communal and choral conditions, and still referring absolutely to present interests of the horde as a whole. There are no traditions, no legends, no epic, no lyrics of love, no hymns to star and sunset. All poetry is communal, holding fast to the rhythm of consent as to the one sure fact.

The Eskimo,[1] despite his surroundings, is in better social case than the Botocudo; while the sense of kind is as great, individual growth has gone further, and song is not limited to festal and communal promptings. The "entertainer" has arrived, although, when he begins to divert his little audience in the snow-hut, he must always turn his face to the wall. Still more, there is no monopoly; as with peasants at the Bavarian dance, where each must and can sing his own improvised quatrain, so here each member of the party has his tale to tell, his song, dance, or trick. The women hum incessantly while at work; but the words are mainly that monotonous air, the repeated *amna aya* of the popular chorus. Individuals have their "own" tunes and songs, which easily become traditional; but the solitary song is not so much an Eskimo characteristic as the communal song, for they are

[1] "The Central Eskimo," by Dr. F. Boas, *Sixth Annual Report, Bureau of Ethnology*, 1884–1885, Washington, 1888, pp. 409 ff.

a sociable folk, and never spend their evenings alone. They sing, as so often was the case in mediæval Europe, while playing ball; but the combination of choral song and dance is a favourite form, and both singing and dancing have in this case one name, with features common to the festivity all over the world, — exact rhythm, repetition of word and phrase, endless chorus, a fixed refrain, — the *amna aya*, — short and intermittent improvisation by solitary singers and reciters. The art of these singers and reciters is in an advanced stage; for they perform alone as well as under support of the chorus. Three phases of their art may be mentioned. First, there is the prose tale with songs or recitatives interspersed, a sort of *cante-fable*. Then there is the tale chanted in a kind of recitative, which Dr. Boas calls poetic prose. Thirdly, there are "real poems of a very marked rhythm, which are not sung but recited," and the reciter "jumps up and down and to right and left" as he speaks his piece. That is, here are tales which have come to such a pitch of art that choral and refrain and repetition of words are a hindrance to the flow of the story. Still, even here the solitary performances stand out against the background of choral singing in which they once formed such a modest part, and on every provocation they slip into it again and are lost in the old rhythm of emotional repetition and communal consent.

The negro slaves of the South, finally, with their traditional dance and song, strangely influenced by one of the few elements of civilization which really came into their life, the religious element, offer another interesting bit of evidence to show how emotional speech, a rude poetry, is born of rhythm by consent of a throng. In those so-called "spirituals" of the negro is the recitative or the chorus to be looked upon as original? Perhaps Colonel Higginson had as good a chance to study this communal song as any one could have;

in an article[1] written soon after the war he described the singing of the "spirituals" by men of his regiment, now in camp, now on the march, now to the fall of the oars. He speaks of the trait so prominent in all primitive song, exact and inevitable rhythm, however harsh the voices and however uncouth the words. "Often . . . I have . . . silently approached some glimmering fire, round which the dusky figures moved in the rhythmical barbaric dance the negroes call a 'shout,' chanting, often harshly, but always in the most perfect time, some monotonous refrain." What was the favourite of all these spirituals, "sung perhaps twice as often as any other"? A song called *Hold Your Light*, "sung with no accompaniment but the measured clapping of hands and the clatter of many feet;" it "properly consisted of a chorus alone with which the verses of other songs might be combined at random."

> Hold your light, Brudder Robert, —
> Hold your light,
> Hold your light on Canaan's shore. . . .

For Robert, another name would be given,[2] then another, and so on for half an hour. This seemed to Colonel Higginson "the simplest primitive type of 'spiritual.'" Next in favour was: —

> Jordan River, I'm bound to go,
> Bound to go, bound to go,
> Jordan River, I'm bound to go,
> And bid 'em fare ye well,

then with Brudder Robert, Sister Lucy, and so on, the well-known cumulative refrain. Now if one had only the text of many of these songs, and knew nothing of the singing and dancing, one would call them rhythmical prose, recitative; for example, a part of *The Coming Day*. One is told, however, that this "was a boat-song and timed well with the tug

[1] *Atlantic Monthly*, XIX. (1867), 685 ff.

[2] See below, on Cumulative Songs.

of the oar." The fact is that here, as in savage and presumably in primitive song, movement of body and rhythm of voice are the main consideration, while the words, on which civilized man imposes individual and syntactic correctness, are of very subordinate value. Syllables may be dropped or added at will, but the rhythm must be exact; and the simplest way to avoid verbal distress is the primitive device of repetition.[1] When the words, and the thought in them, begin to be of overmastering importance in poetry, "scanning" acts as deputy of exact rhythm and song, until at last declamation pushes scanning aside, and rhythm is reduced to the same ancillary function once assigned to thought and words.

Here, then, are the vital elements in the discussion. Rhythm is an affair of instinctive perception transformed into a social act as the expression of social consent. It has been said that beginnings and not origins are the object of our quest; how rhythm in poetry may stand to rhythm in nature, to the breath or the pulse of man, to periodic movements of tide, of star, and so in vaster and vaster cosmic relation, or, again, to infinitesimal rhythms in the cell, in the cell of the cell, — are queries apart from the present purpose. Important, however, is the doctrine held by modern scholars that poetic rhythm is objectively an outcome of human activity, and subjectively a process of human perception.[2] Perhaps the best short study of the wider question has been made by Wallaschek.[3] Insisting that "rhythm is the form

[1] See the marching song, p. 690, *Go in the Wilderness.* Thanks to the repetitions, it "scans" correctly enough, even when it is read.

[2] Meumann's remarks on this subject are good, though they apply no further than the narrow circle of his experiments. See *Untersuchungen*, pp. 26, 35, 77. Grant Allen, *Physiological Æsthetics*, London, 1887, pp. 114 f., 118, is quite wide of the mark; facts of physiology, in this case, need very careful testing by the facts of poetry.

[3] *Mind*, N. S., IV. (1895), 28 ff., "On the Difference of Time and Rhythm in Music," supplementing researches in his *Primitive Music.*

of the objective movement, time-sense (*mesure, takt*) the form of the perceiving subject-mind," noting that "the evenness of time-groups in music arises from the original organic union of dance and music," he goes on to point out a fact which seems to be fundamental for any study of beginnings in poetry as well as in the sister art, although it is music of which he speaks. Vocal utterance merely as result of "corporal stimulus," song like that of birds, is not yet music,— nor, one may add, is the cry of the solitary infant, individual or racial, to be counted as poetry. "The peculiar germ which has alone been found capable of the enormous development actually accomplished in music"—and in poetry—"is the *chorus*, with its framework, the dance." A bird's song or a man's cry is merely vent for emotion; but when several persons sing together, there is more than emotion, there is consent, and consent means that they must observe, group, and order the tones. "They could not keep together if they did not mark periods . . . for there is no concert possible without bars. What they perform is rhythm, what they think is *takt*, and what they feel is surplus of vigour." There may be some error in the details of this analysis. Wallaschek has not done justice to the "genesis of emotion," as Ribot[1] calls it, through unaided rhythm; he may not concede enough to the song of birds, and may be wrong in saying that no one ever heard animals sing in concert;[2] hysteric cries, which tend to be rhythmic and show a maximum of emotion with a minimum of purpose, have doubtless more to say in early rhythm—one thinks of the songs of lament, the *voceri*—than he admits;[3] but his main point about choral beginnings is of

[1] *Psychology of the Emotions*, p. 104.

[2] See his *Primitive Music*, pp. 239, 236, note; and Grosse, *Anfänge*, p. 213.

[3] The theory of breath-lengths, often noted, comes here into play. Under high excitement breathing grows abnormally loud, and the recurring pauses are regular. Play-excitement, festal shouting and leaping, would of course bring this about; but the individual must be studied. Strongly accented verses result from such a

immense importance. Poetry, like music, is social; like its main factor, rhythm, it is the outcome of communal consent, a *faculté d'ensemble;* and this should be writ large over every treatise on poetry, in order to draw the mind of the reader from that warped and baffling habit which looks upon all poetry as a solitary performance. The modern reader is passive; even hearing poetry is mainly foreign to him; active poetry, such as abounded in primitive life, is to him the vagary of a football mob, the pleasure of school children; and to such a reader the words of Wallaschek are salutary indeed, insisting that not the sense of hearing alone is to be studied when one takes up the psychology of music, but the muscular sense as well, and that the muscular sense has precedence. "'Making music' means in the primitive world performing, not listening," a statement which applies as well to poetry. And what sort of rhythm, under leave of Norden and the rest, is one to assume for the primitive consent whether in music or in poetry? Well, earliest music shows "an unsettled melody, an uncertain and constantly varying intonation, a perpetual fluctuation of pitch," but, contrasted with all this, "the strict and ever prevailing rhythm," "the precision and marvellously exact performance of numberless performers."[1] For two facts, then, of great moment in the

process, as any one can see who undertakes to recite poetry during violent but regular exercise, — say, in swinging Indian clubs. Here, too, one learns how rhythm preceded pitch and quantity; the jerked-out accents leave little room for measuring either height or length of tones. But the throng and its consent brought out this rhythm, not oratory; and one must keep in mind the remark of Hamann, after his famous phrase about poetry as the mother-tongue of man, "wie Gesang älter als Declamation."

[1] The ethnological evidence for this statement is given in Wallaschek's *Primitive Music* on nearly every page. Many good things on the origin of rhythm could be quoted from older writers. A. W. Schlegel undertook a physiological and genetic study of rhythm, but, at Schiller's prompting, offered more attractive metal to the Kantlings with "das Beharrliche im Wechsel." One notes, however, the modern tone of passages in the Berlin Lectures; *e.g.* I. 242 ff. Now and then he almost anticipates Bücher's *Arbeit und Rhythmus.* Sulzer's article

study of poetry, there is universal testimony from savage tribes all over the earth. Singing is mainly choral and timed to the dance; and the rhythm, no matter how large the throng, is amazingly correct.

So much for the savages. Arguments from the study of children, as was said in foregoing remarks on method, should be applied with great caution to the history of literary forms. It may be noted, however, that nothing brought out thus far by such studies has worked against the assumption of extremely accurate rhythm as the fundamental fact in primitive poetry. Of course, one must not set a child to tasks that belong in mature stages of poetry. The early efforts of children to make a metrical composition[1] are generally rough and only approximately rhythmic. Repeat a few verses, and ask the child to make verses like them, giving him paper, pencil, solitude, encouragement, and the promise of cake, all the known aids by which an adult poet wins his peerage or the abbey; the child will probably hit a rime or so, more or less accurate, but the verse will halt. This, however, is easily explained. Solitary composition, the process of following a set form of sounds by making sentences of his own to fit the scheme, the combination of thought with rhythm, is a task beyond his powers, and for an excellent reason; it was also beyond the powers of primitive man. But let the same child, with a dozen other children, in an extemporized game, fall to crying out some simple phrase in choral repetition; the rhythm is almost painful in its exactness. Repeat to this child rimes of the nursery; he is sworn foe to defective metre, and boggles at it; indeed, such defects are hard to find in all the amiable nonsense. The child's ear for rhythm is acute; his

in the *Allgemeine Theorie* is very interesting. For early material, see Blankenburg's invaluable *Litterarische Zusätze*, 3 vols., 1796–1798. A good recent discussion is found in the third book of Guyau's *Problèmes*.

[1] Unless it is a succession of inarticulate sounds. See Groos, *Spiele der Menschen*, *Jena*, 1899, p. 42.

execution of it in choral, or in verse learned from the hearing, is precise; his demands upon it are of the strictest; but in solitary composition, a mental effort, he loses his rhythmic way, and grows bewildered in those new paths of thought. A teacher of considerable experience recently made the statement that children in school will turn loose or defective metre, once the idea of rhythm is given them, into accurately measured verse. Indeed, it is probable that the halting verses of an indifferent poet, such as one finds in newspapers, begin in the maker's constructive process as correct rhythm, but lose this cadence in the course of composition.[1] Be that as it may be, however, the rhythmical sense of children is remarkably exact for purposes of choral singing and recital.

It is evident that one is not likely to be embarrassed by a lack of rhythm in early poetry, but rather by a lack of anything else. There is the danger, when one has made so much of rhythm, that this early art will be called nothing more than vocal music, and will vainly claim the title of poetry. Here are dance and music, one is told, and that is all. Wagner[2] believed in the original union of the three arts; but Wallaschek[3] separates poetry from music and dance. Unfortunately, he does not say what primitive

[1] Compare the "meaningless" words so common in savage poetry. The art of combining with exact rhythm a series of syntactic sentences which give a connected story, or express a logical series of thoughts, is no primitive process. Earliest poetry is repetition of sounds, — not meaningless, for they were connected with the occasion, — of words, of sentences, with a diminishing use of the refrain, a diminishing frequency of repetition.

[2] In his "Art of the Future," *Gesammelte Schriften*, III. 82 ff., he tells how dance, song, and poem were at first inseparable. Dance has as artistic material "the whole man from top to toe"; but it becomes an art only through rhythm, which is also the very skeleton of music: "without rhythm no dance, no song." Rhythm is "the soul of dancing and the brain of music." With the human voice comes poetry, all three being woven in one: out of this union of the three "is born the single art of lyric," but they get their highest expression in the drama.

[3] *Primitive Music*, pp. 174, 187.

poetry could have been; recitative he rejects utterly; it is clear, however, that he is thinking of a poetry which no one is disposed to father upon earliest man, that poetry of thought and syntactic statement familiar to later days. Poetry, he says, always depends upon the intellect. Far better, because clearer and in closer accord with ethnological facts, are the brief statement of Ribot and the elaborate theory of Donovan. Ribot,[1] considering as a matter of fact how spontaneous movements pass into creative and æsthetic activity, finds by all evidence at hand that dancing in pantomime was the "primordial" and universal art, and that it was composite, "including the rudimentary form of two acts destined later on to separate in the course of their evolution, — music and poetry. Poor music, indeed, . . . but remarkable for the strictness of rhythm and measure, and poor poetry, consisting in a short sentence incessantly repeated, or even in monosyllables without precise signification." That is a clear statement; but it takes for granted, in some measure, what Donovan tries to prove, — the festal origin of speech.[2] Whether Donovan does prove this or not, he makes it perfectly clear that the vocal music, which Wallaschek separated from poetry without giving an idea what poetry was and how it began, was itself poetry, and had functions which expressed the human emotions of that time as well as the most finished poem expresses modern emotion and thought. With the philological arguments we are not concerned, and, indeed, theories about the origin of language have always been kittle cattle to shoe; we are concerned, however, with these four elements of a primitive festal gathering: bodily play-movements, rhythmical beating, some approach to song, and some degree of communal interest.

[1] *Psychology of the Emotions*, pp. 335 f.

[2] In an article so entitled, in *Mind*, XVI. (1891), 498 ff., and N. S., I. (1892), 325 ff.

Of these, the first and the fourth are fused in dancing, which begins as a celebration of victory, and is found later in the harvesting of a crop and in the vintage. "Communal elation following success in a common enterprise" is the earliest occasion for social consent of the festal type; and it finds expression in imitating that successful act, along with "rhythmic beating,"[1] and with excited individual cries which are brought into rhythm with the steps, the gestures and the "beating" itself. Hence speech and song. In his second article, Donovan tries to trace the process by which meaning got into these cries, and how they led to grammatical forms of speech; what interests us here is the exactness, the prevalence, the dominant force of rhythm as foundation of consent, and so of social act, dance, song, word. As with savages now, so with primitive man, however wild and confused the social mass may be, rhythm is at the heart of their social life. Here is the point of order in the chaos; and one may safely assume that such order and precision of mere sounds would be the obvious stay for all efforts to give them meaning and connection. Language, after all, is communication. This is probably what Donovan means when he makes rhythm the prime social factor, the bridge from merely animal to human; rhythmic forms, he says, are "witnesses of a lower stage of progress than any yet known

[1] The tendency to use hands as well as feet in keeping rhythm is illustrated by the Ba-Ronga of Delagoa Bay (Junod, *Les Chantes et les Contes des Ba-Ronga*, Lausanne, 1897), where the use of sticks may help to explain Donovan's "rhythmic beating." With these people "tout s'y chante et . . . tous ou presque tous les chants s'y dansent" (p. 21). Refrains are sung "ten, twenty, fifty times in succession"; the songs have two elements, the solo and the refrain *en tutti*. A circle is formed, the men holding sticks in their hands; the solo singer leaps into the middle and sings a few words; then all the dancers sing a refrain, raising and dropping their sticks in cadence, though the rhythm is primarily given by their stamping feet. Then the soloist again, only slightly varying his theme; and again the long refrain (pp. 32 f.). The war-songs are almost entirely refrain, sung by all the warriors as they dance, "antique et grandiose choral," says Junod.

to anthropological records," — the "stage of the passage between brute and man"; and he gives modern philology food for thought when he declares that many facts and considerations "run counter to the notion that song, or rhythmical and poetical forms, must be supervening embellishments of speech which imply a certain height of civilization." A chapter in his earlier book[1] goes more into the details of communal poetry under primitive conditions, and answers objections which might be made to this poetical function of the throng. A happily chosen verse from Horace enforces the deprecation of that habit which now makes a poet's muse the poet himself or else an amiable fiction. The earliest "muse" was simply that "music" or rhythm of the throng which held up the singer's tottering personality in his first steps over the burning marle of individual expression before the throng itself — still a nervous matter! — and prompted or sustained his improvisations; for primitive man this muse was the cadence of falling feet, rhythmic cries, social consent. And how came those "higher artistic interests connected with speech out of the pantomimic and choral dance?" Direct evidence, Donovan remarks, is meagre; but of indirect evidence there is a "mighty mass." Hindu words for the drama go back to the word which means to dance. Hellenic drama has an even more definite development of the same sort. European lyric poetry grew out of the choral dance; and folksongs which sprang directly from "the spontaneous elation of the crowd," though rare, still occur even now in Greece, Italy, Russia, Hungary.[2] Accentual verse is "the natural inheritance of poetry which grew from the fusion of rhythms and

[1] *From Lyre to Muse, a History of the Aboriginal Union of Music and Poetry*, London, 1890; Chap. V., "Fusion of Tones and Words."

[2] "It is said that if it is known that anybody in particular composed a song, the people in some of these places will not sing it," *Ibid.*, pp. 138 f. For this vexed question, see below, chapter on Communal Poetry.

tones and words. The words uttered by a rude people spontaneously, and during the elation produced through following the movements of the dance and listening to the accompanying tones, were obliged to assume the natural impulsive element of rhythm." Horace, in a familiar passage, tells how the artist began his work with this choral and communal material[1] now unknown except in survivals like the refrain of harvest songs: —

per audaces nova dithyrambos
verba devolvit,

new words, that is, instead of the old choral repetitions. That these communal songs, however, were poetry in themselves seems sufficiently proved. The objection urged by Wallaschek, that rhythmic sounds were inadequate to the demands of poetry, falls flat for the negative reason that nowhere else can poetry be found under primitive conditions, and for the positive reason that these rhythmic sounds were unquestionably full of communal significance and may well have served as the raw material of speech itself.

So far the theory of social consent as the basis of rhythm and the foundation of poetry has been supported mainly by the dance. This play-theory, this festal origin, may be accepted as probable; but it must leave room and verge enough for the part played by labour. Human society was organized in the spirit of a grim struggle for life; and human labour under social conditions is a main part of the struggle. Professor Karl Bücher's essay on Labour and Rhythm[2] is meant

[1] Of course Horace (IV. ii. 10 ff.) is thinking of Pindar's "new" compounds and fresh expressions; but the quotation agrees as well with the history of the dithyrambic poem.

[2] "Arbeit und Rhythmus," reprinted from the *Abhandlungen d. kgl. sächsischen Gesellschaft d. Wissenschaften, philol. histor. Classe*, XVII. 5, Leipzig, 1896. According to Groos, *Spiele der Menschen*, pp. 57 ff., some of these statements have been modified. In the second edition of the *Entstehung der Volkswirthschaft*, pp. 32 f., a book which the present writer could not consult, Bücher concedes the

in part as a sociological study of the beginnings of poetry; it has been greeted everywhere as an important contribution to our positive knowledge of the case; and a summary of it is unavoidable for the matter now in hand.[1] His argument is clear. Fatigue, which besets all work felt as work by reason of its continued application of purpose, vanished for primitive man as it vanishes now for children, if the work was once freed from this stress of application and so turned to a kind of play. The dance itself is really hard work, exacting and violent; what makes it the favourite it is with savages as with children? Simply its automatic, regular, rhythmic character, the due repetition of a familiar movement which allows the mind to relax its attitude of constant purpose. The purpose and plan of work involve external sources and external ends; rhythm is instinctive, and springs from the organic nature of man; it is no invention.[2] The song that one sings while at work is not something fitted to the work, but comes from movements of the body in the specific acts of labour; and this applies not only to the rhythm, but even to the words.[3] So it was in the festal dance. That primitive man was less impeded in bodily movements than is now the case, and that these movements were more marked; that the rigorously exact movement begat a rigorously exact rhythm, to which at first half meaningless sounds and then words were joined, often lingering in later days as a refrain of field or spinning-room — witness the pantomimic action which goes with the words of that New Zealand planting-song, and a host of sim-

priority of play, and sees in it the starting-point of labour. This, however, does not change the validity of Bücher's main argument for the connection of labour and rhythm, so far as they concern the beginnings of poetry.

[1] A. W. Schlegel here and there hints at this origin of rhythm in labour; so does Sulzer. See note above, p. 101. See also the Abbé Batteux, "Sur les Nombres Poëtiques et Oratoires," *Mém. Acad. Inscript.*, XXXV. 415: "le marteau du forgeron tombe en cadence, la faulx du moissonneur va et revient avec nombre . . . le rhythme soutient nos forces dans les travaux pénibles."

[2] Bücher, p. 101.

[3] *Ibid.*, p. 52.

ilar survivals; that poetry and music were always combined by early man, and, along with labour, made up the primitive three-in-one, an organic whole, labour being the basal fact, with rhythm as element common to the three;[1] and that not harmony or pitch, but this overmastering and pervasive rhythm, exact, definite, was the main factor of early song, — these are conclusions for which Bücher offers ample and convincing evidence. In particular we may look, first, at his conclusion against unrhythmic poetry, then at his theory of rhythmic origins, and finally at his study of individual and social labour. For the first, he remarks, as all students of ethnology have remarked, that primitive folk care little for melody; the main, the only musical element in their songs is rhythm. Rhythm is not bound up with speech as speech, and must come to it from without; for mere observation and development of the rhythmical tendencies inherent in language could not have led to the fact of rhythm as known to primitive man. The main external source of rhythm, then, is the habit of accompanying bodily movements with sounds of the voice, and these bodily movements were primarily movements in man's work. Taking such songs of labour as still remain, Bücher finds that the more primitive these are, the closer relation they have with the labour itself. The rhythm, too, is fixed by the movement; words change at will and are mostly improvised. Briefly, Bücher adds one more answer to that old question about the origins of poetry, and finds them chiefly in the labour of primitive man, where energetic and continual movements of an instinctively rhythmic nature begat "not only the form but the material" of poetry. The same rhythmic succession of rise and fall is common to

[1] "Grundelement dieser Dreieinheit," *Ibid.*, p. 78. Of course, he admits elsewhere similar functions of the dance, which was, after all, a kind of labour, even when not an imitation of labour. Hence Bücher gives priority to labour in its large sense. For primitive man the line between work and play was not too sharply drawn.

labour and to verse; and as for the words, these came not from bodily exertion, but from the sounds produced by the work itself, sounds like the noise of the feet in treading, like the blows of a primitive implement, which irresistibly provoked accompaniment by the voice. That these sounds had a meaning vague at first, then sharper, clearer, and connected with the cause, conditions, and purpose of the work, is lawful inference. Words that so took their places in the regular and inexorable rhythm of work or dance must share in that regularity; recitative, or the rhythm of easy prose, has no place under such conditions, and Bücher rejects it utterly. Again, all human work began with movements of arms and legs "which instinctively move in rhythm." With Bücher's further development of this theory, that beating and stamping, earliest forms of work, plus the human voice which followed the rise and fall of the labour, are the basis of metrical "feet"; that iamb and trochee are stamping measures, spondee a measure of striking or beating, still easy to note where two hands strike in rhythm; that dactyl and anapæst can be heard at the forge of any blacksmith whose main blow on the iron is either followed or preceded by two shorter, lighter blows,—with these attractive but minor considerations one may agree or disagree, but the vital fact of rhythm as the pulse of earliest human labour and play, of earliest poetry, of earliest music, is vastly strengthened by the evidence and the arguments set forth in this admirable essay.

For the matter of individual and social[1] labour, Bücher has inference and hints, but hardly a developed theory. It is easy, however, to infer that stress is to be laid on the social rather than on individual conditions. In play and the dance

[1] A strong support for this social foundation of song is found in observations such as Böckel has made among the peasants of Hesse. "Their song," he says (work quoted, p. cv.), "is nearly all choral; the countryman, when sober, seldom sings alone. It is remarkable," Böckel goes on to say, "how these people, who singly show little capacity for music, can make such an artistic effect in chorus."

this is everywhere conceded. To tread the winepress alone, however the instinctively and unavoidably rhythmic movement might provoke one to song, was a small factor in rhythmic development when compared with the consent of many feet treading in joy of the vintage.[1] For individual labour, songs of women grinding at the mill, once a most wearisome task, are the best example; and hints of these, even scraps of actual song, are found in plenty.[2] But two women and more were often to be found grinding together, and the social consent of such songs must have been at least as frequent as the lonely voice. Bücher points out, moreover, how the solitary act of labour, particularly with heavy tools, tends to be uncertain and unrhythmic, and how the addition of a second workman, say at the forge, or in threshing or in ramming stones, at once induces an exact rhythm, the rhythm born of consent. This is a primitive process and most important. The idea of savages as capricious, and therefore not acting in concert, is a hasty inference, true only to a certain point; for it is civilized folk who work independently, and it is the uncivilized who must cling to rhythm both in work and in play, since nowhere else are men found so dependent on concerted automatic work as in savage life. A man of advanced culture thinks out his own labour, and does it in his own way; his concert of work with other men is a higher synthesis of individual performances which is unknown to the savage. All this opens to our eyes the spectacle of a long evolution, at one end of which, the uncertain, tentative beginnings of social life, we see human beings acting, alike in the tasks and in the pleasures of their time, with a minimum of

[1] Several men, as a rule, trod the grapes with naked feet. Songs directly sprung from this labour survived for long ages. The material is indicated by Bücher, pp. 88 f. The later festal songs, of course, were symbolical and reminiscent.

[2] The famous Greek song, preserved by Plutarch, is matched by recent songs of the Africans, as well as by those of European traditions.

thought and a maximum of rhythm; while at the hither end is a highly developed society, where the monotonous whir of machinery has thrust out the old cadence and rhythm of man's labour, where strenuous and solitary wanderings replace the communal dance, and where every brow is marked with the burden of incessant thought.

The threads of evidence, then, all end in one point close to that blackness of thick darkness which veils the life of earliest man; at this point, the point of social consent, work is not far from play, and art is still in solution with practical life. The arts of movement, of music, dance, poetry, are in evidence only along with the arts of subsistence and tribal life, with the labour, actual or reminiscent, of primitive social conditions; while the arts that take permanent form, such as sculpture and painting, appear only in the results of this labour as rude forms of ornament. What holds together these heterogeneous elements is rhythm, "the ordered grouping of movements, as they occur in temporal succession," so Bücher defines it; and it is rhythm which must count, by his reckoning, as one of the greatest factors in social development, a function, too, not out of date even under existing conditions of life.

So much by way of proof, and it seems conclusive, for rhythm as the fundamental fact of poetry. True, it is not the fundamental fact for modern consideration, which goes below the surface and seeks a deeper meaning, asking for the nobly imaginative and for that mingling of the emotional and the intellectual which submits "the shows of things to the desires of the mind"; it is not even the overwhelming element in modern poetic form. Naked limbs no longer move unimpeded in the dance, no longer stand out free and bold as they tread the winepress; naked and insistent rhythm, too, is, for the most part, so hidden by draperies of verbal expression, that one is fain to call it no essential factor in a poetic process. Modern art, deliberate and intellectual, turns in scorn upon that helpless poetry of the horde, as Prospero upon Caliban: —

> I pitied thee,
> Took pains to make thee speak, taught thee each hour
> One thing or other: when thou didst not, savage,
> Know thine own meaning, but wouldst gabble like
> A thing most brutish, I endow'd thy purposes
> With words that made them known.

Imperious thought is ashamed of this mere regularity, this recurrence, this common gift; where is the art in it? Art, said Schiller, must have something in its work that is voluntary, fresh, surprising; the voice, he said, may be beautiful, but there is no beauty in mere breathing. Has not poetry, then, it may be asked, gained in meaning for mankind, in nobility and dignity, precisely as it has loosed the bands of rhythm, forsworn this ignoble and slavish regularity, receded from the throng, spurned the chorus, turned to solitary places, and cherished the individual, the artist, the poet? Granting the throng, the dance, the rhythm, the shouts, is not all this but poetry in the nebular state, and does not real poetry begin where Aristotle makes it begin, when an individual singer detaches himself from the choral mass, improvises and recites his verses, and so sets out upon that "mindward" way which leads to Sophocles and Dante and Shakspere? We do not dance Shakspere's poetry, we do not sing it, we hardly even scan it; why then this long pother about a lapsing and traditional form?

Well, in the first place, rhythm is there in Sophocles, Dante, Shakspere; it was sung to large extent in the drama of Sophocles, and even with Dante and Shakspere it is subconsciously present in the mind of every sympathetic reader who accepts the verses by those poor deputies of aural perception, the eyes. Not the least of artistic triumphs in poetry are concerned directly with rhythm. Those lines of *Hamlet*, —

> Absent thee from felicity awhile,
> And in this harsh world draw thy breath in pain,—

are poetry through their harmony of rhythmic adjustment, and if divorced from rhythm cease to be poetry. Every good lyric, even in modern times, fairly trembles and prays to be sung, at least to be taken in its full rhythmic force; the "pastel in prose" only serves to send us back to genuine lyric with a new love of rhythmic regularity. In modern dramatic, epic, and incidental poetry, the case is different; but this difference brings no loss to the cause of rhythm. One does not wish to read *Under the Greenwood Tree* in verse any more than one wishes to read *As You Like It* in prose. Meredith's *Egoist*, an epic prose comedy of modern life, is as satisfactory in its way, barring the comparisons of genius, as *Twelfth Night* or *Much Ado*, the dramatic comedy in verse. It is our keen thinking, fastened upon a character like Sir Willoughby, like Malvolio, that is in question; and those soothing cadences which appeal to the consciousness of kind and set the solitary in sympathetic throngs, as in a lyric, we do not need. Satire of emotional traits, to be sure, may require the exaggeration of verse as in *Jump-to-Glory Jane;* but verse is not degraded by this, any more than it is degraded in helping one to remember the number of days in a month. The hold of rhythm upon modern poetry, even under conditions of analytic and intellectual development which have unquestionably worked for the increased importance of prose, is a hold not to be relaxed, and for good reason. The reason is this. In rhythm, in sounds of the human voice, timed to movements of the human body, mankind first discovered that social consent which brought the great joys and the great pains of life into a common utterance. The mountain, so runs a Basque proverb, is not necessary to the mountain, but man is necessary to man. Individual thinking, a vast fermentation, centrifugal tendencies of every sort, have played upon this simple and primitive impulse; but the poet is still essentially emotional, and just so far as he is to utter the great joys and the great pains of life, just so far he must go back to communal emotions, to the sense of kind, to the social foundation.[1] The mere fact of utterance is social; however solitary his thought, a poet's utterance must voice this consent of man with man, and his emotion must fall into rhythm, the one and eternal expression of consent. This, then, is why rhythm will not be banished from poetry so long as poetry shall remain emotional utterance; for rhythm is not only sign and warrant of a social contract stronger, deeper, vaster, than any fancied by Rousseau, but it is the expression of a human sense more keen even than the fear of devils and the love of gods, — the sense and sympathy of kind.

[1] "La sympathie pour les choses," says M. de Vogüé, *Histoire et Poésie*, p. 190, is the "principe et raison de l'art d'écrire."

CHAPTER III

THE TWO ELEMENTS IN POETRY

THE study of rhythm threw one fact of primitive life into very strong relief, — the predominance of masses of men over individual effort,[1] and the almost exclusive reign of communal song as compared with poetry of the solitary artist, with that poetry which nowadays makes sole claim to the title. Does this point to a fundamental dualism? Are there two kinds of poetry, communal and artistic; or must one say that the choral throng and the reading public, the improvising singer and the modern poet, are convertible terms, with refrains, repetition, chorus, as a negligible quantity? Is the making of poetry really one process under all conditions of production; or does the main impulse, in itself everywhere invariable, undergo enough change in its outward relations and conditions to warrant the division of its product into two kinds? Goethe is thought to have answered this question in his discussion of certain Lithuanian popular songs, when he wondered "that folk make so much of these ballads of the people, and rate them so high. There is only one poetry, the real and the true; all else is approximation and show.

[1] Bastian, in his book *Der Völkergedanke im Aufbau einer Wissenschaft vom Menschen*, Berlin, 1881, pp. 8 f., notes that in a modern work of art one looks for traits of the genius that brought it forth, while in the beginnings of society, of institutions, one looks "for the unconscious stirrings, in the organism, of the average man who has realized himself in them." And in an address (same book, p. 172) on the aims of ethnology, he declares that for this science man is not the individual *anthropos*, but the social being, the *zoon politikon* of Aristotle, which demands the social state as condition of his existence. "*Das Primäre ist also der Völkergedanke.*"

Poetic talent is given to the peasant as well as to the knight; it depends whether each lays hold upon his own condition and treats it as it deserves, in which case the simplest relations will be the best." And there an end, cries the critic; what more is to be said? Nothing, if one is discussing poetry merely as an impulse to emotional expression which springs simple and distinct from the heart of man. But there is more to be said when one treats poetry not as the impulse, but as the product of the impulse, a product falling into sundry classes according to the conditions under which it is produced. Setting theory aside, it is a fact that critics of every sort have been fain to look upon the product of the poetic impulse as something not simple, but twofold.

As was the case with rhythm, where a tradition of the priority of verse compared with prose led to extravagant theories of early man as singing instead of talking, and realizing generally the conditions of an Italian opera stage, so with this dualism now in hand; extravagant theories of folk-made epics and self-made songs, have brought it into a discredit absolutely undeserved. In some form, to be sure, this dualism of the poetic product pervades the whole course of criticism, and varies from a vague, unstable distinction to a definite and often extravagant claim of divided origins; its differencing factor now sunders the two parts as by a chasm, and now leaves them with only the faintest line between. Always, however, this differencing factor is more than an affair of words. It has nothing to do with classification of materials or of form, as when Schleiermacher opposes the epos and the drama as "plastic" to the purely lyric or "musical." It is not the dualism of high and low implied in Fontenelle's delightful "Description of the Empire of Poesy,"[1] with its highlands, including "that great city, epic," and the "lofty mountain of tragedy," burlesque, however, in the low-

[1] *Œuvres*, Paris, 1790, III. 165 ff., from the *Mercure* of January, 1678.

lands, and comedy, though a pleasant town, quite too close to these marshes of farce to be safe. It is not the antithesis of definition, not a mere exclusion, — poetry against science, pleasure against truth, imaginative verse against unimaginative, emotional against practical and didactic; not a separation of cheap, shabby verses from the poetry which Ben Jonson thought perfect, and fit to be seen "of none but grave and consecrated eyes." In a loose application, this twofold character of the poetic product takes the form of an antithesis between art and nature, a vague contrast, with terminology yet more vague; and here, again, it is not the rival claims of art and nature in any one piece, — whether

> Natura fieret laudabile carmen, an arte,

or in any one man, — "the good poet's made as well as born";[1] but it is the contrast shown by poetry that is essentially "natural" in origin, over against the rival sprung from art. Often it is impartial: Jonson's learned sock, or the wild wood-notes of Shakspere, — "with Shakspere's nature or with Jonson's art," is Pope's echo of Milton; but Milton's nephew, Phillips,[2] pits "true native poetry" against "wit, ingenuity, and learning in verse, even elegancy itself," — Spenser and Shakspere, that is, against his moderns. So one comes by way of these great "natural" poets to the rural muse herself, who has always been lauded and caressed when eulogy was safe. If mediocrities are versing, "Tom Piper makes us better melodie"; and this is Spenser's honest view, not his "ironicall sarcasmus." Back to the shepherds,

[1] Nowhere better discussed and settled than in Goethe's sonnet, "*Natur und Kunst, sie scheinen sich zu fliehen*," with its concluding lines: —

> In der Beschränkung zeigt sich erst der Meister,
> Und das Gesetz nur kann uns Freiheit geben.

[2] *Theatrum Poetarum*, first published 1675, ed. Brydges, Canterbury, 1800 (who limits it to English poets, so changing the title), p. xxxvi.

says poetry, when it is tired of too much art; rustic and homely and unlettered, is opposed to urban and lettered and polite, song of the fields to verse that looks across an ink-stand at folios of the study. But this tendency in criticism to rebuke poetry of the schools, its rouge and powder, by pointing to the fresh cheeks of unspoiled rustic verse, is hardly to the purpose.

Passing from this loose and popular account of the dualism, one finds the contrast, still mainly unhistorical, but stated with precision, in the æsthetic realm. Schiller, one of the masters in that school which combined metaphysical theory with critical insight, divided poetry into the naive and the sentimental; his famous essay, however, should be read along with his poem on the *Künstler*, and with A. W. Schlegel's review of the poem; unsatisfactory as Schiller thought his verse, it gives a historical comment on his theory, and he used the idea of it for his Æsthetic Letters. It shows how art, — thought and purpose, that is, — slowly took the place of spontaneity, and so it gives a better because a historical statement of the dualism in hand. Still, the phrase of naive and sentimental passed into vogue; this is almost as much as to say objective and subjective; and one knows what riot of discussion followed. Ancient was set against modern, the old dispute, realist against idealist, classic against romantic, conservative against radical; add short and pithy phrases from Goethe, dithyrambs on "om-mject and sum-mject" from Coleridge; drop then, a nine days' fall, to the minor treatises in æsthetics: the thought of a century has been ringing changes on this dualism. They are not to be noted here, and are seldom to the purpose. Moses Mendelssohn's division into the "voluntary" and the "natural" looks at first sight like an oracle from Herder; but it must be borne in mind that Mendelssohn refused to regard as poetry those waifs and strays of song which Herder praised. Masing, in a dissertation[1] of considerable merit, divides into poetry of perception, which is rimeless, answering to the classical or the objective, and poetry of feeling, which is rimed and includes Christian, individual poetry: but there is no great gain in this. Mr. E. C. Stedman[2] thinks poetry is "differentiated by the Me and the Not Me," and thus he obtains his two main divisions of the poetic product. So run some of the purely theoretical contrasts; without stay in historic study, their distinctions are based upon the poetic impulse, and there is of course a far clearer case when one considers poetry in the light of those conditions under which it is produced. Æsthetic writers who apply the tests of sociology, for example, have made a vast gain in their method of treatment and in their results. Poetry to them is no vague, alien substance, a planet to be watched through telescopes; it is an outcome of the social life of man, and social facts must help to explain it. Critic, historian, psychologist, all put new life into the æsthetic discussion; and the artist himself is at hand. Earlier than Taine, Hennequin, and Guyau, and along with Sainte-Beuve, Richard Wagner,[3] in a practical purpose, and full of the ideas of 1848, tried to bring the conditions of artistic production into line with the study of society. It is not nature, he thinks, but the opposition to nature which has brought forth art; man becomes independent of climate; and social, human struggle is the making of this new man, this "man independent of nature," who alone called art into being, and that not in tropical Asia, but "on the naked hillsides of Greece." Primitive man, dependent on nature,

[1] *Ueber Ursprung und Verbreitung des Reimes*, Dorpat, 1866, p. 18. "Anschauung" and "Empfindung" are the terms.

[2] *Nature and Elements of Poetry*, pp. 76 f.

[3] *Gesammelte Schriften und Dichtungen*, Bd. III., three essays, "Die Kunst und die Revolution" (1849); "Das Kunstwerk der Zukunft," a more important work, dithyrambic, but highly interesting and full of the "folk," as against "Ihr Intelligenten"; and thirdly, "Kunst und Klima" (1850).

could never bring forth art, a social product made in the teeth of adverse natural conditions.[1] Wagner, however, goes further. Such is the history of art; but what of its future? Art, literature, have become a solitary piece of performance and of reception. The lonely modern man, pining for poetic satisfaction, has but a sad and feeble comfort in the poetry of letters. Back to social conditions, back to the old trinity of song, movement, poem; back to the *ensemble*, the folk-idea, the poetry of a people; let Shakspere and Beethoven join hands in the art that is to be and that must spring, as it once sprang, from no single individual artist but from the folk![2] Dithyramb apart, here is a theory of social origins with a definite though curious dualism of art and nature; Wagner talks *Jacob-Grimmisch*, it is true, and raves as Nietzsche raved afterward; but he has sociological hints for which one searches the school of Grimm in vain. Even in Victor Hugo's fantastic but suggestive phrases,[3] the new science, the agitation of St. Simon and his school, may perhaps be found; and there is no disguise of any sort in the sociological æsthetics of Guyau,[4] who repeats Hugo's notion in scientific terms, and so gives a precise expression to the dualism once so vague. Primitive art, according to Guyau, is a waking vision, and what we now call invention was at first nothing but a spontaneous play of fancies and images suggesting and following one another in the confusion of a dream. Real art begins when this pastime comes to be work, when thought and effort seize upon the play of fancy.[5]

[1] *Ibid.*, pp. 255 f., 261, 268.

[2] See especially *ibid.*, pp. 133–207.

[3] Preface to *Cromwell*, p. 16: "La société, en effet, commence par chanter ce qu'elle rêve, puis raconte ce qu'elle fait, et enfin se met à peindre ce qu'elle pense," Hugo's well-known sequence of lyric, epic, drama.

[4] *L'Art au Point de Vue Sociologique*, p. 26.

[5] This doctrine is in line with modern psychological notions of the part played by intelligent mental selection upon the instinctive material of consciousness. See Lloyd Morgan, *Habit and Instinct*, pp. 323 f.

These were mainly critical and æsthetic views. Of greater interest and importance is the dualism as it took shape under the hands of that historical school which had the great democratic movement in literature for its origin, Herder for its prophet, and A. W. Schlegel for its high priest. Here the dualism concerns not so much nature and art, uncertain terms at best, but the body of people, the folk, the community, nation, race, as contrasted with the individual artist, the "man of letters." It is poetry of the people over against poetry of the schools. Conditions of this sort had been noted by earlier writers of what one may call the scientific bent, that is, by men like Scaliger, who in this respect was following Aristotle; not, of course, by those who looked upon the oldest poet as divine, a prophet and a seer, the view taken by Platonists like Spenser[1] and Sidney, by the early renaissance, by Ronsard, and by belated followers of Ronsard. He, for example, not only says that earliest poetry was allegorical theology, to coax rough men into ideas of the divine,[2] but, in his preface about music,[3] written for a collection of songs and addressed to the king, he holds to the idea of a spontaneous and sacred perfection in this primitive verse. Later, so he explains in his Poetics, came "the second class of poets, whom I call human, since they were filled rather with artifice and labour than with divinity," — nature and art, again, in pious antithesis. It is different with the scientific school. Scaliger, following Aristotle's hints about the origin of the drama, is for a normal process from the natural to the artistic. Dante had made dualism a

[1] See *Shepheard's Calender*, October, Argument, — a specimen of the doctrine in that never-published *English Poete*.

[2] "Abbregé de l'Art Poetique," in *Works*, ed. Blanchemain, VII. 318.

[3] *Ibid.*, VII. 340. "Aussi les divines fureurs de Musique, de Poësie, et de paincture, ne viennent pas par degrés en perfection *comme les autres sciences*, mais par boutées et comme esclairs de feu, qui deçu qui dela apparoissent en divers pays, puis tout en un coup s'esvanouissent."

matter of rank, of merit, setting the *vulgare illustre* apart from the *humile vulgare*, and bidding spontaneous, facile poets beware how they undertake the things that belong to art;[1] Scaliger is not only historical but comparative, and in the right fashion, assuming, at least for origins, no gradations of rank. He is not for degeneration but for development; instead of dividing the sheep from the goats, he regards nature and art as two phases of the poetic conditions. Looking at the three forms of primitive life,[2] he gives the parentage of verse to the pastoral; hunters were too mobile, and ploughmen too busy, while shepherds had not only leisure for meditation but the songs of birds as lure. In this earliest stage Scaliger assumes two kinds of poetry, which he calls the solitary and the social; and again in the second division he makes a further contrast of the artless or natural, — not, he warns his reader, not to be classed as vulgar, — and the more artistic, such as those amœbean forms which are found in later pastoral verse. In other words, Scaliger hints at a fundamental dualism; and his account of the matter, modern in spirit despite its conventional style and its appeal to the ancients, is better than Herder's cloudy enthusiasm in all respects save one, and that, of course, an exception of vast importance: Scaliger failed to put the rustic and communal verse of Europe on a par with "natural" and social songs of the prime.

This distinction of art and nature as a theory of origins, and with a touch of the historical method in its treatment, is found again and again in treatises on poetry from the renaissance to our own time.[3] It is by no means confined

[1] For writers in the vulgar tongue, Dante reverses the rule of more matter and less art. They are too facile. "Pudeat ergo, pudeat idiotas tantum audere deinceps, ut ad cantiones prorumpant," *de vulgar. Eloq.*, Cap. vi. The *canzone* must not be content with the speech of common life; let it essay an exalted style.

[2] Cap. iv., *Pastoralia*, p. 6.

[3] G. J. Vossius, *de artis poeticæ natura*, 1647, Cap. iii. Many subsequent writers followed Scaliger's account of origins.

to the brilliant and epoch-making writers. Who was farther removed from Herder, so far as notions about poetry are concerned, than Gottsched? But Gottsched, dull dog, as Dr. Johnson would have called him, makes a clear distinction between natural and artistic verse;[1] more than this, he backs his theory of origins by referring to those "songs of the hill folk," heard in his own day, which still show characteristics of primitive poetry. Earlier yet, in the remarkable work of Morhof[2] one finds use of the comparative method and a keen sense of historic values; here is investigation, not theory outright, as with the younger Racine,[3] or mere chronicle, as with M. de la Nauze.[4] It is curious, too, that from the clergy came some of the most rationalistic accounts of the dualism of nature and art, in opposition to the divine and human idea of the renaissance. One must not forget Herder's cloth; Lowth took Hebrew poetry, as poetry, quite out of the supernatural; and Calmet,[5] whose work on the Bible was once valued by scholars, comments at length on the dualism as natural and artificial, not as human and

[1] *Critische Dichtkunst*, 1737, pp. 86, 72.

[2] *Unterricht von der teutschen Sprache und Poesie, deren Ursprung, Fortgang und Lehrsätzen*, Kiel, 1682. This book has been called the first attempt at a history of German, and, indeed, of collective European, poetry. Morhof gives a historic account of rime, compares German verse with verse of other nations, and is the first writer in Germany to name Shakspere.

[3] "De la Poésie Naturelle ou de la Langue Poétique" and "De la Poésie Artificielle," in *Mém. Acad. Inscript.*, XV. 192 ff., 207 ff. (1739). The only interest lies in the titles, the text is all verbal quibbling. In *Mém.*, XXIII. 85 ff., is a plan for a general history of poetry. But Racine Junior is negligible.

[4] *Ibid.*, IX. 320 f. (1731–1733), in a paper on the songs of ancient Greece. He repeats the idea that art comes out of nature, but lays stress on a development of special singers, a sort of guild, as contrasted with earlier universality of song. This is the contrast made afterward by Wilhelm Grimm (*Heldensage*, 2d ed., pp. 382 f.) between "free" and professional song.

[5] *Augustini Calmet dissertatio de poesi veterum Hebraeorum*, . . . Helmstadii, 1723. A French version is in the *Dissertationes qui peuvent servir de Prologomenes de l'Ecriture Sainte*, . . . Paris, 1720, 3 vols., I. 128 ff. See particularly 15 ff. of the Latin: "Duo habentur Poeseos genera: naturale et artificiale," etc.

divine. Improvisation seems to be his test for the natural sort, submission to rules and deliberation, his test for artificial verse; and in the first case it is wrath, joy, sorrow, hate, love, some natural outburst of passion, which is poetry by the mere fact of its utterance. Moreover, this poetry of nature is found in every clime;[1] and inseparable from it, in early stages, is the natural music, song, which itself in course of time must be tamed by art. Like Budde in our own day, Calmet points out "natural" songs in the Bible. It was left, however, for Herder to bring forward all natural, artless poetry not as a regret but as a hope, or rather as a disinherited exile come back to claim his own; how the German pleaded for his client, and with what success, is matter of common fame. At the historical school of which he is the conspicuous exponent in matters of poetry we must give a closer look.

Herder, in point of fact, was before a larger tribunal than that of poetry, and in his plea for communal verse he was joining the great democratic movement which ran through European thought at large, no less active because less conspicuous in science, art, letters, religion, than in affairs of state. A passion for democracy had gone from literature into politics and again from politics into literature, begetting this notion of creative power in the people as a whole; about the time that philosophers discovered the people in politics, Hamann and Herder discovered the folk in verse. The earlier eighteenth century, like all the preceding Christian centuries from the time of St. Augustine,[2] when saint or prophet or king was the embodiment of progress, still turned history into biography,

[1] "Non incommode ergo dicimus, Poesin methodicam artem esse, accurate et studiose exprimendi passiones, naturalem vero, quae sine arte, sine meditatione praevia, eas sistit. Omnis populus, omnis terra, omne temperamentum, omnis affectus sua non destituitur rhetorica aut poesi naturali. . . . *Natura semper producit rudius aliquid, quod ars perficere conatur.*"

[2] See Barth, *Die Philosophie der Geschichte als Sociologie*, Leipzig, 1897, I. 202.

and human development into a series of individual inventions; any movement in social life, whether of war or of peace, was due to the great man, — general, king, orator, poet, — who began or led the movement. Pascal's pleasantry about Cleopatra and her nose became a serious system of history and philosophy. Even as late as Turgot,[1] for example, one pinned one's faith to great men, to genius, for the advancement of mankind. The seventeenth century had asked for *raison;* the eighteenth sought *esprit.*[2] Genius was already a watchword when the democratic movement began, and it was not discarded by the new school; the Rousseaus and Herders clung to genius, but with a new interpretation of the word, and added that larger idea of "nature." Critics are apt to forget that the return to nature was preceded by a return to genius. The next step was to substitute natural genius for the great man, to separate genius from the individual; and here the democratic movement found help at hand in the progress and gains of science. Science was now clear of the church, and began to work into the domain of law, causes, force; it sought the impersonal both in natural and in supernatural things. Cold and analytic in the earlier decades, science in the later eighteenth century grew emotional, synthetic, romantic, and full of zeal for what the Germans call "combination." What a change from the earlier mood, represented, one might say, in Shaftesbury's letter on enthusiasm! "Good humour," he writes in 1707,[3] "is not only the best security against enthusiasm, but the best foundation of piety and true religion." Even as late as 1766, when the spirit of enthusi-

[1] "Sur les progrès successifs de l'esprit humain," *Œuvres,* II. 597 ff.

[2] On this change in poetic criticism, see Von Stein, *Entstehung der neueren Aesthetik,* p. 97. It must be remembered, however, that while Turgot clung to the individual in this sense, his search for laws of progress, movements, tendencies, was really preparing ruin for individualism, and making Condorcet's and Herder's task more easy.

[3] *Characteristics,* 5th ed., Birmingham, 1765, I. 22.

asm was again abroad, aristocratic Horace Walpole sounds the old note against the new communalism in his account of a sermon which he heard Wesley preach at Bath; the preacher "exalted his voice, and *acted very ugly enthusiasm.*" Enthusiasm, however, was now rife in science itself; still blocked on the theological side, it turned to nature and what lay undiscovered in her domain. No talk as yet of a struggle for existence, no distinct lapse of faith in humanity as main object of cosmic solicitudes; but a disposition to find in the sweep and conflict of natural forces sufficiently good answer to any question about the history of man, and a tendency to force upon individual men a transfer of values to the race. Not the individual, but the mass, and behind this mass the currents of life at large, were to interpret history. The great man disappeared, or else served simply as mouthpiece for the national and popular genius; and it was at this point that Herder appeared with his *Thoughts for the Philosophy of the History of Mankind*, — thoughts that here and there foreshadow the doctrine of evolution. Down to the extreme theories of Buckle, this point of view was taken by historians and philosophers. True, much is said of the individual; Rousseau, Goethe in his *Werther*, Herder, even, and Hamann, all glorified the free, individual man; it is not individual man in the old sense, however, but rather man himself as type of the human brotherhood, as one of a throng, the "citizen" whether high or low. More than this, it was a glorification of primitive man himself without the differencing and individualizing work of culture; the eighteenth century, and not merely in Rousseau's sentimental fashion, discovered the savage on one side, and, on the other side, unspoiled men of the prime. In literature there was an outbreak of gentle savages and a very mob of Robinson Crusoes; while for philosophy and science, the alchemy of human perfectibility, a desire to reconstruct society by the elixir of primitive life and a study of man as he ought to be, preceded the chemistry of modern anthropological and sociological researches, which aim at an analysis of earliest social conditions and the science of man both as he was and as he is.

This democratic thought of the eighteenth century had an outer and an inner circle, answering in great measure to the notion of humanity and the notion of the people or "folk." It was Vico who put men upon the first trail, who reformed scientific methods, and who, with all his antiquated theories, is often so surprisingly modern. He bade men look for the mind of humanity, the soul of it, as revealed in history, poetry, law, language, religion. He traced something of the inner circle as well, tossing aside Homer's personality, and saying that Homer was the Greek people itself as it told the story of its deeds. He set up the antithesis between imagination and reason, and gave the formula of culture as a decrease of the one and an increase of the other. Herder said these things seventy years later, and indeed his mere plea for humanity and nationality [1] adds little to the ideas of Vico; what the German added of his own was on the larger scale a substitution of people for race, and on the smaller scale a plea for the actual folk about one, the community of rustics, the village throng, not idealized shepherds and subjects of the Saturnian reign. From Vico to Herder, then, democracy was in the air, pervading the rationalism that so easily turned into sentiment and the naturalism that so readily fabled a new supernaturalism. Particularly in its theories of poetry the eighteenth century responded to the democratic impulse along three lines, the scientific, the historical, and what one would now call the ethnological and sociological.[2] A detailed

[1] *Stimmen der Völker*, Dedication: *Euch weih' ich die Stimme des Volks der zerstreueten Menschheit.*

[2] Leslie Stephen, *History of English Thought in the Eighteenth Century*, II. Chap. XII. § vii., divides the general course of thought into sentimental, romantic, and rationalistic tendencies.

account of these three currents of thought in their effect upon the study of poetry would be of interest and profit in the present work, but demands too much space; it must be reserved for separate treatment. We must confine our attention to the movement for communal or popular verse, and even that must be described in merest outline.

The first man in Europe to recognize poetry of the people, and to make it a term of the dualism now in hand, was Montaigne. He discovered the thing and gave a name to it, — *la poésie populaire;* he praised it for its power and grace; and he brought it into line with that poetry of savages then first coming into the view of European critics. The specimen which he gave of this savage verse remained for a long time the only one commonly known in Europe; in like manner, a Lapland *Lament*, published in Scheffer's Latin, came to be the conventional specimen of lowly or popular song. Montaigne, however, spoke boldly for the critical value of both kinds, savage and popular, bidding them hold up their heads in the presence of art. He praises the two extremes of poetic development, nature and simplicity on the one hand, and, on the other, noble artistic effort; for what Cotton translates as "the mongrets" he has open scorn.[1] Along with the savage verses which he quotes in another essay[2] he makes shrewd comments on the refrain and the dancing, shows an interest in ethnology, and even names his authorities, — "a man in my house who lived ten or twelve years in the New World," and in smaller degree natives to

[1] *Essais*, I. liv., near the end: "La poësie populere et purement naturelle a des naifvetez et graces par où elle se compare à la principale beauté de la poësie parfaicte selon l'art: comme il se voit ès villanelles de Gascoigne, et aus Chançons qu'on nous raporte des nations qui n'ont conoissance d'aucun sciance ny mesmes d'escriture. La poësie mediocre qui s'arrete entre deus est desdeignée, sans honur et sans pris."

[2] On Cannibals, I. xxx. "Ce premier couplet, c'est le refrain de la chanson. . . . Toute la journée se passe à dancer."

whom he talked at Rouen. Now this insight, this outlook, of Montaigne are unique. Sidney, whom a German scholar[1] praises for catholicity of taste equal to that of Montaigne and not derived from him, is too academic; he notes the *areytos* of America, by way of proof that rudest nations have poetry, and bursts out in that praise of "the old song of Percy and Douglas," only to take away from its critical value by a limitation quite foreign to the spirit of Montaigne. Neither Sidney nor Puttenham,[2] in their notice of savage and of communal poetry, came anywhere near the Frenchman's point of view.

The catholicity and discernment of Montaigne, the careless approval of Sidney, the comparative vein in Puttenham, had really no following in Europe until Herder's time. Poetry of the people remained a literary outcast; and as late as 1775 a German professor "would have felt insulted by the mere idea of any attention" to such verse.[3] Englishmen, to be sure, began long before this to collect the ballads, to print them, and even to write about them in a shamefaced way; but this was eccentricity of the kind for which, according to Matthew Arnold, continental folk still make allowance. Ambrose Phillips, or whoever made the collection begun in 1723, is very bold in his first volume; he "will enter upon the praise of ballads and shew their antiquity;" in the second volume he weakens, and will "say as little upon the subject as possibly" he can; while in the third volume he actually apologizes for the "ludicrous manner" in which he wrote the two other prefaces. He had suggested that the ballads were really "written by the greatest and most polite wits of their age"; but nobody in England paid much heed to the subject of origins, barring a little powder burnt over the thing by

[1] Fresenius, *Deutsche Litteraturzeitung*, 1892, col. 769 ff.

[2] Or whoever wrote the book. See Arber's ed., pp. 26, 53.

[3] So says Ferdinand Wolf in his famous essay on Spanish ballads.

Percy and Ritson; and the making of a theory, the founding of ballad criticism and research as a literary discipline, was left to German pens.

It has been said that Herder was the prophet of the faith in communal poetry. Herder's "origins," so far as this doctrine is concerned, are interesting enough. That the individual is child of his time, child of his race, child of his soil; that he is not only what "suns and winds and waters" make him, but what long ages and vast conspiracies of nature and the sum of human struggle have made him, — strand by strand of this cord can be brought from Hamann, from Blackwell, Lowth, Robert Wood, Hurd, Spence, from Condorcet, Montesquieu, Rousseau; but all that does not make up Herder. It was his grasp of this entire evolutionary process, his belief in it, his fiery exhortation, in a word, his genius, that made him the only begetter of the modern science. Full of scorn for closet verse of his day, he held up the racial or national, the "popular" in its best sense, against the pedantic and the laboured, — poetry that beats with the pulse of a whole people against poetry that copies its exercises from a dead page and has no sense of race. He sundered poetry for the ear from poetry for the eye, poetry said or sung from poetry that looks to "a paper eternity" for its reward. Under his hands, in a word, the dualism became real, a state of things impossible while one was juggling with an adjective like "natural" or with a phrase like "naive and sentimental." He gathered and printed songs of the folk, as he calls them, or by another title, voices of the nations.[1] Here, of course, is lack of precision; a peasant's song and a soliloquy of Hamlet, one because really "popular," the other because really "national," are ranged alike as folksongs. But the dualism stands. Oral, traditional, communal poetry, and whatever

[1] *Stimmen der Völker* and *Volkslieder*. *Volkslied* is original with Herder. See note, p. xxvi., of the author's *Old English Ballads*.

springs from these, are set clearly against poetry of the schools. Naturally, Herder was unjust to the cause of art, or rather he seems to be unjust. What he does is to bid the artist stand for a community or race and reflect their life, or else fall, a negligible and detached thing. Poetry is a spring of water from the living rock of community or nation; whether Moses, Homer, Shakspere, dealt the unsealing blow, or whether the waters gushed out of their own force, Herder cared not a whit.

This doctrine of a dualism in poetry was still further elaborated by A. W. Schlegel, who brought to the task not only his unerring literary tact,[1] his critical insight, his astounding sympathy for foreign literatures, but his method of historical and genetic research. In his early essay on Dante, he broke away from the method then in vogue, and used historical tests instead of that philosophical analysis so dear to Schiller. No one has stated the dualism of communal and artistic poetry so clearly as Schlegel has done;[2] and yet, owing to a curious lack of perspective in modern criticism, he is credited with the achievement of crushing the dualism to naught. Leaving the details to another occasion, we may give a brief outline of this case, which has so distinct a bearing on the question of poetical origins. In his lectures and in sundry essays, Schlegel states the historical dualism, and repeats Aristotle's account of early communal and improvised verse, adding, however, what Aristotle refused to give, recognition of this as poetry and respect for its rude nobility of style. As Schlegel left the matter in his lectures, there was nothing to which one could raise an objection; and the same is true of a temperate statement, made by Wilhelm von Hum-

[1] "Nicht jeder versteht Poesie zu wittern," is a remark of his still in some need of emphasis, *Lectures* (*Neudruck*), III. 141.

[2] "We shall treat first the poetry of nature, and then the poetry of art. We shall follow this development historically." . . . *Lectures* (*Neudruck*, etc.), I. 25 f.

boldt,[1] which may be quoted here at length. "In the course of human development," he says, "there arise two distinct kinds of poetry, marked respectively by the presence and the absence of written records. One, the earlier, may be called natural poetry; it springs from an enthusiasm which lacks the purpose and consciousness of art. The second is a later product, and is full of art; but it is none the less outcome of the deepest and purest spirit of poetry." One sees it is not the communal bantling that has to be praised and defended here; not rude, uncivil verse that once found an advocate in Herder, but now needs no advocate; it is the poetry of art that must be lauded and protected as even-christian with "natural" verse. Democratic ideas had put the poetry of nature above all else; the pantheistic doctrines of Schelling, carrying even Schlegel off his feet, had made a school for the universal, general, communal, absolute, in verse; and a wholesome reaction had set in. Humboldt's modest words could have been signed by nearly every critical warrior, Trojan or Tyrian, who took up his pen in the long dispute; the trouble had begun when scholars tried to give details about the origin of natural or popular verse and essayed to draw close lines of definition between the people and the artist. Jacob and Wilhelm Grimm, full of romance, piety, and pantheism, laid stress upon this kindly word "natural" and dogmatized it into a creed.[2] A song sings itself; a "folk" can be poet; nations make their own epic; the process is a mystery: these and like phrases are now regarded by short-sighted critics as a fair summary of the democratic or communal doctrine of poetry, and are thought to have been blown into space, along with the doctrine, by a clumsy jest of Scherer about the Pentecost. Scherer, indeed,

[1] *Verschiedenheit des menschlichen Sprachbaues*, a part of the introduction to his researches on the Kawi language, § 20, *Werke*, VI. 249.

[2] See the introduction to the author's *Old English Ballads*.

has given a history of this movement, with what seems to him a closing of the account, in his admirable book on Jacob Grimm; but neither this nor his jest can be regarded as final. He appeals to Schlegel as the great literary critic who really killed this doctrine of the folk in verse as soon as it was born, although the great reputation of the Grimms gave it an appearance of life and vigour down to the time say . . . of Scherer. Now it is a fact, overlooked by German scholars, that A. W. Schlegel laid down a theory of communal origins, almost identical with that of the Grimms, at a time when Jacob was barely fifteen and Wilhelm fourteen years old. In an essay on Bürger,[1] whom he loved and admired, Schlegel asks whether this man of genius was really what he thought he was, a poet of the folk, and whether his poetry could be called poetry of the people. To answer the question, Schlegel makes a study of old ballads, and says that these were not purposely made for the folk, but were composed among the people, — "*composed, in a manner of speaking, by the folk itself as a whole.*"[2] This community which made the old ballads was of course homogeneous; the style of them is without art or rhetoric; they come spontaneously. In short, "the free poetic impulse did that with ease and success to which the careful artist now purposely returns." Here is the later doctrine of Jacob and Wilhelm Grimm in a nutshell; how much of it did Schlegel reject fifteen years later in that famous criticism[3] of the Grimms' *Old German Forests*, where he turns state's evidence against his fellow conspirators for demos? Simply its extravagances, but by no means its reiteration of a dualism in the poetic product springing from conditions of production.

[1] A. W. Schlegel, *Werke*, ed. Böcking, VIII. 64 ff., written in 1800. See particularly pp. 79 f.

[2] "Deren Dichter gewissermassen das Volk im ganzen war."

[3] Reprinted, *Werke*, XII. 383 ff., from the *Heidelberger Jahrbücher* of 1815.

That idea stands intact; for all of Schlegel's historical studies are based upon it. Moreover, the Grimms said far more than Schlegel had said, and went into deeper extravagances of romance. He denied their assumption that the great mass of legend, song, epic, which one finds or surmises at the beginnings of a national literature, is the authoritative and essentially true deliverance of the nation itself. Nor is there a pious mystery — and here Schlegel touches the quick — in the making of such songs. A poem implies a poet. In brief, the Grimms were not to furbish up the idyll of a golden age, bind it in a mystery, and hand it over to the public as an outcome of exact philological studies. This process, he said in sum, is all theory and no fact; and here lies the stress of Schlegel's criticism, which really involved only a partial and superficial recanting of his own doctrine. He was always wont to turn from theory to fact, and in the Grimms' wild theory he found no facts at all; he protests against the self-made song, the folk-made song even; but he would have been the first to give ear to any plea for a difference between songs of art and songs of the people that was based on facts and that might bring out those social conditions which determine the poem as it is made. He had himself repeatedly brought out these conditions, these facts, and he nowhere recants the doctrine which he founded on them. He unsays, perhaps without consciousness of any change of opinion, his old saying about the folk as a poet; he does not unsay his belief in the dualism of poetry according to the conditions under which it is produced. "All poetry," he declares, "rests on a union of nature and art; without art it can get no permanent form, without nature its vitality is gone." True; but there is communal art and there is individual art, or rather there are two kinds of poetry according as art and the individual or instinct and the community predominate; and this dualism he had repeatedly affirmed, just as Aristotle had hinted it long before him. Schlegel does not reduce it to a mere matter of record,[1] as modern critics do when they seize upon Humboldt's saying that the difference between oral and written is the "mark" of the dualism — he does not say its essence; for it is treated, even in this critical essay, as a matter of conditions of production. The scholar who took up poetry on the genetic and historical side, who followed brutish and uncivil man slowly tottering into the path of art, is not lost in the critic who simply refuses to see primitive poetry bursting by miracle out of a whole nation into an Iliad, a Nibelungen Lay, a Beowulf.

This, then, is particularly to be borne in mind; the dualism of the poetic product based on the difference between communal and individual conditions of production does not rise and fall with the dualism as it took shape in the theory of the Grimms.[2] Aristotle had set aside all unpremeditated, artless verse of the throng, and had regarded it at best as mere foundation, no part of the poetic structure. Jacob Grimm went to the other extreme, and set off from poetry all laboured, premeditated, individual verse; he accepted modern poetry, to be sure, but explained away the poet; the superstructure was nothing save as it implied that unseen foundation. Or, to put it in different phrase, the old doctrine of imitation as mainspring of poetry had yielded to the idea of a power, an informing energy; one turned, like Addison, to the imaginative process, or else to deeper sources. Herder told men to seek this source, this poetic

[1] Oral and communal literature, it is almost superfluous to point out, are not one and the same thing. See Max Müller on "Literature before Letters," *Nineteenth Century*, November, 1899, pp. 798 f.

[2] Such an assumption takes most of the value from Berger's detailed account of the controversy over popular song, "Volksdichtung und Kunstdichtung," *Nord und Süd*, LXVIII. (1894), 76 ff., an account which is often inaccurate and quite incomplete. Berger's conclusion that there is no essential difference between poetry of the people and poetry of art confuses, as is usual in this school of Germans, the poetic impulse with the poetic product.

power, in the people, with their primitive passions and their unspoiled utterance. Herder was general, often merely negative, and exhorted; the Grimms were positive and dogmatized, teaching that the whole people as a whole people once made poetry. But this extravagance must not drag down in its death those sober facts about which criticism has always hovered with its hints or statements of the twofold nature of poetry. Moreover, just as these facts are to be held in plain view, and not lost in the haze of an impossible theory, so, too, they are not to be rationalized and explained away into a facile, unmeaning phrase about the difference between oral and written record. It is a question of the difference in poetic production due to varying conditions under which the poetic impulse has to work; and some difference of this sort, not of mere record, is recognized in the whole range of criticism, mostly, however, by expressions about art and nature which leave much to be desired in the way of precise statement. Nature and art are terms of æsthetics; even when used in a more or less historical sense, the historical comprehension of them is uncertain; can they not be transferred then, to terms of sociology, of ethnology, of literary conditions, so as to correspond with the actual facts of poetry and with the actual history of man,— transferred in good faith, and for the interests of no theory, but to provide clear tests for an investigation which studies communal poetry in order to determine whether it can throw light upon the conditions of primitive song? There is certainly such a dualism of conditions apart from the record. Even the most intrepid monist allows the dualism of the term "mankind" according as one takes man social or man individual, the solitary man of reflection, ethics, judgment, and the same man as one of a crowd of madmen — mad for the nonce, mad gregariously, but mad. M. Tarde has recently drawn this picture in very bold outlines. There are two men in the juryman,— the individual and the juryman. Does this, then, hold in poetry? It is a fact that poetry made by a throng, or made in a throng, or made for a throng, or made in whatever fashion but finding its way, as favourite expression, to a throng — and every theory of communal verse may be referred to one of these cases — is a quite distinct kind of poetry from that which is made by the solitary poet for the solitary reader. Nowadays nearly all poetry is written and read, but once upon a time nearly all poetry was sung and heard; a very hasty glance at this antithesis will show that it concerns production at least as much as it concerns the record. It serves as basis for the division of poetry into one class where the communal spirit and environment condition the actual making, and into another class where the artist, the individual, has upper hand from the start.[1] It sets primitive poetry, at least in some important characteristics, over against the poetry of modern times. If, then, communal poetry still exists in survival; if the sense of literary evolution, the facts of literary evolution, the facts of ethnology, the conclusions of sociology, all assert that primitive poetry was communal rather than individual in the conditions of its making; then it is clear that a study of the survivals ought to be one of the best ways by which one could come to reasonably sure conclusions about poetry of the prime.

[1] As direct, unqualified fact. One is dealing here with no phrases, no illustrations, such as the editor of Brantôme employs when he says (preface to the *Vie des Dames Galantes*, p. x), "dans un siècle, il y a deux choses, l'histoire et la comédie : l'histoire, c'est le peuple, la comédie, c'est l'homme."

CHAPTER IV

THE DIFFERENCING ELEMENTS OF THE POETRY OF ART

NOBODY will deny that the modern man does more thinking and less singing than the man, say, of Shakspere's time; and nobody will deny that thinking needs solitude, while singing — real, hearty singing — asks the throng and a refrain. Thought, M. Anatole France[1] declares in his vivacious way, "thought is the acid which dissolves the universe, and if all men fell to thinking at once, the world would cease to be." "Lonely thinking," says Nietzsche, "that is wise; lonely singing, — stupid." In the same fashion, a solitary habit of thinking has made itself master of poetry, particularly of the lyric; while the singing of a poem is going fast out of date. Poetry begins with the impersonal, with communal emotion, and passes to a personal note of thought so acutely individual that it has to disguise itself, wear masks, and prate about being objective. For objective and even simple poetry may be highly subjective at heart; and to define subjective as talking about one's self, what Bagehot, in his essay on Hartley Coleridge, calls self-delineation, is by no means a sufficient account of the trait. When the folksong runs: —

> A Nant's, à Nant's est arrivé,
> *Saute, blonde, et lève le pied,*
> Trois beaux navir's chargés de blé;
> *Saute, blonde, ma joli' blonde. . . .*

[1] *La Vie Littéraire*, II. 173.

and Béranger sings:—

Une plainte touchante
De ma bouche sortit;
Le bon Dieu me dit, Chante,
Chante, pauvre petit!

it is not only wrong to take simplicity as the differencing factor of the communal song, for Béranger is quite as simple, but it will not do to fall back on mere self-delineation as end of the matter in art. Half of the folksongs of Europe are self-delineations of the singing and dancing crowd, in mass or by deputed "I." The real difference lies in the shifting of the point of view; song, once the consolation and expression of the festal crowd, comes to be the consolation and expression of the solitary poet. "I do not inquire," Ribot remarks,[1] "whether this sort of isolation in an ivory tower is a gain or a loss for poetry; but I observe its growing frequency as civilization advances, the complete antithesis to its collective character in the earliest ages." To study such a change in the long reaches of poetic progress would be an almost impossible task even if the material were at hand; it is best to take a comparatively short range of time and a definite place,—say the literature of modern Europe from its beginning in the Middle Ages down to the present time. The extremes are fairly sundered. Europe had lapsed from civilization to a half barbarous state, from the height of the Roman empire to the depth of the dark ages, with a corresponding decline of intellectual power and a great inrush of communal force. Out of these communal conditions, individual and intellectual vigour made its difficult way; how difficult, how tortuous that way, every one knows; and it is along this route, and about the time of the renaissance, that one may best watch the differencing elements

[1] Work quoted, p. 340.

of artistic and individual poetry as they come slowly into view.

As the individual[1] frees himself from the clogs of his mediæval guild, in literature as in life, there begins the distinctly modern idea of fame, of glory, as a personal achievement apart from community or state; and there, too, begins the idea of literary property. Fame of the poet had its classical tradition, and was asserted in a conventional, meaningless way by mediæval poets, chiefly in Latin; but the market value of a poem is something new.[2] From this time on there is a pathetic struggle in the poet's mind whether he shall regard his poem as offspring to cherish or as ware to sell. Randolph, writing to his friend, Master Anthony Stafford, takes the nobler view: —

> Let clowns get wealth and heirs: when I am gone . . .
> If I a poem leave, that poem is my son.

There is pretty antithesis, too, between the director and the poet in Goethe's play before the play in *Faust*, — one for his box-receipts, and the other for the solitudes of poetry and the gods. A happy solution has been found of late for this dilemma; over the naked contradiction of love and merchandise one throws the cloak of the artist. The artist begets in pure love of his art; and he sells for Falstaff's reason, — it is his vocation. Until poetry got this market value, however, it was common goods; poets had written generically,

[1] For the psychological study of individuality in art and letters, see Dilthey, "Beiträge zum Studium der Individualität," *Sitzungsberichte*, Berlin Academy, 1896, I. 295 ff. For a historical study, with sociological leanings, see the admirable work of Burckhardt, *Cultur der Renaissance in Italien*, ed. 1898, I. 143 ff. ("der Mensch wird geistiges Individuum"), 154 f., 178; II. 29 f., 48; and Brunetière, *Évolution des Genres*, pp. 39, 167 (Rousseau and individualism), and *Nouveaux Essais*, pp. 66, 150, 194.

[2] If one had the materials, a similar emancipation of the poet could be noted in Latin, beginning, perhaps, with Ennius — *volito vivus per ora virum* — and Naevius, down to Horace, his fountain made famous *me dicente*, and the *non omnis moriar*.

as members of a class or guild,[1] and any member might use the common stock of expressions and ideas. A translator was as great as his original.[2] The eighth chapter of Dante's essay on composition in the vernacular opens with a curious discourse about artistic property, as if the new idea and the new phrase needed a gloss. "When we say, 'this is Peter's *canzone*,' we mean that Peter made it, not merely that he uttered it!" Such an explanation, however, seems timely enough if one remembers that "a mediæval writer held it to be improper to join his name to any literary composition,"[3] and that Dante, "first of the moderns" as he is, and personal as his work seems to be, actually names himself but once in the whole *Commedia.* Here is the dying struggle of that clan ownership[4] which had ruled from the days of the primitive horde; for it is clear that intellectual property would be the last kind to be developed, and even if the poet liked to see his name graven on the colder side of the rock, this was not an isolated, personal distinction, but was merged in the register of the guild like the names on a soldiers' monument. Horace's "write me down among the lyric poets" was an intelligible ambition to mediæval minds; but the purely personal triumph of his *non omnis moriar* and its splendid context was alien to their way of thought. Barring the degree of genius in each, one may say that Dante and Victor Hugo were equally strong in their intense individuality; here is a case where Gautier's phrase holds good that the brain of an artist was the same under the Pharaohs as it is now; yet that conditions change the product, that the

[1] Vossler, *Poetische Theorien in der italienischen Frührenaissance*, Berlin, 1900, p. 3: "Im Mittelalter hatte jede Gesellschaftsklasse ihren eigenen zünftigen Sänger (*rimatore* oder *dicitore per rima*), der nur von ihr verstanden und anerkannt wurde."

[2] Lounsbury, *Chaucer*, III. 14.

[3] Nyrop, *Den oldfranske Heltedigtning*, p. 288.

[4] On the individual poet as mouthpiece of the clan, see Posnett, *Comp. Lit.*, pp. 130 ff., and Letourneau, *Évolution Littéraire*, p. 78.

individual note, piercing in the modern, becomes almost communal and generic in the older poet, that a distinct curve of evolution to the personal extreme, even in artistic poetry, can be drawn between them, is clear to probation for any one who will compare two famous passages which a hasty inference would probably declare to be on the same straight individual line. If one looks at the whole passage where Dante speaks of his poetic achievement,[1] and if one neither isolates a phrase nor yet sentimentalizes it all to suit modern ideas; if one notes the satisfaction which the poet feels with his work in and for the guild, and how he passes the time of day with a brother craftsman; then one will find in it not only a touch of artlessness, of what is called, rightly or wrongly, the mediæval, the communal, but an effacement of personality in the very act of asserting it. He shows, as it were, his diploma from the guild of poets. To bring this artlessness into clear relief, one has only to compare the thirty-second of Hugo's *Chants du Crépuscule*, where the poet, alone in an old tower, addresses the bell which hangs there, its pious inscription insulted by the obscenities, blasphemies, and futilities written over it; he is no exile, this poet, but proudly and contemptuously isolated from his kind, whose brutishness he has just deplored; and he speaks thus to the bell, — of all survivals the most characteristic of mediæval thought, the veriest symbol of communal religious life: —

> Sens-tu, par cette instinct vague et plein de douceur,
> Qui révèle toujours une sœur à la sœur,
> Qu'à cette heure où s'endort la soirée expirante,[2]

[1] *Purgat.*, xxiv. 52 ff.: —

> Io mi son un che quando
> Amor mi spira, noto, ed a quel modo
> Che ditta dentro, vo significando.

But it must be read with what precedes and what follows.

[2] It is almost impertinent to remind the reader of Dante's famous verses, *Purgat.*, viii. 1 ff. Perhaps Hugo remembers his Dante here. Compare Section iv. of this same *Chant.*

Une âme est près de toi, non moins que toi vibrante,
Qui bien souvent aussi jette un bruit solennel,
Et se plaint dans l'amour comme toi dans le ciel ?

Then the superb lines of comparison: life has written on the poet's soul base and irreverent inscriptions, like those on the bell; but a touch of the divine, a message, and like the bell, so his soul breaks out into harmonies in which even the audacities and futilities perforce take part. Compare all this introspection, this immense assumption of individual importance, with the objective, communal tone of Dante, despite that "I am one who sings whenever love inspires me," — so like Hugo's assertion, and yet so different. In each of these passages one can see artistic individuality; but between them stretches a long chain of development in which each link is a new emphasis on the individual in art. One of the earliest and strongest of these links was forged by the renaissance; although it must be borne in mind that Dante represents not simply his guild of singers, but behind them a singing community of peasants, the songs of field, spinning-room, and village dance, still dominant among unlettered folk and not yet shamed into silence by print and the schoolmaster.

The change, however, was there; the tide had turned against communal sentiment, and individuals were feeling a new power. Not only fame and glory fled from the guild to the great man; individual disgrace, the lapse, the shortcoming, find a record. Once the flyting was carried out before the folk, rose and fell with the occasion, and was a thing of festal origin, like the Eskimo poem-duel, or the earliest amœbean verse, or the German *schnaderhüpfl;* but Aretino now appears as the father of journalism in our pleasant modern sense, as the arch reporter, the discoverer and publisher of personal scandal.[1] In painting, too, one notes the sudden

[1] The emancipation of woman as an individual begins here in Italy. See M. de Vogüé's study of the Sforza (in *Histoire et Poésie*), and the general statement of Burckhardt, *Cult. Ital. Ren.*, I. 144, note 3.

rage for portraits; and it is the portrait of the individual for himself, not simply of pope, or of abbot, or of prince, as the head and type of a corporation, although a trace of this influence lingers in the setting of the picture, witness one of Holbein's merchants, with his bills, pens, memoranda, and a dozen mercantile suggestions scattered about him. Poetry, of course, felt the change first of all, both in subject-matter and in form. For the latter, there is the founding of the sonnet, that apartment for a single gentleman in verse. One thinks at once of Petrarch, rightly called "the first modern man," and deserving the title better than Dante, who was quite as mediæval as he was modern,[1] while Petrarch belonged to the new world; besides his sonnets, his correspondence and his confessions show that he not only felt the need, as none of his predecessors had felt it, to reveal and analyze his personality, but also recognized an interest on the part of the public to which these revelations could respond. The mediæval poet sought his public, did not call the public to himself; and the artistic form of his poetry is the utterance of common feeling in a common and often conventional phrase. The May morning, the vision,[2] the garden and the roses and the blindingly beautiful young person, the allegorical birds and beasts, — this was the late mediæval tether; although allegory helped the poet to escape the throng and hedge his personality with some importance, even allegory is in the service if not of the throng, at least of the guild. Allegory

[1] "Ego velut in confinio duorum populorum constitutus simul ante retroque prospicio," a saying of Petrarch, would apply better to Dante. The *Vita Nuova* has psychological analysis enough for ten moderns; but the mediæval in it all conquers the modern, as one feels the moment one turns to Petrarch's correspondence. Perhaps Norden, *Antike Kunstprosa*, II. 732, lays too much stress on Petrarch's backward gaze; he did look backward to the classics, but he was not mediæval. See the charming extracts given in Robinson and Rolfe's *Petrarca*.

[2] Hardly borrowed from the classics, as Gautier hints in general, and asserts for Old French epic. See Benezé, *Das Traummotiv in der mhd. Dichtung bis 1250, und in alten deutschen Volksliedern*, Halle, 1897, pp. 53 ff.

as a poetical form mediates between the old communal ballad, or the *chanson de geste*, and the new lyric of confidences. The modern poet cut loose from it all, and cast about for the gentle reader, soon to be his portion by the happy intervention of print. Ronsard strikes this note of separation from an unappreciative throng, and so does many another humanist; while Chaucer's contempt for the masses is not so much artistic as mediæval and aristocratic. Dunbar, our first really modern poet, the first to take that purely individual attitude, was also first of our poets to see his work in printer's ink. Even when the form of literature demanded objective treatment, the interest began to be individual. We now laud our poet or playwright for the fine individuality of his folk, and flout those masterless tales, songs, ballads, where even the hero is a mere type, or, worse, a mere doer of deeds. This doer of deeds answered the desire for poetic expression at a time when an individual was merged in his clan; the excess of interest in action is proportioned to the excess of communal over individual importance. As the artist develops, as he begins to feel his way toward individualism, his genius is spent first upon allegory, and then, as real life grows more imperious, upon the type, a compromise between individual and community. Here stands Chaucer. Like Dante he looks both ways; his squire, for example, deliciously clear and individual as he seems, has as much reminiscence of Childe Waters as prophecy of Romeo. It is characteristic of the two periods in which Chaucer and Shakspere respectively worked, that while one named his masterpiece, the study of a vulgar woman, "a wife of Bath," the other called a like masterpiece "Mrs. Quickly of Eastcheap," — a very pretty little curve of evolution in itself; and when the portrait of the merchant is drawn, — and what a portrait! — that careless "sooth to sayn, I noot how men hym calle," as compared with Shakspere's treatment of Antonio, is suggestive not only of the aristocrat, but also of the mediæval point of view. Even the setting of the Prologue is in point, — these pilgrims, each a representative of his class or corporation, their common lodging, their association, even if temporary, as in a guild, their jests, courtesies, and quarrels, all in the open air. A century later, people had come indoors. Professor Patten,[1] alert to note the connection between æsthetic change and a change in economic conditions, points out the alteration thus wrought in the passage from communal to individual life. Window-glass, the chimney, bricks, all improvements of the home, changed this home from a prison to a palace, from something shunned and undesired to the focal point of happiness. Outdoor communal amusements yielded to indoor pleasures shared by a few. The dances and the license of May-day, uproarious and often questionable rejoicings once common to all, were now left to the baser sort, while quiet, reputable folk turned to their homes. Knight and prioress, too, no longer rode beside the miller and put up with his *gros rire*, his drunken antics, and his tale.

The main expression in poetry brought about by that new power of the individual is the confidential note, the assumption of a reader's interest in the poet's experience, what J. A. Symonds called "the lyric cry," begetting on the part of this reader or hearer a sense at first confined to such mutual relations of the poet and the sympathetic soul to which he spoke, but spreading little by little until it is now fairly to be called the medium, the atmosphere, of poetry at large; one names it sentiment. The history of modern verse, with epic and drama in decay, is mainly the history of lyrical sentiment. Where does this first appear in European poetry?[2] Answers

[1] *Development of English Thought*, pp. 81 f.

[2] Déor's song, first in point of time of English lyrics, is a *vox clamantis in deserto*. The breezy personality of it, the individual confidence, the appeal to

to such a question are made with melancholy forebodings, seeing that a first appearance in literary annals is as unstable as the positively last appearance of a favourite singer; but French criticism has pitched, with considerable show of right, upon that amiable vagabond, Villon. Certainly the *Grand Testament* is as familiar in its tone to the modern reader as it is difficult and obsolete in its speech; and Sainte-Beuve, in a pretty bit of criticism, has undertaken to show why Villon's most famous ballade touches this modern sense, while verses seemingly like it are scorned as monkish prattle.[1] Throughout the Middle Ages a favourite form of communal sentiment, or rather of theological and professional reflection, was to ask where this and that famous person might now be found. The mediæval poet could string together interminable rimed queries like these of St. Bernard:—

Dic ubi Salomon, olim tam nobilis?
Vel ubi Samson est, dux invincibilis?
Vel pulcher Absolon, vultu mirabilis?
Vel dulcis Jonathas, multum amabilis?

and so on, with pagans like Cæsar, Tully, Aristotle. A capable Frenchman traced this sort of poem far back, and on his heels came a tireless, not to say superfluous, German;[2] but it was Sainte-Beuve who did the one important thing. He sees in Villon's queries about those fair ladies dead and gone little more than the old conventional question, and finds Villon's originality in the exquisite refrain, with its light, half-

great names and great things to prop Master Déor's own hope that something good will turn up,—all this is discouragement to the critic who likes to go about pasting labels on various epochs of literature. But there is Déor's rival, Wīdsīð, the typical singer lost in the guild, or rather a dozen singers rolled into one,—communal triumph.

[1] *Causeries du Lundi*, XIV. 296 f. Learned research on the *ubi sunt* formula is noted by Professor Bright, *Modern Language Notes*, 1893, Col. 187.

[2] Classical parallels go for little here; changes rung upon the *memento mori*, like Horace's *quo pater Æneas*, a statement, are not in line with these mediæval queries.

mocking pathos: *But where are the snows of yester year?* The Latin simply failed to add: —

> Ast ubi nix vetus, tam effusibilis?

Yet Sainte-Beuve did not quite touch the quick. Even this refrain is no more original than the queries; for it not only echoes a popular phrase, and perhaps is itself nothing more than a communal refrain,[1] but it continues a theme of the mediæval poet even better known than the *ubi sunt.* The real change is not in words or phrase, but in a shifting from the professional to the personal point of view. The poet of the sacred guild could put this fact of mortality either as a question or as an "example," — witness a thirteenth-century poem,[2] where the prospect of dissolution is fortified by the roasting of St. Lawrence, the beheading of John the Baptist, and the stabbing of Thomas à Becket; while the same manuscript which holds this "example" has a charming little poem of questions, the *Luve Ron* of Thomas de Hales, often quoted as forerunner of Villon's ballade. "A maid of Christ," — and we note this touch of the guild, — "asks me to make her a love-song. I will do it. But the love of this world is a cheat; lovers must die, and men fade all as leaf from bough. Lovers, quotha? *Where, indeed, are Paris and Helen; where Tristram, Ysolde, and the rest; where, too, are Hector and Cæsar?* As if they had never lived at all!" At first sight this lyric of the guild seems a counterpart to the pagan cry of Villon, as if the latter were a parody of the old formula without the piety and with a vague touch of

[1] Chaucer, *Troilus*, V. 1174 ff.: —

> From hazel-wode, ther Ioly Robin pleyde,
> Shal come al that that thou abydest here;
> Ye, farewel al the snow of ferne yere!

Boccaccio has instead an allusion to the "wind of Etna." Chaucer's phrase is "a reference to some popular song or saying," in Skeat's opinion.

[2] Printed by Morris, *Old English Miscellany*, pp. 90 ff.

genius in the refrain; but the difference is more than this. Villon transfers sentiment from the guild to the individual.[1] It is a supreme and triumphant and epoch-making attempt to do what the individual poet had always essayed to do and found impossible, — to leap communal barriers entirely, and tear himself free from the guild. The monk could not doff his cowl; his face is hidden; his song asks the organ, the choir, the general confession, the litany, for a background, even when it seems fairly Wordsworthian: —

> Winter wakens all my care!
> Now these trees are waxing bare,
> Oft I sigh and mourn full "sair,"
> When it cometh in my thought
> Of this earthly joy, how it all goeth to naught.[2]

Not so with Villon. He knows no guild, save that of the jolly beggars; and he can do with ease what even Ronsard does only with difficulty, and leaning on a classical staff: —

> Sous le tombeau tout Ronsard n'ira pas, —

paraphrase of Horace. But these ladies pass in line before Villon for his own whim;[3] they are there to throw a more intense light upon his own personality; and the cry of the refrain, subtle but absolute touch of individual sentiment, is the new lyric cry.[4] Across the channel this cry is echoed in what at first hearing sounds like the veriest poem of a guild,

[1] Not, of course, merely in this ballade. Among other examples of the quality, see stanzas 28, 29, 38 ff. of the *Grand Testament.* See other ballades; passages in the *Petit Testament:* —

> "Au fort, je meurs amant martir,"

and of course the *Regrets de la Belle Heaulmiere.*

[2] About 1300; modernized, of course. Compare the sweep and firm individual control of Wordsworth's *Loud is the Vale,* — lines on the expected death of Fox.

[3] M. Gaston Paris, *Poésie du Moyen Age,* II. 232, contrasts Villon with Charles of Orleans, the "dernier chanteur du moyen age," while the other is "premier poète moderne," and that "par le libre essor de l'individualisme." See the rest of this admirable summary.

[4] The Lorelei legend would once have been given for its own sake; now it is merely a reason, which the poet imparts to his reader, "dass ich so traurig bin."

Dunbar's *Lament for the Poets*,[1] and in its refrain, superficially so mediæval, *Timor mortis conturbat me!* But for English lyric, Dunbar is the first poet of sentiment, in its modern meaning, as Villon is for the French. In brief, the more one studies these changes, which could be detailed to the limits of a book, the clearer one sees that Europe learned from Villon, Dunbar, and their fellows, to take sentiment[2] instead of the old morality, and to regard lyric verse as the bidding to a private view of the poet's mind. The poet now makes himself the central point of all that he says and sees; he lays all history, all romance, under tribute to support the burden of his own fate and frame his proper picture; he is the sun of the system; he serves no clan or guild, and admits his readers only one by one to an audience. The advance from Villon's time is chiefly to add the intellectual to the individual, an obvious process. Emotion has come so thoroughly under individual control that the art is now conscious and the artist supreme, and so thoroughly under intellectual control that the feelings, however common and widely human their appeal, must own the mastery of thought. The one involves the other; for consent of emotions is a far easier affair than consent of opinions and agreement of reasoning. Emotion is the solvent of early superstition, traditional beliefs and affections, in a community, as it is in an individual. "I felt," says Rousseau, "before I thought; it is the common lot of humanity."[3]

[1] *Lament for the Makaris* (dead poets for dead ladies), *quhen he wes Seik*,— a significant situation, like Tom Nash—again with dead lords and ladies—and his "I am sick, I must die: Lord have mercy on us!" For the imitation of Villon by Dunbar, see the notes by Dr. Gregor in Small's edition of Dunbar's *Works*.

[2] Mr. Sidney Lee has surely gone too far in divorcing sentiment from Elizabethan sonnets; as in the case of dance and ballad, literary bookkeeping can be overdone, and borrowing may too easily obscure production.

[3] See Ribot, *Psychol. Emot.*, p. 267, on arrested development of emotion. He allows, by the way, p. vi., not only a physiological basis of emotion, but, pp. 7, 12, gives autonomy to the emotional states, and allows them to exist independently of intellectual conditions.

In societies custom is a consent of instincts, an unconscious law; legislation, definite and conscious, is a consent of thinking individuals. A creed has always been easy to change, for it is matter of thought; a cult, a form, a superstition, communal instincts, in a word, go not out even with prayer and fasting.

Objections against all this have little weight. One is told that the renaissance brought uniformity and not diversity of poetic form and thought. But that rationalism, so called, which then came in, and which made reason superior to emotion, worked for the individual and not, as critics say, for the social forces in art.[1] It is true that all this rational activity, this intelligent study and discussion of the classics, led to a certain uniformity in poetic work; but every advance in rationalism really accents the individuality, the artistry, the intellectual power of the poet, and leads him further from the communal and instinctive emotional level. Keen emotion brings men closer; keen thinking separates their paths, even if it leads them to one destination. Communal emotion is still the mine whence a poet gets his gold; but where the gold was once current in mere bulk, or at best in weight, it must now be stamped with the sharpest possible impression of artistic thought. Or, again, one may be more precise in one's objection. Attacking this idea that emotion, or the mass, rules in one age, and the individual, or thought, in another, as something akin to Comte's discredited evolutionary drama in three great acts, — feeling, fancy, reason, — one may insist on the piercing emotional individualism and subtle thinking of the church at a time when the communal note is assumed as dominant in mediæval life. Here again we must protest against the tyranny of terms. What does Haym mean by the individualism of the Middle Ages, and precisely what was

[1] The tyranny of terms mars some of the conclusions in Professor Francke's valuable book on *Social Forces in German Literature*, and the "individualism" to which he often refers has divers meanings.

this individualism of the church? According as one looks at the church, one may say that it was individual or that it was communal in its influence. There are really three elements in the case. The people of the Middle Ages in Europe were to a great extent organized in a communal system, for the unlettered community kept many features of the clan, not to say of the horde, and social growth itself was a matter of the guild. In such relations the individual had little to say; and it was out of these conditions that the renaissance, working first through the Italian commonwealths, began to draw the individual into his new career. Here, then, was the communal life of the Middle Ages. The second element in the case is the church as a huge guild, organized for the communal life out of which it grew, and subordinating individual thought, emotion, will, to the thought, emotion, and will of this whole body. These two elements, long in undisputed power, slowly yielded to a third. Within the church itself, and at first unable to exist outside of it, lay this intellectualized and individualized emotion which in later times found the church to be its implacable foe; whether the Hebrew psalms be congregational or personal,[1] it is certain that the monk in his cell felt them to be intensely individual, and in the hymns which he wrote, largely by inspiration of these psalms, one finds much of that spirit which fills a modern lyric. A hymn has two meanings for the Christian. One is its communal meaning, as the Scottish kirk could prove; and probably no one but a Scot, with "the graves of the martyrs" in mind, can fully appreciate this meaning of a congregational hymn. But to most people a hymn has the individual note of *Jesus, Lover of my Soul;* this is the note of early Christian hymns, and is due to a protest against communal conditions[2] made by that

[1] See next chapter.

[2] Becker, *Ursprung der romanischen Versmasse*, Strassburg, 1890, pp. 6 f., notes that a mediæval hymn by no means expressed mediæval life; it was an

spirit of Christianity which has been its chief force in modern times, that certification of value given to the humblest single life, that lifting of the chattel serf into a soul; a spirit which began and fought the long battle against tradition of race and clan and guild. De Vigny, in his exquisite *Journal of a Poet*,[1] points out the importance of the confessional in literary growth, and derives from this source the "romance of analysis," with its exaggeration of the value of a single soul. This new accent upon the individual, due to the spirit of a new faith, was strengthened in the Middle Ages by what one understood of the spirit of classic poets; and when the two forces had worked into the heart of mediæval life, mediæval life ceased to be; modern life stood in its place, modern art, letters, statecraft even, all inspired by the individual principle.[2] Now the mistake made by men who talk of the individualism of the Middle Ages is that they confuse this germ of intense personal emotion, mainly confined to the cell of the mediæval monk, with the conditions of mediæval life at large, conditions, by the way, which had little record in documents. One forgets that the records, mainly made by studious monks, would give an exaggerated importance to this personal element, this inner life, and would ignore to a great extent the life without. Müllenhoff did well to insist that the Middle Ages neither spoke the speech nor wore the garb of a monkish chronicle, — still less, it may be added, of a monkish

individual affair, as was proved at length by Wolf, *Lais*, pp. 86 ff., who calls the hymns "kunstmässige Gedichte (*carmina*)" by known and named churchmen. These often had classical models in mind. Later the hymns were suited to congregational purposes.

[1] See p. 172; and cf. the passage about the solitary way of the poet, p. 175: "Les animaux lâches vont en troupes. Le lion marche seul dans le désert. Qu'ainsi marche toujours le poëte."

[2] Gervinus thinks that the individual came to his rights in the crusades, when Christian ideals were substituted for ancient ideals. But the classical traditions of authorship, if not of wider issues, were one with the individual spirit of Christianity. The struggle was against communal conditions of life in general.

hymn. With Christianity emphasizing the value of a single soul, with the emancipation of the individual from state, guild, church, and with the secularization of letters and art, this habit of referring wide issues of life to the narrow fortunes of an individual made itself master of poetry. The emotion of a clan yielded to the emotion of a single soul. A progress of this sort is seen in *Sir Patrick Spens*, *Macbeth*, and Matthew Arnold's *Dover Beach.* Chronology in its higher form makes the ballad a mediæval and communal affair, the play a thing of art. Each deals with a Scot as centre of tragedy. In the ballad not a syllable diverts one from a group made up of the sailor, his comrades, and their kin. The men put to sea and are drowned; the ladies who will sit vainly waiting, the wives who will stand "lang, lang, wi' their gold kaims in their hair," give one in belated, unconscious, and imperfect form a survival of the old clan sorrow, a coronach in gloss. The men are dead, the women wail, and that is all. But Macbeth, as the crisis draws near, bewails along with his own case the general lot of man;[1] "der Menschheit ganzer Jammer fasst ihn an." Finally, in *Dover Beach*, modern subjectivity wails and cries out on fate from no stress of misfortune, but quite *à propos de bottes* and on general principles. Subtract now the changes due to epic, dramatic, lyric form; the progress and the curve are there. The constancy of human nature, yes; but there are two worlds in which this constant human nature finds varying expressions: one is the mediæval, where St. Francis can say "laudato sia Dio mio signore con tutte le creature, *specialmente messer lo frate sole*" . . . and so on, with his joy in nature; and one is the modern, where Wordsworth must strike that other note, *my heart leaps up*, or whatever else. Here, indeed, are two distinct worlds, even if it is the same human heart.

So, too, what one calls objective in modern poetry is not

[1] "To-morrow and to-morrow and to-morrow. . . ."

objective in the communal, mediæval sense; and what one thinks to be sentimental or even subjective in the ballads or other communal song is not subjective or sentimental in any modern way. A throng in those homogeneous conditions was unsentimental in its poetical expression for the good reason that a throng has emotions distinct from the emotions of an individual; this, too, is why sentiment and individualism have kept step in the progress of poetry. Tennyson is objective enough in his verses about the widow of a slain warrior and her rescuing tears when her child is brought to her. But this is not really objective, not communal; it is sentiment, of a high order to be sure, but sentiment. What a different point of view in the commonplace of the ballads! Was the head of the house slain and the widow left lamenting, invariably, —

> Up spake the son on the nourice's knee,
> "Gin I live to be a man, revenged I'll be ;"

that is true communal and objective emotion. Scott, who was saturated with ballads and ballad lore, was the last of English poets who could write in an impersonal and communal way. After him always, as mostly before him, the subjective and sentimental note came canting in even where severest objectivity is supposed to reign. If one wishes to feel this in Scott, — for it is a thing to feel and not to prove by syllogisms, — one has only to read the final stanza of *Bonnie Dundee;* not great verse, indeed, but full of a certain unforced simplicity, a large air, a communal vigour, an echo of unpremeditated, impersonal, roundly objective song.[1]

There is another process in the poetry of art which serves to disguise the real tendency toward individual instead of communal emotion. Communal poetry had a wide, free, out-

[1] A pretty study in communal feeling, as compared with artistic and individual sentiment, could treat the use of a supernatural element in the ballad *Clerk Saunders* and in Keats's *La Belle Dame sans Merci.*

door life; the modern poet is bounded in a nutshell, — but he has his dreams. With intense subjectivity comes the need to cover a vast range of space and time; in place of the clan or the community, its grief and joy, set forth by the communal song, one finds a solitary poet, a sort of sick king in Bokhara, dealing with the universe, and putting into his lines that quality which is best expressed in general by the often abused name of *weltschmerz*, and in particular by those countless passages in modern lyric like the poem which Shelley wrote "in dejection," or that verse of Keats which expresses so admirably the modern lyric attitude in contrast with a singing and dancing throng: —

On the shore
Of the wide world I stand alone and think.

For this lyric daring, this voyaging through strange seas of thought alone, this blending of personal reflection with the whole range of human thought and human emotion, makes poetry cosmic, but does not make it communal or even objective. The sudden interest in savages, and the glorification of primitive virtues, even the reasoning against reason and the emotion for emotion, are part of the subjective process. Jean-Jacques, Ossian, the *bésoin de rêverie*, cosmopolitan sentiment and sensibility set in vogue by Sterne,[1] — all these details of the romantic movement need no emphasis; but it is significant that this subjective search for the objective brought genuine communal poetry into view, and it is by no means to the glory of the critic that he so often puts romantic zeal and poetry of the people upon the same plane of origins. The scientific triumphs of a century and more have added external nature to the poet's province; they have put a new sympathy for natural things along with zeal for humanity and that sense of the individual and the artist which were due to the renaissance, justifying to the full

[1] See Texte, *Rousseau*, pp. 330 ff.

Bacon's definition of art as *homo additus naturae.* Poetry now means the emotional mood of a thinker alone with his world; we forget that it ever meant anything else.

The subjective and the sentimental in such excess must each beget a reaction; they roll back upon themselves, and the shock has two results, which the critic is tempted at first sight to call objective. One is the sharp dramatic study, where the poet puts himself into the place of another person. The second is that great reaction of sentiment which is called humour. As for the dramatic element, there is no question that a would-be communal reaction, "the need of a world of men," follows naturally upon excess of the subjective note. But the communal reaction cannot restore communal conditions. The *we* of throng poetry has yielded little by little to the lyrical *I-and-Thou*, and finally to the *I*, pure and simple. An obvious reaction is to put the *I* into the personality of another. This device, now so common, began in the early renaissance by the identification of the poet, not with another person, but with another class of persons. Burckhardt notes the *Canzone Zingaresca* of Lorenzo as "one of the earliest products of the purely modern impulse to put one's self, in a poetic and conscious manner, into the situation of a given class of people." The "objectivity" of later poets runs into this mould; it is a conscious process, however well done, and is quite different from the lack of all subjective interest which marks early song. One is reminded of the splendid efforts of Horace to bring back the courage and simplicity and austerity of old Roman life to the Rome of Augustus. Nietzsche may bid us build our cities on Vesuvius, and Stevenson may revive that old love for "the bright eyes of danger"; but it is not the old lover that the Scot revives, and the *silva antiqua* is of modern planting. The transfer of persons brings one no nearer to communal objectivity; it is a reaction

[1] *Cult. Ren. in Ital.*, II. 72.

against individual sentiment, which only throws into stronger relief the prevailing tone of a poetry overwhelmingly lyric, individual, and sentimental.

Again, growing out of the same change of heart from the communal to the personal and artistic, is that essentially modern quality of humour, which really springs from an intensely subjective, not to say introspective, state; it is sentiment in disguise. One of the surest tests of communal poetry is the lack of conscious sentiment and of conscious humour. When we say that a ballad is pathetic, either the pathos and sentiment are in solution with the material of the ballad, or else we read them into the ballad outright.[1] So, or nearly so, with the humour. Communal humour is cruel; as religion, now a matter of love, began with abject fear, laughter, so unkind scientific folk assert, began as exultation over the torture of a conquered foe, just as children are often amused at the suffering of man and beast, until they take the cue of pity from their elders. Fielding, in his reaction against overdone sentiment, also went back to the communal idea of humour. Parson Adams is cudgelled and abused within an inch of his life, and in *Tom Jones* bloody heads and broken bones make for merriment on all occasions. The squire of the picaresque novel, — Lazarillo de Tormes for an early case, or for a late and trivial example of tremendous adventures of this sort, Trufaldin in Pigault-Lebrun's *Folie Espagnole* — like the poor hero of Cervantes, even like Mr. Pickwick, like all the breed, may look to bear unmerciful beatings by way of contributing to the fun. In the later ballads of Robin Hood, tinkers and beggars trounce the hero again and again; and it is a concession to the yokel's point of view when the subtle humour of Falstaff in *Henry IV* yields to those indigni-

[1] Even Icelandic sagas, which show considerable artistic skill, make the diction of their heroes anything but pathetic, whatever the situation. See Heinzel, "Beschreibung d. isländ. Saga," *Sitzungsberichte Wiener Akad.*, XCVII. 119.

ties of pinchings and the buck-basket at which modern readers boggle in the *Merry Wives.* Burckhardt again lays under obligation the historian of literature in general, and the champion of this antithesis in particular, when he points out[1] the clannish and communal note of what in the Middle Ages passed for humour. It was a thing not of individuals but of classes, guilds, cities, towns, villages,[2] countries, — collective altogether. Jests at Scotchmen or at our own Jerseymen, and the exchange of civilities between rival colleges, are jaded survivals of this honest but obvious merriment. Scholars, chiefly Teutonic by birth,[3] have a way of praising this sort of thing as sound, old, wholesome fun, *derber humor;* but it is an acquired scholastic taste, and, as a rule, one does not lay down his Uncle Toby to listen to mediæval banter. If modern humour is an antidote against modern sentiment, both come from the same source, and *similia similibus* was never more true than here; sentiment is individualized emotion in excess, and humour is the recoil. Walpole had this in mind when he said that life is a tragedy to one who feels, but a comedy to one who thinks. The humour which springs from exces-

[1] Work quoted, I. 167.

[2] Northall, *English Folk-Rhymes,* prints a number of these; for example, p. 34, in Lancashire, Gorton lads sing: —

The Abbey Hey bulldogs drest i' rags,
Dar' no com' out to the Gorton lads.

One thinks, too, of the Scottish feuds, and a favourite tune like that of Liddesdale: —

O wha dare meddle wi' me?
O wha dare meddle wi' me?
My name it is little Jock Elliot,
And wha dare meddle wi' me?

See Chambers's *Book of Days,* I. 200.

[3] Vilmar, in his little *Handbüchlein,* p. 5, is full of righteous enthusiasm for an old cutthroat ballad, and full of righteous scorn for Heine's cynical lines, "Spitzbübin war sie, er war ein Dieb;" the modern reader, for his sins, prefers Heine and chances the moral turpitude involved in his choice.

sive thought, from sentiment in reaction, is at the world's end from that rough and boisterous communal fun; it is equally removed from delight in tragedy, itself a sign of youth.[1] To trace the course of modern poetic humour from Chaucer, Villon, Dunbar, down to Heine, who does in verse what Sterne did in prose, would be "a journey like the path to heaven," in whichever sense one chooses to take the comparison,—delightful or difficult; enough in this place to point out the flickering humour that plays across the subjectivity and sentiment of Heine's *Death Bed*,[2] with its parody of Homer, its scorn for the public, and all the rest.

Such are the chief differencing factors of the poetry of art as they appear in process of evolution from the Middle Ages to the present time. They belong to poetic material; a further result of the process appears in poetic style. Individual and sentimental poetry has developed a poetic dialect and widened the gap between the speech of a poet and the speech of common life. This goes deeper than conventional phrases and epic repetitions, which at first sight induce one to assert precisely the opposite view and call modern poetry a return from the conventional to the simple in expression. Emotion, however, that is spontaneous, communal, direct, and without taint of reflection, will catch the nearest way and avoid deliberate or conscious figures of speech, the trope or "turning" peculiar to our verse; and there is a steady progress in poetry from the simple or natural[3]—which does not exclude the metaphorical, if

[1] Interest even in the great tragedies has come to be duty rather than inclination. In the Abbé Dubos's day tragedy was still preferred; but he says that whereas he read Racine with keenest delight at thirty ("lorsqu'il etoit occupé des passions que ces pièces nous dépeignent"), at sixty it was Molière.

[2] *Der Scheidende.* Sentiment naturally turns to the cadence of rhythm, while humour feels at home in prose; hence it is easy to see that humour in verse, as with Heine, is ancillary to sentiment; while sentiment in prose, as with Sterne and even Lamb, is ancillary to humour.

[3] See below, Chap. VII.

only metaphor be the outcome of unconscious processes of speech — to the tropical; poetry little by little makes its own dialect.[1] Of course there are excesses and subsequent returns to simplicity, witness the metaphysical school of poets in England; but the tendency is always to the individual, which is the unusual and unexpected, and hence to the metaphorical. Precisely, too, as sentiment turned upon itself, so the metaphorical turns upon itself and makes a metaphor out of the literal; for example, Professor Woodberry in his sonnet on a portrait of Columbus: —

> Is this the face, and these the *finding eyes?*

But this simplicity and objective force of poetic language, rarely so successful as here, and rare in any case, is itself subjective and the outcome of individual assertion.

It is now in order to look at survivals of communal and primitive verse, and to learn from a study of their differencing factors no longer what the beginnings of poetry were not, but what they really were.

[1] See the author's *Old English Ballads*, p. xxx, and reference to Wordsworth's famous preface. See also Gray's letter to R. West, April, 1742, "The language of the age is never the language of poetry," and what follows.

CHAPTER V

THE DIFFERENCING ELEMENTS OF COMMUNAL POETRY

Survival of primitive and communal poetry as it can be detected in the ballads and the popular rimes of Europe, in the songs of those savage tribes which seem to come nearest to conditions of prehistoric life, and in the beginnings of national literatures so far as any trustworthy record remains, must now be studied analytically, not as poems, but rather with a view to the elements which difference poetry of the people from the poetry of individual art. That a considerable body of verse, European as well as savage, represents the community in mass rather than the solitary poet, is universally conceded; it is generally but not universally conceded that the making of such communal poetry is under modern conditions a closed account. If this view is correct, a curve of decline and extinction can be drawn corresponding to that curve of the developing artistic and individual type considered above. With this assertion of a closed account, however, must go a caution of great weight; the actual traditional ballad of Europe is not to be carried back into prehistoric conditions. A process of this sort brings ridicule upon arguments which ought to be made in rational terms; and it is to the elements of prehistoric poetry surviving in a ballad, and in kindred verse, that one must look, not to the whole poem, which is a complex of communal and artistic materials. One may say without fear of a contradiction in terms that the ballad has in it elements which go back to certain conditions of poetic production utterly unknown to the modern poem of art. These elements also occur as fragments in popular rimes; but the ballad has drawn chief attention because it is a complete and readable poem in itself.

These ballads of Europe have a large literature both of collection and of criticism;[1] and in some cases, notably the English, collection of material has the melancholy advantage of being final. Despite arguments of Mr. Joseph Jacobs and Dr. John Meier,[2] the making of ballads is a closed account; that is, a popular ballad of to-day, even if one allows the term to pass, is essentially different from a ballad such as one finds in the collection of Professor Child. Conditions of production in the street, the concert, the *café-chantant*, even in the rural gatherings[3] controlled by that "bucolic wit," are different from the conditions of production which prevailed in a homogeneous and unlettered community of mediæval Europe. A. E. Berger, in a popular essay[4] which may go with that of Dr. John Meier as representing an extravagant rationalism now in vogue about poetry of the people quite as extreme as the extravagant

[1] See the author's *Old English Ballads*, Boston, 1894, Introduction (on terminology, origins, criticism), and Appendix I. (*The Ballads of Europe*). For collections, see, of course, the material in the tenth volume of Child's great work. On the relations of this communal ballad to the other kind of ballads, see Holtzhausen, *Ballade und Romanze*, Halle, 1882, and Chevalier, *Zur Poetik der Ballade*, Programme of the Prague *Obergymnasium*, in four parts, Prague, 1891–1895.

[2] "Volkslied und Kunstlied in Deutschland," Beilage zur *Allgemeinen Zeitung*, Munich, Nos. 53, 54, March, 1898,—a paper first read in October, 1897.

[3] Only the narrative song is here considered; for popular lyric see below.

[4] "Volksdichtung und Kunstdichtung," in *Nord und Süd*, LXVIII. (1894), 76 ff. It may be noted here that the temptation to take this easy attitude toward poetry of the people, as toward a fictitious and fanciful affair, is largely due to a misunderstanding of the evolutionary side of the case. The distinction is not one of coexistent forms of poetry so much as of successive stages of evolution. It is no hard matter to take so-called popular poetry of the day and reduce it to terms of art—the lowest terms, of course; but with poetry of the people treated as a closed or closing account, and with historical evidence about it in former times, a very different problem is presented. An important hint to this effect was given by Dr. Eugen Wolff in his paper "über den Stil des Nibelungenliedes," *Verhandlungen der vierzigsten Versammlung deutscher Philologen*, etc., Leipzig, 1890, pp. 259 ff.

romanticism of Grimm, limits the difference between this poetry and the poetry of art to the difference of oral and of written record; but he quite concedes the closed account. Here, however, the two rationalists get into a deadlock. Dr. Meier will not allow the closed account, goes back to Steinthal, and against the modern view asserts that *dichten des volks*, the ownership of a poem by the folk at large, who sing it into a thousand changing forms. The process according to Meier is now what it always has been, first an individual composition, then oblivion of the individual and popularity for the song, which is felt by the people — "a necessary condition of folk-poetry" — to be their own, with manifold changes due in no case to any artistic purpose or deliberation. Now in all this Dr. Meier puts himself at odds with the defenders of oral poetry as held apart from written and printed verse, a distinction which he ignores. He agrees with them that, in the words of Berger, "there is no organic difference between poetry of the people and the poetry of art;" but the difference that does exist for Meier prettily contradicts the difference assumed by the others, Berger and the rest regarding the ballad, a thing of oral tradition, as now out of date. Not only does one test neutralize the other test, but both parties to this deadlock take a point of view fatal to any real mastery of the subject. They fail to look at the conditions under which communal poetry was produced, and they fail to study it in its essential elements. From this proper point of view, however, it is clear that traditional ballads were not made as a song of the street or the concert-hall is now made, and it is clear that ballads of that communal kind are not made under modern conditions. It has just been shown that the difference between mediæval poetry at large and poetry of the day may be best expressed in terms of the guild and the community as against the individual and subjective note. Poetry of the guild, if the phrase will pass, was composed by poets of the guild and found a record; we are wont to think that sort of thing made up all mediæval poetry; but the community itself had a vast amount of song which was composed in public and for the occasion, found no written record, and is recovered only in varying traditional forms. The conditions of modern life forbid the old communal expression, free and direct; but of course the throng is still bound to voice its feelings, and takes the poetry of art, masters it, owns it, changes it, precisely as Dr. Meier contends, but with no very edifying results. Every collection of ballads, even of folksongs, with their dignity, their note of distinction, compared with sorry stuff of the streets, bears witness to this difference between old and new. Landstad[1] in 1848 noted that ballads were fast vanishing from Norway. Bujeaud[2] complains that in France "new" and fatuous verses supplant traditional song; and he gives as example a "chanson nouvelle dédiée à une jeune fille." Ralston,[3] for Russia, comments on the new popular verse "laboriously produced in the towns and unblushingly fathered upon soldiers and gypsies." Save in a few dialects, the old runes, and with them the power to make popular song, are dying out in Finland; communal poetry there is going to pieces, and the process confirms what was said above about the relations of feeling and thought in verse.[4] Throughout Germany[5] the current ballads and folk-

[1] *Norske Folkeviser*, Christiania, 1853, pp. iii f.

[2] *Chants et Chansons Populaires des Provinces de l'Ouest*, Niort, 1895, I. 12. For the authorship, Le Braz remarks, *Soniou-Breiz-Izel, Chansons Pop. d. l. Basse-Bretagne*, Introd., p. xxv, "à mesure que les productions populaires deviennent plus médiocres, leurs auteurs se font un devoir de conscience de les contresigner."

[3] *Songs of the Russian People*, p. 40.

[4] Krohn, "La Chanson Populaire en Finlande," Proceedings Internat. Folk-Lore Congress, 1891, pp. 134 ff., a valuable paper. "La poésie s'est refugiée dans la pensée, mais elle n'a pu se maintenir intacte de trivialité." See also Comparetti, *Kalewala*, pp. 16 f.

[5] E. H. Meyer, *Volkskunde*, pp. 327, 331.

songs are seldom even traditional; hardly anywhere are they made in field and spinning-room as they were made half a century ago. At the annual dinner of the border shepherds, held at Yetholm in the Cheviots, so Sir George Douglas[1] relates, "there is no longer any thought of native inspiration; the songs sung after dinner are of the type familiar in more vulgar localities, and known as 'songs of the day.' Even the old ballads are neglected." Traditional native songs of the countryside have vanished from the fields and villages of Europe, and are replaced by opera airs, sentimental ditties, and the like; Loquin's attempt[2] to refer the old songs to similar sources is anything but a success; indeed, as one hears the new and thinks of the old, one is reminded of an ignoble analogy in the habit of many farmers here in eastern America, who sell their fresh fruit and vegetables, or neglect to raise any, and use with relish and a kind of pride the inevitable "canned goods." On many farms the kitchen-garden has vanished like the old songs.[3] Apart from these base respects, however, it is clear that the throng is powerless to revive even mediæval conditions; and the traditional ballad, as every competent editor either asserts or implies, is no longer to be made. Ferdinand Wolf, Grundtvig,[4] Talvj, and a number of others, declare that the homogeneous and unlettered community, now no longer with us, is the only source of a genuine ballad. True, communities can still be

[1] *James Hogg* (Famous Scots Series), p. 25.

[2] In *Mélusine*, IV, (1888–1889), pp. 49 ff., and continued.

[3] It is significant that the vogue of singing-clubs in German rural districts, which would seem to make for communal ballads, really drives them out. See Dunger, *Rundâs u. Reimsprüche aus dem Vogtlande*, Plauen, 1876, p. xxx.

[4] The introduction to Rosa Warrens's *Schwedische Volkslieder*, 1857, is by Wolf, and Grundtvig did a similar favour for her *Dänische Volkslieder*, 1858; opposed as regards authorship, the two are agreed on the source of a ballad in the homogeneous community. This even Comparetti recognizes: *Kalewala*, p. 21. See, too, Liliencron, *Deutsches Leben im Volkslied um 1530*, p. xi., and Baring-Gould, *English Minstrelsie*, Vol. VII. Introduction ("On English Song-Making"). But it is useless to pile up these references.

found which have something of the old conditions and of the old power. Mr. Baring-Gould notes that in divers places English folk still sing, perhaps even make, the good and genuine song. A correspondent of the *New York Evening Post*, in a pleasant letter[1] describing the Magyar dance and song, notes that these people prefer singing to talking, and makes the statement that "there is scarcely a stable-boy or a kitchen-maid who has not, at some time, been the creator of at least one song — both words and music. The favourite time for launching these ventures on the part of the young women is when they gather to spin in the evenings." Sir George Douglas, in the note already quoted, says that ballads of tradition have retreated from shepherds to "a yet shyer and less sophisticated set of men, to wit, the fishermen of the smaller fishing towns." It is said, too, that conditions quite analogous to those of the old Scottish border, and ballads of corresponding quality, some of them, indeed, very ancient ballads of tradition, may be found in the mountains of Kentucky. But this is all sporadic and dying activity. In favoured places it is still true, as Professor E. H. Meyer says of Germany, that communal singing lingers,[2] but even this is moribund; and communal making, so he admits, is dead.[3] More than this: no modern poet, however great, has yet succeeded in reviving the ballad in imitation. Scott, not to

[1] January 27, 1900.

[2] Of course, one community may still sing, while another has forgotten. Beaurepaire, *Étude sur la Poésie Populaire en Normandie*, 1856, pp. 24 f., notes this, as well as the fact that some kinds of songs linger while others die. He found no *vocero* left in Normandy, but old choral wedding songs still were heard. The dance is going — the old village dance, the *ronde*: pp. 30 f.

[3] Böckel, *Deutsche Volkslieder aus Oberhessen*, Marburg, 1885, has an introduction of great value, which shows how utterly German folksong is a closed account. Traditional ballads are still sung, but none are made; what is now made is mainly "Schmutz und Rohheit." Factories, singing-schools, are putting an end to communal song. The process of decay, he thinks, began as early as 1600. For description of modern communal songs, see p. cxxviii. Folksong, he says (p. clxxxiii), is dead throughout civilized Europe.

speak of the failures of Leyden and Sharpe, made poems in some respects as good as the old ballads, and made a beautiful bit of verse — *Proud Maisie is in the Wood* — very like a folksong; but they are not the real ballad, the real folksong, and Scott would have been first to deny the identity. As for the street songs and that sort of verse, from the wheezing sentimental ditties down,[1] one has only to compare them with genuine old ballads to see how utterly they fail to meet any test of really communal poetry. Even three centuries ago, when earth was nearer the ballad heaven than now, broadsides, "garlands," trash of the street and the hawker's basket, all balladry of trade, were sharply sundered from the good old songs. One knows what Ben Jonson thought of "ballading silk-weavers" and the rest; one also knows the saying attributed to him by Addison that he would rather have been author of *Chevy Chace* than of all his own works.[2]

A word is needed, however, before one passes from this matter of the closed account, in regard to a notion that people hold about modern communal song. It is still made, they say, by the lower classes, but it is too indecent for currency, and is conventionally unknown. Now it is

[1] See John Ashton, *Modern Street Ballads*, London, 1888. For the French, see C. Nisard, *Les Chansons Populaires chez les Anciens et chez les Français, essai historique suivi d'une étude sur la chanson des rues contemporaine*, . . . Paris, 1867, 2 vols. Vol. II. treats street songs. This is really a continuation of Nisard's *Histoire des Livres Populaires*, 2 vols., 1854, on almanacs, prophecies, divinations, magic, etc. Nisard's account of origins is ridiculous, — or perhaps it is meant to be playful. See I. 69.

[2] In addition to the material quoted in the introduction to *Old English Ballads*, see Nash, Harvey, and the other pamphleteers on nearly every page. Chettle, *Kind-Harts Dreame* (Percy Soc., 1841), particularly pp. 9 ff., has a lively account of ballad making, printing, selling, singing, in this lower stratum. What is so lewd, he asks, that it has not been printed "and in every streete abusively chanted"? For the state of things somewhat later, see a curious publication, *Whimzies, or a New Cast of Characters*, London, 1631; it describes in alphabetical order, "almanach-maker," "ballad-monger," and so on, down to "zealous brother"; for ballad-monger, see pp. 8–15.

a fact which may well get emphasis here, that the real ballad of tradition, while it never boggles at a plain name for things now rather understood than expressed, is at a vast remove from the obscene, and from those hulking indecencies which, along with the vapid and the sentimental, make up the bulk of modern unprinted and unmentioned song. Herd printed a few high-kilted ballads,[1] but even age refuses to lend them the appearance of communal and traditional; and the chasm grows wider when one deals with an audacious collection like that of Mr. Farmer,[2] where "high-kilted" is a mild name for nearly all the specimens. Here, now, are those "songs of Burns" — to which Blémont appealed for proof that the popular muse is still prolific — running to a favourite tune, but on the forbidden ground; here are obscenities, drolleries, *facetiae*, such as grooms and the baser sort still sing everywhere, and such as the Roman scratched on a wall. Here are the songs in cold print, and with the label "national"; it is no answer to ignore them. But when some one nods his head shrewdly, and stands with arms encumbered, and says one could, if one would, show this same old ballad still made by bards of the people and sung up and down the land as aforetime, only it is not fit for ears foolishly polite, and all the rest, — then, indeed, it is well to bring the matter to book. For these songs are not really traditional ballads, and never belonged to the community as a whole; the ballad of old oral tradition did belong to the community as a whole. Quite apart from ethics, with no rant after the manner of Vilmar, it is to be remembered that communal poetry, sung in a representative throng, cannot well be obscene; made by the public

[1] *Ancient and Modern Scottish Songs.*

[2] *National Ballad and Song: Merry Songs and Ballads Prior to the Year 1800;* 5 vols., privately printed for subscribers only, 1897. The fourth volume of the Percy Folio teaches a like lesson.

and in public, it cannot conceivably run against the public standard of morality. Australian songs such as Scherer studied shock the European; maypole songs of older England were an offence to the Puritan; mediæval doings on Shrove-Tuesday night were not to edification; crowds as well as individuals even now like at times to give voice to their belief in cakes and ale; but notwithstanding all these allowances, it is clear that a song made and sung by a really communal crowd will give no room to private vices and to those events and situations which get their main charm from a centrifugal tendency with regard to public morals. This hole-and-corner minstrelsy is no part of communal song; for further proof, one may note the few genuine old ballads, quite free from indecencies, which Mr. Farmer prints, and which are such a foil to the superfluity of naughtiness before and after. They are of a different world. In short, the main thing is to remember the protest made so strongly by Herder and by Richard Wagner. "Folk, — that does not mean the rabble of the street," ran Herder's formula[1] for the past; while Wagner[2] describes the united "folk" of the future for whom and from whom alone art of a high order may be expected. But Wagner's folk of the future can never be that homogeneous, unlettered folk of a mediæval community from which sprang our communal verse of tradition. "Many epochs," says Bruchmann,[3] "give one the impression as if in old times singing and the making of poetry were universal gifts. This is psychologically conceivable. The more uniform the intellectual life of individuals . . . *the more we may expect uniform utterance of that life. So the poetry of such a time would be entirely*

[1] *Werke*, ed. Suphan, XXV. 323.

[2] See above, p. 121.

[3] *Poetik* (well called *Naturlehre der Dichtung*, and an excellent piece of work), pp. 99 ff.

poetry of the people." It is clear that such conditions are far removed from the present,[1] and that the making of communal poetry in any appreciable quantity or quality must now be a closed account.

So much for the curve of evolution by which these communal elements of poetry decline as they approach our time, and increase as one retraces the path of poetry and song. But one is by no means to suppose that the ballad of tradition, as it lies before one now, can be taken as an accurate type of earliest communal song. *Sir Patrick Spens* and *Innsprück, ich muss dich lassen* are not perfect examples of the songs which primitive man used to sing, not even of the original mediæval ballad such as the women made about St. Faro in France or as those islanders made a hundred years ago about the frustrated fisherman. Improvisation in a throng cannot give the unity of purpose and the touch of art which one finds in *Spens;* that comes partly from individual and artistic strands woven in with the communal stuff, and partly from the process by which a ballad constantly sung in many places, and handed down by oral tradition alone, selects as if by its own will the stanzas and phrases which best suit its public. What one asserts, however, is that in this ballad of *Spens*, although in less degree than with other ballads, the presence of artistic elements is overcome by the preponderating influence of certain communal elements. These communal elements are to be studied in all available material, and consist, taken in the mass, of repetitions of word and phrase, chorus, refrain, singing, dancing, and traces of general improvisation; and all these elements, except for imitative purposes, are lacking in the poem of art, or if present, are

[1] When folk read and write, they cease to improvise poetry, and the folksong really ceases; that the æsthetic impulse, however, abides with them, even in low levels, but has other results, is shown by Gustav Meyer in an interesting passage of his "Neugriechische Volkslieder," *Essays*, p. 309.

overwhelmed by the artistic elements. Even in the ballads which have gone on record, and are made artistic to some degree by this very act, — killed with kindness, — there are still more traces of the throng than of the individual artist; this transfer from conditions of communal making and tradition to conditions of artistic record must always be taken into account. The collector of oral tradition, particularly ballads, finds it nigh impossible to write them down in their uncontaminated state; he gathers flowers, but what he puts into his book is only a *hortus siccus*. Anecdotes in proof of this abound; one may be quoted from the account given by Hogg[1] of a visit from Scott in 1802, soon after the publication of the *Border Minstrelsy*, where Scott printed some ballads which the Ettrick shepherd had taken down from his mother's singing. Now the mother was face to face with Scott, and sang him the ballad of *Old Maitlan'*; delighted, Scott asked her if it had ever been in print. No, she said; never one of her songs had been printed till Scott had printed them, and in doing so he had entirely spoiled them. "They were made for singing an' no for reading; but ye hae broken the charm now, an' they'll never be sung mair." And Hogg adds: "My mother has been too true a prophetess, for from that day to this, these songs, which were the amusement of every winter evening, have never been sung more." — And now to these vanishing or vanished songs themselves.

We are to examine the European ballad or traditional narrative song, and compare its elements with such shards of communal verse as are still found here and there, and with ethnological material; lyric of the people and refrains for the dance will be studied in another place. The lyric, though simple and "popular" enough, is mainly an affair of the lover and his lass, and has the centrifugal more than the

[1] Sir George Douglas, *Hogg*, pp. 38 f.

communal tendency even in that jolly little song, now six or seven hundred years old, which jumps so easily into English, the *Du bist mîn:*[1] —

> Thou art mine, I am thine,
>   Of that right certain be!
> Locked thou art within my heart,
>   And I have lost the key:
>   There must thou ever be!

Refrains for the dance,[2] of course, are communal and express communal joy; one of them, with both the interjectional and the full refrain, leaves no doubt at all; it is a song for the dance of May:[3] —

> A l'entrada del tems clar, — *eya,*
> per joja recomensar, — *eya,*
> e per jelos irritar, — *eya,*
> vol la regina mostrar
> qu'el' est si amoroza.
> *Alavi' alavia, jelos,*
> *laissaz nos, laissaz nos,*
> *ballar entre nos, entre nos.*

To these refrains of the dance we shall return in due time; the bulk of popular lyric is simple, rural, but not communal. There remain the epic survival, the ballad, and popular rimes. Epic in the larger sense is not to be considered here; for it comes down to us at the hands of art, communal as it may have been in its beginnings, and it is not a simple contemporary note of deeds which have a merely local and social interest, a stage of development common to most

[1] See the context of it in Lachmann u. Haupt, *Minnesangs Frühling*, pp. 221 ff.

[2] Jeanroy, *Origines de la Poésie Lyrique en France*, Paris, 1889, Part III., shows conclusively the origin of these songs in the public dance.

[3] "Balade" of the twelfth century: Bartsch, *Chrestomathie Provençale*, p. 107. *Alavia* = "away from us, begone," the *procul este profani* of the dancers. See also G. Paris, *Origines de la Poésie Lyrique*, etc., a review of Jeanroy, Paris, 1892, pp. 12 ff. The rimes in *-ar* running through this stanza and the rest, and certain touches of art, show the changes in record; but the refrain and the spirit of the piece are quite communal.

traditional ballads.[1] One sees, if one will glance at the actual ballad, why theories of Niebuhr and of Buckle about the foundation of history in artless chronicles of this communal type must be taken with great reserve[2] and reduced to very slender assertion. Not in early history, not even in the great epics, not even by help of the Homeric question, can one study communal elements to the best advantage, but rather in simple ballads of tradition, in the communal narrative song.[3] It is sung, danced, — hence the rhythm of it; it tells of some communal happening — "the germ of folksong is an event," says Böckel,[4] — hence the narrative.

[1] Quellien, *Chansons et Danses des Bretons*, Paris, 1889, p. 11, notes that one event is not likely to be treated both in the song and in the tale: "ce qui est tombé dans le domaine de la narrative prosaïque est par cela même exclu desormais de la chanson." Communal song must seize present things; in the tales it was "once upon a time."

[2] Buckle, *Hist. Civ. Engl.*, I. Chap. vi., calls ballads "the groundwork of all historical knowledge," and says they are "all strictly true" at the start. The use of writing, he thinks, put an end to their value.

[3] This traditional, narrative song is called ballad throughout the present book, — unfortunately an equivocal term. The terminology of the whole subject is notoriously bad, and "ballad" is no exception to the rule. See *Old English Ballads*, pp. xviii ff.; Blankenburg, *Litterarische Zusätze u. s. w.*, I. 387 ff., under "Dichtkunst"; for modern "ballad," Werner in the *Anzeiger für deutsches Alterthum*, XIV. 165 ff., 190 f., XV. 259; for German names, Erich Schmidt, *Charakteristiken*, pp. 199 ff.; on *balada*, Jeanroy, *Origines*, etc., p. 403, who shows the passage of the word from its meaning as a dance-song to the technical term for a fixed form of verse. In Corsica a *ballata* can be a lament (see below under *vocero*), and derives from the dance round a corpse: J. B. Marcaggi, *Les Chants de la Mort*, etc., Paris, 1898, p. 121, note on the *caracolu*, "a sort of pantomime danced about the corpse by the mourning women, with gestures of grief," but now fallen out of use. Of course, the only point here is to separate the ballad from songs like *Greensleeves*, from journalism (for the so-called "ballad" under Elizabeth shows that her folk were as anxious to get into print, or to keep out of it, as we are in days of the newspaper), from occasional poetry, scurrilous rimes, hymns, and all the rest. "Sonnet" was a word that then not only meant any short poem, but occasionally made a little competition with "ballad"; several of the ballads in the Rawlinson Collection, Bodleian Library, are called "sonnet" either by title or in the text.

[4] Work quoted, p. lxviii. Critics look at this narrative and treat it as the only element in the ballad; but at every turn they should remember that the original ballad was always property of a throng, was always sung, was always danced, and was never without a dominant refrain.

What, now, are the tests and characteristics about which writers on the ballad are agreed? All agree that it is a narrative song usually preserved by oral tradition of the people. With few and unimportant exceptions, it is agreed that a ballad must be the expression and outcome of a homogeneous and unlettered community;[1] the dispute is about origins. Grimm and sundry of his day declared that the community itself made the ballad; Grundtvig said the same thing, and Ten Brink, following certain modifications of Steinthal, held the people, and not an individual poet, responsible for the making as well as the singing. Ferdinand Wolf[2] was sturdy enough in his scorn for the "nebulous poet-aggregate called folk," although he clung to the homogeneous community as absolute condition; and his task was to find a representative who could make the ballad to express such a community. Since ballads deal mainly with knights and persons of rank, he concluded, as Geijer had done, that they were due to "a person of quality"; Prior, the translator,[3] went even a step farther and was inclined to think that for Scandinavian ballads, and presumably other poems of the class, one is indebted "to the ladies." Prior is negligible. But Wolf was careful in his statement; and when he noted the predominance of aristocratic persons in the deeds which these ballads sing, he knew that it was a common trait in all heroic and early epic. Germanic poems of this class, the *Béowulf*, the Hildebrand Lay, what not, regard only such characters and not the common man. As Dr. R. M. Meyer points out, this is even carried into the lifeless world, and all things are in superlative; all is splendid, unusual, extreme.[4]

[1] Even Kleinpaul, sarcastic enough against Grimm, implies this condition in his nine characteristics of popular poetry: *Von der Volkspoesie*, published anonymously, 1860, and as supplement to his *Poetik*, 1870. See p. 29.

[2] Introduction to Rosa Warrens's *Schwedische Volkslieder*, p. xix.

[3] *Ancient Danish Ballads*, 1860, I. ix.

[4] *Altgermanische Poesie*, p. 118. See also p. 52.

Even Icelandic sagas deal only with the representative man, with distinguished and notable folk.[1] So Wolf simply said that the ballad was made in this class of society, in a homogeneous class, a *volk von rittern* as he calls it,[2] who mainly "sang their own deeds," — an important concession. Even if one granted this, and allowed the court poet himself to appear in an impersonal way as deputy of the knights in singing about their deeds, it would still be far from individual and deliberate poetry of art, but rather poetry of the guild with a definite theme, traditional form, and recurrent phrases from the common poetic stock.[3] However, the homogeneous and unlettered conditions of a ballad-making community are in themselves enough to account for this preference of rank; the knight, chieftain, warrior, represented his folk, and was hardly raised above them in any intellectual way. Not only were all the members of a community consolidated, at first, against hunger, cold, and hostile tribes, the primitive homogeneity of the horde, but even later, in mediæval civilization, the same roof often covered the knight and his humblest retainer, the same food fed them, and both were marked by the same standards of action, the same habit of thought, the same sentiments, the same lack of letters,[4] of introspection, of diversified mental employment. Even in rural England

[1] Heinzel, "Beschreibung d. isländ. Saga," *Sitzungsberichte*, Vienna Acad., phil. hist. class, 1897, p. 117.

[2] Said of the Castilian and Aragonese ballads in Wolf's *Proben portug. u. catalan. Romanzen*, Vienna, 1856, p. 6. Here, too, he opposes the idea, presently to be considered, that ballads are degenerate epic or romance.

[3] A broader account of the origin of ballads is given by Comparetti, *Kalewala*, pp. 282 f. He refers them to the romantic and chivalric sentiment of the late Middle Ages — beginning, say, with the eleventh century — which passed from the "Romanic-Germanic centre of Europe" into various tongues, was delivered to oral tradition as popular verse, spread and flourished down to the sixteenth century, where it was collected as *romancero*, *romanze*, *kæmpevise*, ballad. But Comparetti neglects the communal conditions.

[4] Of course it was the revival of learning, the humanistic spirit, dividing lay society into lettered and unlettered, which really broke up the communal ballad.

such conditions lingered long; Overbury's franklin[1] "says not to his servants, Goe to field, but Let us goe;" and at the harvest home, where old songs prevail even in modern times, there is "no distinction of persons, but master and servant sit at the same table, converse freely together, and spend the remainder of the night in dancing and singing, on terms of easy familiarity."[2] How this state of things is intensified in the Highland clan, every one knows; and in going back to the horde there can be no doubt in regard to the sharp curve toward communal conditions and communal expression. Now as to those aristocratic personages of the ballad, the canticles of love and woe which come from such a community would of course put in the foreground of action persons who actually filled the foreground of its life. The ballad represented a compact communal life, and this passed into song in the person of its best representative; hence the panegyric found in all early poetry, the praise of great men who are made one with "the fathers who begat us," not to be explained away as work of Scherer's primitive minstrel, liar and entertainer passing about his hat for primitive pence. It is with modern conditions of life, and with the diversity of modern thought, that art comes down to the middle classes,— what throes were needed to bring the domestic or citizen tragedy to light!—then to the artisan, to peasants, and finally to the outcast, the criminal, the degenerate, as in sundry clever sketches of Alexander Kielland. Homogeneous conditions are first broken by cities, and linger longest in the country; they were particularly strong in primitive agricultural life;[3] and it is in communities of this sort, remote, islanded in the sea of civilization, that most of the traditional ballads

[1] *Characters*, "A Franklin."

[2] Brand-Ellis, under Harvest Home. The "mell-supper," may not derive its name from *mesler*, as suggested, but the fact is clear enough.

[3] Grosse, *Formen der Familie*, pp. 134 f.

have been found. When one thinks of this poetry at its best estate, one must have the old continent and not these sinking islands before one's thought. Nor is the lowest form of culture, degraded and sordid, even when of this homogeneous kind, to be taken as model for the past. One is loath to think of the old ballad community in terms of Zola's *Terre.*

There is, however, another way by which one could account for aristocratic personages and doings of the ballad; this wayside strolling muse may be dressed in the clothes cast off by her high-born sisters of epic and romance. This, as was said above, F. Wolf[1] denied; but J. F. Campbell[2] defines the ballad somewhat in such terms. Mr. Newell[3] thinks the folk-tale a degenerate form, in low levels of culture, of something composed on higher levels and at an earlier time; as if once D'Urberville, now Durbeyfield. Often true for the material of an individual ballad, this is not true of its real elements, of the ballad *qua* ballad, and of its form and vital characteristics. The pattern of ballads whence one will;[4] the stuff of

[1] *Proben*, etc., p. 6, as above, and also p. 31.

[2] *Popular Tales of the West Highlands*, new ed., IV. 114 ff.

[3] *Proceedings*, Internat. Folk-Lore Congress, 1891, p. 64.

[4] Even in the material itself there is a shading from highly artistic down to communal. *Thomas Rymer* undoubtedly comes from a romance. *The Boy and the Mantle* has the flippancy of its origin in the *fabliau;* Jeanroy, *Origines*, p. 155, declares such a touch of the cynical to warrant one in taking the ballad out of that class which he calls popular. *King Orfeo* is a distorted tale from the classics. Plain kin-tragedies, however, like *Babylon*, *Edward*, *The Twa Brothers*, are simple enough for one to leave them to communal origins, and not go source-hunting. Even where the motive seems international, details may be home-made; how much of *Hero and Leander* is left in that Westphalian ballad, *Et wasen twei Kunnigeskinner?* This story of the lovers and the lighted taper is found in many folksongs. See Reifferscheid, *Westfälische Volkslieder*, pp. 127 ff. In the classics and modern poetry, — witness Musæos and Marlowe, — it belongs to art. Comparative mythology laid hold of it, followed it back to India, and from India to the skies, — spring-god, sea, stars, autumn storms, and the rest. But this is needless bewilderment of a plain case; we have only to deal with the way in which Westphalian peasants sing of prince and princess. In three stanzas the story is told; all the rest deals with the situation so given, and here the communal elements (see below, p. 196) come in. The point is that study of subject-matter in ballads

the ballad is communal. If the ballad as a form of poetry were a mere ragbag of romance, one would find in it tags of old phrases, ambitious figures, tricks and turns of speech, change in metrical structure, and all manner of crumbs from the literary table; but these are conspicuous by their absence. The ballad as ballad is original. Count Nigra[1] gives an important reason for this point of view when he notes that the materials of a ballad go anywhere, pass all borders, while metre, rime, and form in general, are borrowed only from *popoli omoglotti*. The ballads employ speech at first hand, no borrowed phrases, a simple, living language; and always the feeling and the expression are coördinate. The ballad is no foul and spent stream that has turned millwheels, run through barnyards, and at last found its way to a ditch; it is wild water, and not far from its source in the mountains. One proof lies in the drinking of it. Ballads still hold their own as the nearest approach to primitive poetry preserved among civilized nations, scanty as the records are; and after infinite discussion of Homeric and other theories, the ballad remains in its old position at the gates of every national literature.[2] The farther one comes into the conditions which made for the ballad, this homogeneous community, this unlettered and undeliberative habit of mind, so much wider one finds diffused the power of improvising and singing verses in a style which is easy to bring into line with the style of traditional ballads. For the ballad in its purity was always sung, and singing is a primary process; romances were re-

is distinct from the study of ballad elements. These are constant in good ballads, whether the subject be borrowed, or be local history, as in *Bessy Bell and Mary Gray*, and the Border ballads generally. In addition to the studies of ballad migration (e.g. *Sir Aldingar*) by Grundtvig and by Child, see a close piece of investigation by Professor Bugge, "Harpens Kraft," in the *Arkiv for Nordisk Filologi*, VII. (1891), 97 ff.

[1] In his introduction to the *Canti Populari del Piemonte*, p. xviii.

[2] On the chasm between ballads of the collections and the recorded beginnings of national literatures, see *Old English Ballads*, p. lxxi.

cited. In other words, power to make poetry of this sort does not begin with the rich and foremost few, and spread slowly among the lower classes; it begins, this is beyond all doubt,[1] as a universal gift, and only with the rise of classes and the diversity of mental training, lettered against unlettered, is the power restricted to a narrow range.

Well, the ballad as species is no making of mediæval aristocrats, ladies or knights, no shards of chivalry and romance; but what of the minstrel? Bishop Percy, Scott, and of late Professor Courthope and Mr. Henderson, have looked to the minstrel to explain the ballad and all its ways. Doubtless many a minstrel made ballads, or rather sang them into modern shape; but the minstrel is merely a link between later artistic poetry and older communal song. He cannot explain this communal song, for he cannot explain the elements of it, — festal crowd, dance, singing, rapid and universal improvisation, repetition, refrain; he inherits what these leave as they vanish from living poetry; and that is all. He does not explain them, but they explain him. Professor Child distinguishes between the "minstrel ballad" and the "popular ballad";[2] but one is willing to hand over better stuff to this amiable rover and allow him a share in many good songs, without prejudice of any kind to the real communal theory. Gustav Meyer, however, one of the ablest scholars that modern Germany has produced, puts[3] the wane of balladry at the point where improvisation by men and women in the fields and round the village linden ceases, and where the minstrel brotherhood, whether blind singers, rhapsodes, or what not, begins.[4] The minstrel ballad is only a stage on that broad road which ends in the stalls; while, conversely,

[1] See below, under Improvisation.

[2] See remarks on "Crow and Pie," *Ballads*, II. 478.

[3] *Essays*, pp. 309 f.

[4] See appendix on minstrels in the author's *Old English Ballads*.

a ballad of the stalls may often hide real poetry of tradition under an ignoble garment. It is clear, then, that the "I" of a ballad ought to disturb the idea of communal origins as little as the borrowed subject does; but when one forgets the singing, dancing, improvising crowd, and thinks of poetry only in terms of modern literary composition, inference is made that ought not to be made at all. Professor Francke,[1] for example, thinks that the "I" of a German folksong, or that tag at the end which declares the song to have been made by a student, a pilgrim, a fisherman, is proof positive that ballads had individual authorship. The song is a folksong, he says, simply and solely because folk take it up and sing it; thus the often quoted *Limburg Chronicle* noted that "this year" the folk sang so-and-so, and all men know that in 1898 the American "folk" sang by preference *There'll be a Hot Time*. Böhme,[2] indeed, thinks that a leprous monk [3] mentioned in the *Limburg Chronicle*, whose tunes and songs had such a vogue five hundred years ago, brings to light the secrets of the origins of popular poetry. It is odd, however, that Böhme goes on to show how popular poetry differs from the poetry of art, and asks, with great *naïveté*, why one should ever ask for the author of a folksong, seeing that it was never really composed at all! "It was a masterless and nameless affair," he says; and proceeds to quote — Jacob Grimm. But

[1] *Social Forces in German Literature*, p. 117. Talvj draws similar conclusions: *Charakter.*, etc., pp. 339, 405.

[2] *Altdeutsches Liederbuch*, p. xxii. The personal theory is much more temperately set forth, and with a better idea of throng-conditions, by Jeanroy, *Origines*, p. 396.

[3] This leprous monk has been a godsend to the writers on ballad origins. But one might as well appeal to the *ego* in a passage from Thomas Cantipratensis, written near Cambrai, in 1263, and often quoted: Quod autem obscoena carmina finguntur a daemonibus et perditorum mentibus immittuntur, quidam daemon nequissimus qui . . . puellam nobilem . . . prosequebatur, manifeste populis audientibus dixit: "Cantum hunc celebrem de Martino ego cum collega meo composui et per diversas terras Galliae et Theutoniae promulgavi" . . . Here are individual authorship — or collaboration: "I and a colleague of mine," says the demon, — aristocratic origins, and Prior's lady in the case.

for serious answer, it is plain that folksong is an equivocal term. Most of the popular songs, by their nature, must be individual; the universal appeal, the fact that all the world loves a lover, does not make them communal. It was a lad and a lover who sang *Innsprück, ich muss dich lassen;* and it needs no signature. But from this *ich* to the "I" of the tags which one finds at the end of narrative ballads of tradition, is a far cry; indeed there is a gulf between them. When one comes to the refrain, which always expresses or implies a "we," there is absolutely no chance for "I"; but writers on ballads give the refrain a wide berth. However, leave this refrain out of the reckoning; even in actual ballads the "I" is oftenest a mere recorder's signature, and simply mediates between the reader and communal origins. With most English and Scottish ballads there is no "I" in the case; but even if one could find for each and all of these ballads signs of such a singer, editor, recorder, there would still remain behind this "I" certain facts, certain elements, which demand a totally different explanation. Let us look at another declaration of authorship. A Breton song,[1] called *The Good Old Times* and sung by workingmen, ends with these verses: —

> This song was made on the eve of Lady Day after supper.
> It was made by twelve men dancing on the knoll by the chapel.
> Three are ragpickers; seven sow the rye; two are millers.
> And so it is made, O folk, so it is made, and so it is made, this song!

Suppose, on the other side of the account,[2] one should proclaim this as a great find to offset the leprous monk; here, by explicit statement, is a ballad made by twelve labourers of one

[1] Villemarqué, *Barzaz-Breiz*, Paris, 1846, II. 285. *Le Temps Passé* begins p. 273.

[2] Or suppose one should pin the *ego* folk to a belief in the statement found in so many ballads that they are written by the person of whom they sing! This statement is a favourite in Basque songs. See F. Michel, *Le Pays Basque*, pp. 320 f.

mind,[1] here is the communal song, — and so forth! But the statement, interesting as it is, does nothing for any theory of authorship; what concerns one here is the evident dance, the folk assembled, the knoll by the chapel, the repetition, and the refrain, which is more prominent in other parts of the long ballad: in a word, the communal elements. Let us hear what these elements really are. "So," runs Villemarqué's note to this ballad, "so the mountain folk sing, *holding one another by the hand, and continually making a half-circle from left to right, then right to left*,[2] raising and dropping their hands in concert to the cadence, and leaping after the fashion of the *ritornello*." In fact, as Villemarqué had already said in his preface, "the greater part of these songs and ballads of the people are made in the same way. Conversation stirs the throng to excitement; 'let us make a dance-song!' cries some one, and it is done. . . . The texture, due to the general mood, has unity, of course, but with a certain variety of parts. Each one weaves in his flower, according to his fancy, his humour, his trade." This matter will be regarded more closely under the head of Improvisation; but the *gemeinsames dichten* is a fact, and the communal background is cleared of at least a part of the haze which hides it from modern view. In any case, these signatures[3] prove nothing either way; one must go below the surface and behind the signature, if one will come at the differencing qualities of communal poetry. Once more be it said that the present object is not to assert communal author-

[1] Or take the *Schloss in Oesterreich*: —

> Wer ist, der uns dies Liedlein sang?
> So frei ist es gesungen;
> Das haben gethan drei Jungfräulein
> Zu Wien in Oesterreiche.

[2] Compare the dance and singing of the Botocudos, above, p. 95.

[3] No one now pretends that "Expliceth, quod Rychard Sheale," at the end of the Ms. of the old Cheviot ballad, makes Sheale the author of it.

ship, in any literal sense, for the ballad of the collections, but to show in it elements which cannot be referred to individual art, and which are of great use in determining the probable form and origins of primitive poetry. True, one might go farther; there are some strong statements made by scholars of great repute which definitely deny individual authorship, in any modern sense, for the ballad. Böckel,[1] speaking of more recent ballads, rejects, of course, the theory of Grimm, but makes the ballad spring from improvisation of a stanza or so in connection with traditional stanzas of the communal stock. That one ballad has one author, and is made in the way of modern composition of poetry, Böckel, who has studied the remains of rustic balladry with great care and thoroughness, denies again and again. Count Nigra, in the work just quoted, is very emphatic on this point. "This popular narrative song," he says, "is anonymous. *It is not improvised by a popular poet more or less known.*" It requires "a period of incubation, upon which follows a long elaboration, which goes on with divers phases and changes, until the song falls, little by little, into oblivion, or else is fixed in the record." All popular verse, he declares, like language, "is a spontaneous creation, essentially racial."[2] M. Gaston Paris, too, would not lay much stress upon the "I" of a ballad; early popular poetry, he asserts,[3] is "improvised and contemporaneous with its facts"; and such songs[4] are not only "composed under the immediate impression of the event, but *by those and for those* who have taken part in it." In line with evidence to be set forth below, he[5] cares little for the professional minstrels as a source of

[1] Work quoted, p. lvii. The implied protest against Grimm, p. lxxxii, must be read along with the passage just cited.

[2] "Una creazione spontanea essenzialmente etnica."

[3] *Histoire Poétique de Charlemagne*, p. 2.

[4] *Romania*, XIII. 617.

[5] *Ibid.*, p. 603.

early popular song, and doubts their existence among the primitive Germans; for the skill to make and sing verses was as common then as the skill to fight, and warriors sang the songs which they themselves had made.[1]

But there is not only this negative evidence to dispose of the "I" in ballads. Hebrew poetry has been thought to touch the highest individual note in the "I" of the Psalms; but the best Hebrew scholars[2] now accept to a greater or less extent the notion that in many places, if not in all, this "I" is communal, and means the house or congregation of Israel. Smend[3] goes so far as to take the "I" throughout in this sense, and doubtless he goes too far; Budde[4] is on safer ground. But the consent of the best scholars is that "I" often means the community, and this, so Smend insists, not as a deliberate "personification" of Israel as a church, but in the unconscious and communal spirit of a homogeneous and intensely emotional body of people. So the Greek chorus, not simply the leader but the whole chorus,[5] speak often as "I"; and Smend quotes a stanza to the same effect from Horace's *Carmen Sæculare*. It is clear that one is on the traces of a primitive habit which seems impossible to us only because we have no homogeneous conditions to bring about

[1] *Hist. Po. Charl.*, p. 11.

[2] Driver, *Introduction to the Literature of the Old Testament*, p. 389, sums up for a modified acceptance of this theory. It seems clear that some of the Psalms are distinctly individual in every way, and as clear that many others are congregational and communal.

[3] "Ueber das Ich der Psalmen," *Zeitschrift für die alttestamentliche Wissenschaft*, VIII. (1888), 49–148. Against him *in toto* is Dr. Robertson, *The Poetry and the Religion of the Hebrews*, 1898. See pp. 20 ff., 260 ff.

[4] *Religion of Israel to the Exile*, p. 198.

[5] Robertson's objection to this is trivial (work quoted, p. 283), and shows a total lack of insight into the conditions of old communal song. "It is becoming more and more plain," says Donovan, *Lyre to Muse*, p. 162, "that individuals could have had little to do with forming the fashions and manner of Hebrew song." It sprang from the choral dance of the people, which later times called "idolatrous."

such a state of mind. Now and then a hint is gained from some survival, however faint, of these conditions. It is said that a Scot of the Border coming home to find his house plundered, could tell by sundry signs what hostile band had done the deed, and would invariably call them by the place where they lived: "Ettrickdale has been here!" One thinks of the tribes of Israel and of the way in which their names were used. Reuben, runs the text, "Reuben had great searchings of heart." But here is theological ground, and we hasten back to the "I" of folksong. To this subject Professor Steenstrup devotes the third chapter of his book on Scandinavian ballads,[1] which are mainly heroic and strongly objective, in contrast to the more subjective and deliberate ballads of Germany. Now many of the Scandinavian ballads begin with the familiar phrase, "I will sing you — or tell you — a song," and proceed in the second stanza with actual narrative; a comparison of manuscripts, however, shows that it is mainly late copies which begin with this "I" stanza, while earlier copies omit it. In English ballads the "I" is quite as separable and negligible; sometimes, in songs and catches, it is used for mystification:[2] —

> He that made this songe full good,
> Came of the northe and of the sothern blode,
> And somewhat kyne to Robyn Hood, —
> Yit all we be nat soo.

And the refrain follows. In the *Gest of Robin Hood*, and in the other ballads of this cycle, "I," that is to say, the singer, now bids hearers "lithe and listen," or throws in an aside or a gloss, — "I pray to God woo be he," about the "great-headed monk"; with which compare the delightful ejaculation in *Young Beichan*, "And I hope this day she sall be his bride,"

[1] *Vore Folkeviser fra Middelalderen*, Copenhagen, 1891, an admirable book. See particularly, p. 39; also Talvj, *Charakteristik*, p. 340.

[2] Wright and Halliwell, *Reliquiae Antiquae*, I. 248 f.

— now notes the end of a canto, as in the *Cheviot*, "the first fit here I fynde";[1] and makes other detached and alien remarks of the sort. In Russian ballads, as Bistrom[2] points out, the singer addresses his hearers only at the beginning and at the end, often not at all. Evidently, here is a mere singer and recorder, a link between the old singing and dancing throng and the new listening throng; in no case is he a maker, so far as traditional ballads go, and in Scandinavian ballads Steenstrup has proved him to be an impertinence.[3] This is said with due allowance for the functions of a leader in communal dance and song, where the "I" little by little got his foothold and his importance; he steps forward with uplifted beaker and begins a new movement, singing a subjective verse or two, then effaces himself from the narrative ballad which now goes with the dance.[4] "I bid you all dance," he cries, "and we will sing of so-and-so." This introductory stanza, of course, has got into the ballad; and the lyric opening of many a ballad, often touching on the time of year, the place, what not, and often, too, of great beauty, is in most cases to be referred to such an origin. When the ballad is recited, the leader turns recorder, editor, improver, commentator, improvising bard. That damnable iteration in long-winded epics and romances and in later ballads, "this is true that I tell you," belongs to the reciting stage;[5] it is an alien

[1] Sc. *fine*, — finish, end?

[2] *Zeitschrift f. Völkerpsych.*, V. 201. He notes a curious close found in many ballads: —

Danube! Danube!
Thou shalt sing no more.

[3] The opening or close of Germanic epic is often of this "I" character. So the Hildebrand Lay, the *Béowulf*, the *Nibelungenlied* at its end. Later epic shows a poet in the case, who has his own wares to announce. See R. M. Meyer, *Altgermanische Poesie*, pp. 357 ff., and his references.

[4] Steenstrup, work quoted, pp. 43, 28 f.

[5] Often the reciter remarks that it is night; that he is tired, thirsty; let the hearers come again on the morrow and each one bring a coin with him,—and so on. See A. Tobler, *Zeitschr. f. Völkerspsych.*, IV. 175, quoting from *Huon de Bordeaux*.

in balladry. More than this, it is to be pointed out that historical ballads, meant to be recited and not sung, are no ballads at all in the communal sense.[1] They are on the way to epic, and no better study of this process can be made than in the *Gest of Robin Hood.*

So much for the absence of any direct trace of personal authorship in the ballad. It is strange to see critics going everywhere to fetch a reason for this fact, except to the most obvious place to find a reason, — in the singing and dancing throng, where at least the elements of a ballad were made. The subjective, the reflective, the sentimental, are characteristics impossible in throng-made verse. Even now when throngs are to be pleased, say in the modern drama, there is a strange mixture of communal bustle and "situation" with those sentimental ditties meant to touch the private heart. Such a play is a monstrosity, to be sure, sheer anarchy of art; but in its formless, purposeless racket it hits communal taste and excites the Dionysian sense, until the crowd is shouting, leaping, and singing by deputy. Going back, now, to the active throng, and to the ballad which in many ways represents that throng, let us see what communal elements are to be noted in its diction, its form, and its surroundings. The diction of a traditional ballad is spontaneous, simple, objective as speech itself, and close to actual life. The course

[1] It was noted that the Botocudos had no legends, no song of the past. A narrative song in the legendary sense is unknown to primitive folk; what they sing is the event of the day, an improvised song of sentences almost contemporary with the facts, cadenced by the communal dance. The sense of time past is so slender even among North American Indians (Powell, First Annual Report of Bureau of Ethnology to Smithsonian Inst., 1881, pp. 29 ff.), that while they admit that grass grows, they "stoutly deny that the forest pines and the great sequoias were not created as they are." Now this primitive trait of poetry is preserved in communal ballads; and from this strictly communal class, long historical ballads, like those in German collections, should be excluded. Kögel, *Geschichte der deutschen Litteratur*, I. 111, notes that "the epic song . . . is one of the later kinds of poetry. . . . It cannot even be regarded as belonging to the common Germanic stock." But the communal narrative song is another matter.

of artistic poetry, as was shown in the preceding chapter, is away from simplicity of diction and toward a dialect. According to the temper of the time, this dialect of poetry will be broadly conventional, as with Waller, Dryden, and Pope, narrowly conventional, as in the puzzle style of the Scandinavian scaldic verse and in certain mannerisms of Tennyson, or individual, as with Tennyson in his main style and with Browning; but in any case it will be a good remove from the speech of daily life. True, certain features of both primitive and ballad poetry seem to make against this assertion. Dr. Brinton[1] says that all the American languages which he examined had a poetic dialect apart from that of ordinary life; but these records are clearly not of the communal type, not spontaneous, but rather fossil forms and ceremonial rites. Peasants in France, so Bujeaud notes, compose few ballads in their *patois;* Hebel pointed out the same fact for German song;[2] and there is other evidence. But this is no objection whatever to the theory of ballad simplicity; for as these writers concede, peasants do make their improvised songs, their couplets, *schnaderhüpfl*, *rundâs*, songs of labour, songs of feasts, in their own dialect and in nothing else. The traditional songs are often retained, as refrains or the like, in incomprehensible or difficult phrase; but that is another matter, and so far as one deals with communal elements, so far one finds simple and everyday speech, entirely different from the conventional or individual dialect of the poetry of art. Lack of simplicity is held to be a proof of false pretences, of forgery. More than this. The ballads lack figurative language and tropes; they rarely change either the usual order of words or the usual meaning. They lack not only antithesis, but even the common figure of inversion,[3] the figure which

[1] "On American Aboriginal Poetry," *Proc. Numismat. and Antiquar. Soc. Philadelphia*, 1887, p. 19.

[2] See Böckel, work quoted, cxix.

[3] Steenstrup has some good remarks on this point, work quoted, pp. 188 ff., 203 ff.

one would most expect to meet in ballad style. In the ballad itself, inversion is vanishingly rare, and in the refrain, significant fact, it is as good as unknown. Again, any wide word, any mouth-filling phrase, even such a term as "fatherland," which opens a glimpse into the reaches of reflection and inference, is alien to the ballad of the throng. Now it is significant that this lack of tropes, characteristic of ballads no less than their stanzaic form, sunders them from our old recorded poetry; earliest English poetry is a succession of metaphoric terms.[1] All Germanic verse, in fact, laid main stress upon the trope known as "kenning"; the ocean is the "whale's bath," the "foaming fields," the "sea-street"; a wife is "the weaver of peace"; so, in endless variation, the poet called object and action by as many startling names as he could find in tradition or invent for himself.[2] Like the recurring phrase of the ballad, these are often conventional terms; but they differ in quality from it by a world's breadth. For the mark of this trope, in its deliberate or conscious stage,[3] is a palpable effort of invention, a refusal to catch the nearest way; the ballad is rarely figurative. What figures one does find in it, and they are few enough, are unforced and almost unconscious. As Steenstrup says, the Scandinavian ballad "talks like a mother to her child," and has "scarcely a kenning." Faroe and Icelandic ballads, to be sure, have a few kennings,

[1] Of far earlier date than ballads, this poetry is in a later stage of evolution. *Widsið*, the oldest recorded English poem, shows more art and more poetic dialect than many a bit of Scottish verse picked up a century ago.

[2] See R. Heinzel, *Ueber den Stil der altgermanischen Poesie*, Strassburg, 1875; W. Bode, *Die Kenningar in der angelsächsischen Dichtung*, Darmstadt u. Leipzig, 1886; R. M. Meyer, *Altgermanische Poesie*. See too Uhland, *Klein. Schrift.*, I. 390.

[3] A kenning, with many branches in Anglo-Saxon poetry, calls survivors of battle "the leavings of weapons." This may once have been literal; but in its context it looks as deliberate as Lamb's phrase for a resuscitated victim of the gallows, — "refuse of the rope, *the leavings of the cord*" (*Inconveniences Resulting from Being Hanged*).

but they are not frequent. J. F. Campbell[1] speaks of the simple Gaelic ballads as poor in figures, while the epic made from these lays riots in trope. The ballad hardly essays even personal description.[2] A modern Greek song ventures no farther than the conventional comparison of the maiden with a partridge; and no English ballad undertakes to give a picture of the heroine, — only a traditional epithet or so. The heroes are fair or ruddy, have yellow hair; and that is all. There is no realism, as one now calls it. Minute description of nature increases in direct ratio to the increasing individuality of the poet; and one distrusts those German folksongs which bring the sunset, or a fading leaf, or more subtle processes of nature, into line with the singer's feeling, — a trait of German *minnesang*. One will search ballads in vain for a superb touch like that word for the disturbing sunrise which Wolfram puts into the watcher's call to the lovers, "his claws have struck through the clouds," — as if a bird of prey to rob them of their love;[3] for in the ballads nature is a background and rarely gets treatment in detail. Save in chronicle song like the *Cheviot*, it is spring, summer, evening, it is the greenwood, no more definite time or place; and so too it is bird or beast, not a special kind, until conventional rose and lily and deer and nightingale come to their monopoly. It is

[1] *Pop. Tales*, IV. 152.

[2] The general testimony for all ballads. For example, Fauriel, *Chants Populaires de la Grèce Moderne*, I. cxxix; these, he says, are full of commonplaces and recurrent phrases; the diction is "simple, nervous, and direct, that is, it has few figures, almost no inversions, and progresses in short periodic and nearly equal passages." Remains of oldest Greek folk song show the same traits: Usener, *Altgriech. Versbau*, p. 45.

[3] *Wolfram von Eschenbach*, ed. Lachmann, p. 4.

Sîne klâwen
durh die wolken sint geslagen,
er stîget ûf mit grôzer kraft,
ih sih in grâwen . . .
den tac . . .

not communal verse, but poetry of art, which, without mythological intent, transfers a distinctly human motive to nature, as where Romeo sees those "envious streaks" in the east, or where, in the *Béowulf*, old Hrothgar describes the abode of Grendel, with that picture of the hounded stag, and with the "weeping" sky. In the ballads, reference to nature is conventional, though by no means insincere. Though the natural setting is often an irrelevancy, as in *Lady Isabel:* —

> There came a bird out o' a bush
> On water for to dine,
> And sighing sair, says the king's daughter,
> "O wae's this heart of mine," —

still, there are touches of nature, sincere and exquisite and appropriate, to be found in sundry ballads, notably at the opening of *Robin Hood and the Monk.*[1] However, ballads are mainly for the action, not the setting of the stage, and a throng of festal dancers would not care for a bill of particulars. It is the poet, fugitive from throngs, who turns to nature and studies her charms with a lover's scrutiny.

On the other hand, what ballads lack in figurative and descriptive power, they supply in an excess of iteration, of repetition, of fixed and recurring phrases. The recurring phrase, along with the standing epithet, one finds, to be sure, in the great epic as well as in the ballad of tradition; repetition in the simpler sense, however, is peculiar to the ballads. Epithets in the ballad are of a modest type; the steed is "milk-white" or "berry-brown," the lady is "free," — that is, "noble," — while now and then an adjective cleaves to its substantive in defiance of fact, as when the "true-love"

[1] This may well go back to the summer songs, May-day songs, chorals, and so on, of festal crowds; so Bielschowsky, *Geschichte der deutschen Dorfpoesie*, Berlin, 1891, p. 13, concludes for the songs of Neidhart. So, too, with songs on the conflict of summer and winter. Latin poets of the Middle Ages led the way in regular description of nature. See Wilmanns, *Walther*, p. 409. For the general case, Burckhardt, *Cultur d. Renaissance*, II. 15; Uhland, *Klein. Schrift.*, III. 388, 469.

is palpably false, or when the newborn infant is called an "auld son." As for the phrases, when a little foot-page starts off with his message, when two swordsmen fall to blows, when there are three horses, black, brown, and white, to be tested, any reader of ballads can shut his eyes and repeat the two or three conventional lines or even stanzas that follow. Of course, as poetry grows artistic, recurring phrases vanish; the artist shuns what is traditional and evident, seeking to announce by independence and freshness of phrase the individuality of his own art. Tobler notes that while the more communal epic of old France used the same terms and the same general apparatus for a fight here and a fight there, Ariosto contrives, however one fight is like another, to give an individual character to each.

To say that these recurring phrases are due to the need of the improvising singer for a halting-place, a rest, in order to think of new material, is distortion of facts. Undoubtedly the minstrel used these traditional passages for the purpose, but they are due to the communal and public character of the poetry itself, and belong, so far as the question of origins is concerned, to that main fact in all primitive song, the fact of iteration. This is now to be studied not so much in the actual recurrence of identical passages, as in that characteristic of ballad style which may be called incremental repetition. One form of this is where a question is repeated along with the answer, a process radically different from that of Germanic epic, where the zeal for variation has blotted out this primitive note of repetition, and, against all epic propriety, forced a messenger to give his message in terms quite different from the original. Again, each slight change in the situation of a ballad often has a stanza which repeats the preceding stanza exactly, save for a word or two to express the change. Lyngbye[1] found the Faroe ballads

[1] *Færøiske Qvaeder*, p. 74.

so laden with this kind of repetition that in the record he omitted many of the stanzas, giving them all only here and there, to show the general style. Side by side with incremental repetition, which is usually found in sets of three stanzas, runs a refrain, either repeated at the end of each stanza or sung throughout as a burden. Moreover, with all this iteration goes a tendency to omit particulars and events which modern poetry would give in full, so that a very ill-natured critic might define ballads as a combination of the superfluous and the inadequate. But these traits can best be seen in an actual ballad, *Babylon, or the Bonnie Banks of Fordie*, familiar not only to Britain, but "to all branches of the Scandinavian race." [1] It is an admirable specimen of communal elements and traditional form blended with incipient art: —

There were three ladies lived in a bower,
Eh vow bonnie,[2]
And they went out to pull a flower
On the bonnie banks o' Fordie.[2]

They hadna pu'ed a flower but ane,
When up started to them a banisht man.

He's taen the first sister by the hand,
And he's turned her round and made her stand.

"It's whether will ye be a rank robber's wife,
Or will ye die by my wee pen-knife?"

"It's I'll not be a rank robber's wife,
But I'll rather die by your wee pen-knife."

He's killed this may,[3] and he's laid her by,
For to bear the red rose company.

He's taken the second ane by the hand,
And he's turned her round, and made her stand.

[1] Child, *Ballads*, I. 170.
[2] Refrain or burden, not printed with the other stanzas, but sung throughout.
[3] Maid.

"It's whether will ye be a rank robber's wife,
Or will ye die by my wee pen-knife?"

"I'll not be a rank robber's wife,
But I'll rather die by your wee pen-knife."

He's killed this may, and he's laid her by,
For to bear the red rose company.

He's taken the youngest ane by the hand,
And he's turned her round, and made her stand.

Says, "Will ye be a rank robber's wife,
Or will ye die by my wee pen-knife?"

"I'll not be a rank robber's wife,
Nor will I die by your wee pen-knife.

"For I hae a brother in this wood,
And gin ye kill me, it's he'll kill thee."

"What's thy brother's name? Come tell to me." —
"My brother's name is Baby Lon."

"O sister, sister, what have I done!
O have I done this ill to thee!

"O since I've done this evil deed,
Good sall never be seen o[1] me."

He's taken out his wee pen-knife,
And he's twyned[2] himsel o his ain sweet life.[3]

[1] Of = by.

[2] Deprived, parted.

[3] The incremental repetition of this ballad could be matched by many other cases. Typical is the combination of simple and incremental repetition, also in triads, at the end of a French ballad, "Sur le Bord de l'Ile," Crane, *Chansons Populaires*, p. 28. Typical, too, is the interesting Westphalian ballad, already noted, of the Hero and Leander story: Reifferscheid, *Westf. Volksl.*, pp. 2 f.; see *ibid.*, Nos. 2, 5. "Mother, my *eyes* hurt me, — may I *walk* by the sea?" — "Not alone; take thy youngest brother." Reasons follow against and for this. Then repetition: my *eyes* hurt me, may I not *walk*, etc. "Take thy youngest sister," — and incremental repetition of the reasons. Then: —

"O mother," said she, "mother,
My *heart* is sore in me;
Let others go to the churches, —
I will *pray* by the murmuring sea."

The simple "plot" of this ballad might be wrought into a long romance after the mediæval fashion, might be made a modern drama, a modern short story, — Maupassant tells something of the sort in a pathetic but repulsive sketch; the manner of *Babylon*, however, is all its own, carrying one miles from romance and drama and tale back into the communal past. Two stanzas open with the ballad commonplaces, — ladies in bower, the conventional summons of an outlaw by breaking a branch, pulling a flower, or otherwise disturbing the peace, and his appearance on the scene. Then comes swift action; then the lingering, fascinating incremental repetition; then the crash, and the leap into tragedy. True, the sudden turns and the lack of connecting and explaining passages are less marked than in other ballads, say at the end of *Child Maurice*, where the almost bewildering swiftness, the daring omission, roused Gray to enthusiasm beyond his wont;[1] but the trait is evident enough and strong enough, even here, to show that one is far from the garrulity of the romances,[2] far from the forward-and-back

Usually each increment has a stanza, but now and then compression takes place, as in Motherwell's version of *Sir Hugh*: —

> She wiled him into ae chamber,
> She wiled him into twa,
> She wiled him into the third chamber,
> And that was warst o't a' . . .
>
> And first came out the thick, thick blood,
> And syne came out the thin,
> And syne came out the bonnie heart's blood . . .

So with three horses, and what not. This triad is not necessarily sprung from the "Dreitheiligkeit in der Lyrik," of which Veit Valentin discourses in the *Zeitschr. f. vgl. Lit.* (New Series) II. 9 ff. "Dreitheiligkeit in der Lyrik," comes rather from communal iteration in primitive song and dance.

[1] See his letter to Mason, *Works*, ed. Gosse, II. 36.

[2] Professor Earle confuses, in a very uncritical way, the garrulity of romances with the garrulity of epics and of ballads: see his *Deeds of Bēowulf*, p. xlix. A "voluble and rambling loquacity," he says, is the "natural character of the lay, and still more of the epic, which is a compilation of lays." And presently he

of a Germanic epic. It is not to be explained by any abbreviation in the record. Zell long ago pointed out[1] that this habit of leapings and omissions is characteristic of what may be regarded as the remains of Hellenic popular verse. Like the ballad repetition, which is incremental, the ballad omission is progressive, and has nothing of that strain and doubling which makes Germanic epic, in Ten Brink's phrase, spend such a deal of movement without getting from the spot. Yet it is chiefly in the incremental repetition that the ballad shows its primitive habit as compared with the merely retrospective repetition of the romances. The ballad stands close to that spontaneous emotion which rises in a throng and relieves itself in a common, obvious, often repeated phrase; it stands close to the event, and hence the abruptness, the process, due to sight at close quarters, of immediate expression. The æsthetic value of repetition is high when interest is held and concentrated upon a single strong situation, as in *Babylon;* its value is low when the action is a trivial sequence of details, as in a Russian ballad quoted by Bistrom:[2] "He set up his linen tent; when he had set it up, he struck fire; when he had struck fire, he kindled [the camp-fire]; when he had kindled, he cooked the porridge; when he had cooked the porridge, he ate it: when he had eaten it, he lay down," — and so on, in the strain dear to children.[3] Another variety of incremental repetition, which brings one closer to the conditions under which ballads were made, is found in the account of Porthan[4]

says that the romances are "the nearest extant representative of that unwritten literature which from the very nature of things was undisciplined and loquacious." Confusion could hardly go beyond this.

[1] *Ferienschriften*, I. 87.

[2] "Das russische Volksepos," *Zeitschr. f. Völkerpsych.*, V. 187.

[3] See above, p. 69.

[4] See Porthan, *Opera Selecta*, III. 305–381. I quote from the original dissertations *de Poesi Fennica* 1778, pp. 57 ff. He begins by lamenting the decay of old national song near the coast and under clerical influence; intimates that

about the singing of Finnish songs by a leader who improvises, and a second singer, a sort of echo, a dwindled chorus, who joins him and helps to carry the ballad along its way. The leader[1] sings a line; but before he comes to the end of it, his partner catches the idea and joins him in the final measure,[2] — a word or two; then, while the other is silent, this helper repeats the whole line, often with a slight change of words, mainly an adverb or the like thrown in,— "surely," "in truth,"—and with an even slighter change of tone; then the leader sings another verse, the helper falls in, repeats, and so to the end of the song. The two sit face to face with clasped hands, and round them are the people *arrectis auribus*. It is fair to conjecture that the folk were not always silent hearers, and that the helper is deputy of a choral throng which has come to silence in the enjoyment of a superior art;[3] Porthan admits that all sorts and conditions of Finns were once able to make these ballads, and he goes on to tell of the universal custom of the women to improvise little

song was a universal gift and was improvised, although sundry bards are now eminent. Memorable events slip into song, now convivial, now satiric; and there is great store of proverbs. The description of dual singing begins with § XI.

[1] "Præcentor, *Laulaja* . . . adjungit sibi alium socium sive adjutorem, *Puoltaja* sive *Saistaja* dictum."

[2] "Quod facile jam ex sensu ipso, atque metri lege, reliquum pedem conjectando definire licet."

[3] "Rarissimi stantes canunt; et si contingit aliquando, ut musarum quodam afflatu moti stantes carmen ordiantur, mox tamen, conjunctis dextris sessum eunt, et ritu solito cantandi continuant operam." They observe the rules of the game. Porthan, to be sure, notes the absence of dancing as a national and pervasive affair; but the statement must not go unchallenged. Long before this, Olaus Magnus (*Hist. de gentibus Septentrion.*, Romæ, 1555, Cap. VIII. lib. IV. 141) said of the Lappland and other northern folk that they were often moved to dance, — "excitentur ad saltûm, quem vehementius citharoedo sonante ducentes, veterumque heroum ac gigantum præclara gesta patrio rhytmate et carmine canentes, in gemitus et alta suspiria, hinc luctus et ululatum resoluti, dimisso ordine in terram ruunt," a parlous state. Scheffer, to be sure, discredits this statement of the archbishop (*Lapponia*, 1673, p. 292); but Donner, *Lieder der Lappen*, p. 38, believes it, and says it is confirmed by the report of a recent Russian traveller.

songs as they grind at the hand-mills. The trick of singing in pairs is not uncommon, and is seen elsewhere upon a historical background of choral song; Castrén says that the Samoyedes improvise their magic songs in the same fashion, a conjurer of the first class beginning the verse, and joined in the final words by the humbler shaman, who then repeats the whole alone. The song consists of but a few words.[1] Similar methods, on a higher plane, are found in Denmark and Iceland. Ethnological evidence, too, is at hand; in Africa, Captain Clapperton heard two singers sing an artless ballad, one doing the verses, the other the refrain.[2] Often two dancers lead a dance.[3] It is only a step, moreover, from the twain with clasped hands, to the two singers of a flyting, Eskimo song duels, strife between Summer and Winter, amœbean verse of all kinds; see, for example, the Carlin and little boy in the Swedish ballad, or Harpkin and Fin in the English,[4] where one verse suggests the reply in the next. From these to the *schnaderhüpfl*, when one after another steps out and sings, and so back to the chorus, as in Lyngbye's case of the Faroe fisher, is but another easy inference; in short, it is clear, by overwhelming proof, that the individual performers are a survival of the singing, dancing throng with its infinite repetitions and its unending refrain.

Still another form of incremental repetition will occur to the reader as based on old custom but bare of all save the rawest æsthetic ministrations, and nowadays used only for jocose ends. The same line or stanza is sung indefinitely, with the use of a new name, number, fact, in each repetition; or else the repetition is cumulative, a test of memory, some-

[1] Castrén, quoted by Comparetti, *Kalewala*, p. 66, note.

[2] Talvj, *Charakteristik*, p. 87; Steenstrup, pp. 85 f.

[3] *Ibid.*, pp. 23 f.

[4] Child, *Ballads*, I. 21.

what as in "The House that Jack Built."[1] There is a German student song, still popular, where the names of those present are rimed, one after the other, into a fixed formula; while degenerate and silly verses of one's youth, nursery songs,[2] counting-out rimes and the like, will occur to one by the dozen, and seem less negligible, get, indeed, an æsthetic lift, when one finds in them distinct hints of some old incantation, some choral song to bless house and field, as well as echoes from the dance and the labour of primitive man. Counting-out rimes in Germany are often epic,[3] with a spice of adventure, thus working into ballad territory; and these, as with children's games at large, hold to the dance. F. Wolf sunders the dramatic dances of the Catalan peasantry, with lives of saints, battle of Christian and Moor, robber tales, and

[1] See "Hans Michel," and the notes to it in Reifferscheid, *Westfälische Volkslieder*, pp. 47, 175. The song "Drüben auf grüner Haid," pp. 51, 176, is used in the spinning-room, old home of communal minstrelsy, to stir the women to their work. Further, see Coussemaker, *Chants Pop. des Flamands de France*, p. 129, for a pious chanson: One is one, One is God alone, One is God alone, And that we believe. Two is two, Two Testaments, One God Alone . . ., etc. Three is three, Three Patriarchs, Two Testaments . . . and so on, up to the Twelve Apostles. *Ibid.*, pp. 333, 336 ff., 353, are comic songs of the kind; and these are highly important, for they are songs of the dance, and still in vogue for communal processions. Their main features are repetition — and the refrain.

[2] See Halliwell, *Nursery Rhymes*, p. 197: —

John Ball shot them all.
John Scott made the shot, —
But John Ball shot them all.
John Wyming made the priming,
And John Brammer made the rammer,
And John Scott . . ., etc.

This is cumulative. But an old song of the fifteenth century is incremental, a jolly bit of verse withal: Wright-Halliwell, *Reliquiae Antiquae*, I. 4 f. —

The fals fox camme into owre croft,
And so owre geese ful fast he sought;
Refrain: With how, fox, how, with hey, fox, hey,
Comme no more into oure house to bere owre gese awaye.

The fals fox camme into *oure stye* . . ., etc.

[3] E. H. Meyer, *Deutsche Volkskunde*, p. 124.

so on, as their theme, the work of professional singers, from those simple dances of the country folk and of the children, some of which are of the type now under discussion. He gives[1] a pretty little incremental specimen of this latter sort. But labour is also in the game. In Gottschee[2] there is a ballad of a servant maid who served one year and earned a chicken; chicken hatched chickens: served second year and earned a duck; duck stands on big, wide feet, chicken hatches chickens: served a third year and earned a turkey; turkey said *Long Ears*, duck stands, and so on: and then lamb, kid, pig, calf, pony, little man (the husband) who says *Love Me*, and finally "a youngster" who says *Weigh Me*, — and then back through it all to the chicken. This is sung of course by the girl; but from the cumulative song, with more or less refrain, it is an easy step to the choral song of labour, which is naturally incremental. Such is the song[3] of women weeding the millet, which combines the old refrain of labour in the field with the incremental repetition of a hardly coherent ballad. Prettier is that song[4] which the playmates of a bride sing during the weaving of her bridal wreath.

To-day a maiden has been joyous, —
Joyous she now nevermore;
Joyous surely she shall yet be, —
But as maiden nevermore.

[1] *Proben*, p. 34: "La Mina de Puigcerdá."

[2] K. L. Schröer, "Ein Ausflug nach Gottschee," in *Sitzungsber.*, Vienna Acad., phil.-hist., LX. (1868), 165–288. See pp. 231 ff. One is distantly reminded of the cumulative song (Chambers, *Popular Rhymes of Scotland*, p. 35) of "Katie Beardie," — for the dance: —

Katie Beardie had a coo,
Black and white about the mou';
Wasna that a dentie coo?
Dance, Katie Beardie!

Katie Beardie had a hen, —

and cock, "grice," so on, — probably as many animals as were won by her distant cousin in Gottschee. See also the "Croodin Doo," p. 51; "My Cock, Lily Cock," p. 31; "The Yule Days," p. 42; and others.

[3] Schröer, p. 274.

[4] *Ibid.*, p. 277.

To-day a maid has handed garlands,[1] —
Hand them shall she nevermore;
Hand them shall she surely yet, —
But as maiden nevermore.

The third stanza simply puts "binding" for "handing." Here is the incremental repetition along with the fixed refrain, — not a very difficult communal feat, by the way, and, as in all these cases, getting its rhythm from the work or the dance, its meaning from the event or deed in hand. So, too, when the bride goes away, she is again besung, and the events are occasion of the quite contemporary words; thus, as she is lifted upon the husband's horse, —

She is seated, she has sobbed!
She has ridden away, she laughed![2]

The better known collections are full of these simple cumulative songs, which it would be superfluous to record. In Algeria women sing an endless song of the sort with fixed refrain and incremental stanza. A combination of the counting-out rime and the song of labour is found in many places, for example, a Gascon ballad[3] sung by women as they wash clothes and beat the linen in cadence; the feature of dropping a number with each new stanza reminds one of those *Ten Little Indians* of one's youth: —

[1] To the young men invited thus to the wedding.

[2] The Armenian bride does the singing herself, combining incremental repetition with a refrain in which the crowd may join (Alishan, *Armenian Popular Songs*, Venice, 1852: the third edition, 1888, omits the name of the translator):

Little threshold, be thou not shaken;
It is for me to be shaken,
To bring lilies.

Little plank, be thou not stirred;
It is for me to be stirred,
To bring lilies.

[3] Bladé, *Poésies Populaires de la Gascogne*, II. 220 ff. In the *Chants Heroiques des Basques*, p. 48, Bladé tells how the Basques use these songs of number.

Nine are washing the lye,
  Nine.
Nine are washing it,
Nine are rubbing it,
Pretty Marion in the shade,
  Pretty Marion, —
Let us to the fountain go.

Then "eight are washing," then seven, and so on, one woman dropping out at each break. Again, soldiers on the march sing the interminable song of increments with a refrain:[1] —

Ma poule a fait un poulet,
Filons la route, gai, gai,
Filons la route gaiment.

Ma poule a fait deux poulets . . .

Bücher[2] traces all these marching songs back to a primitive form such as one still hears in Africa, where "for hours at a time" the natives on the march keep singing a half-dozen words or phrases in monotonous repetition, and with no increments. The development hence through incremental stanzas up to the Tyrtæan lyric of battle, verses of the *Chanson de Roland*, and so on, is evident enough. Repetition of the incremental and cumulative sorts, moreover, is easily connected with religious rites. "It seems a fair inference," says Mr. E. B. Tylor,[3] "to think folklore nearest its source where it has its

[1] *Ibid.*, same page. Herd, *Ancient and Modern Scottish Songs*, I. 117 (reprint of 1869), among a number of marches more or less artificial, prints a chorus:

Little wat ye wha's coming,
Little wat ye wha's coming,
Little wat ye wha's coming,
Jock and Tam and a's coming,

to which an indefinite series of incremental stanzas can be added, — as: —

Duncan's coming, Donald's coming,
Colin's coming, Ronald's coming . . .

and so the chorus, and again another stanza, and so on. A different kind of song for the march is "Un wenn nu de Pott en Lock hett," printed by Firmenich, *Germaniens Völkerstimmen*, p. 187.

[2] See his references, *Arbeit u. Rhythmus*, p. 71.

[3] *Primitive Culture*, I. 86.

highest place and meaning." At the end of the book of Passover services used by modern Jews, as Mr. Tylor and others have noted, there is a poem which curiously resembles the nursery tale of the old woman and her pig; the angel of death is dignified enough, and is slain by the Holy One, but cat eating kid, dog biting cat, and so on, are something ludicrous. Mr. Tylor thinks all this the original of the nursery tale itself. Again, in the same book there is a solemn counting poem; one is God, two are the tables of the covenant, and so on up to thirteen, when all is reversed in order back to one. Watchmen's songs counting the hours will occur to every reader. Germanic heathendom, doubtless, had this counting song in its ceremonial rites;[1] while incremental repetition in the charms, that oldest form of recorded poetry, is often found, witness the highly interesting charm against a stitch in the side, or rheumatism, from an English manuscript of the tenth century;[2] here are not only the recurring line of incantation, and the epic opening usual in charms, but a trace of something like the repetition with increments: "There sat a smith and made a knife," and again, "six smiths were sitting, warspears working;" why not *caetera desunt?*

Repetition is not an invention and grace of artistic poetry, as the books are fond of saying; it is the most characteristic legacy, barring rhythm, which communal conditions have made to art. Its artistic expression, in which, to borrow Emerson's phrase, it comes back to the passive throng "with a certain alienated majesty," no longer the simple iteration of a refrain or an incremental ballad, takes noblest form in tragedy and monody, shading down into artifice, however effec-

[1] Tacitus, *Germania*, c. 10. Liliencron u. Müllenhoff, *Zur Runenlehre*, Halle, 1852. Simple iteration, of course, is everywhere in charms: *ter dices* is the stage direction.

[2] Grein-Wülker, *Bibliothek*, I. 317 ff.

tive, in Maeterlinck's *Princesse Maleine* and *Pelleas et Mélisande*[1] where it almost makes rhythm of the prose, and into clever but legitimate tricks in Molière's famous *galère* passage and in his other passage, almost as famous, of the *sans dot.* It is used to give simple effects; probably it constitutes the charm of Hiawatha, as well as of that imitated ballad by Hamilton, the *Braes of Yarrow*, which Pinkerton ill-naturedly called "an eternal jingle." We may therefore divide poetic iteration into two great classes,—one natural or primitive, which is as much as to say communal, the other artistic, with a No Man's Land or Siberia whither one banishes the artificial. This artificial iteration of poetic style is perhaps nowhere so insistent as in those interesting but exasperating oddities known as *Greenes Funeralls*,[2] published "contrarie to the author's expectation." Of course, the step from art to artifice is not too obvious. Every one knows the smoothness, the fluidity, as Arnold calls it, which Spenser gave to his verse, often by this delicately managed iteration—say in *Astrophel;*[3] Donne softens his roughness with it in many a poem; but it becomes a tiresome trick at R. B.'s hands:—

> Ah, could my Muse old Maltaes Poet passe
> (If any Muse could passe old Maltaes Poet),
> Then should his name be set in shining brasse,
> In shining brasse for all the world to show it,[4]

[1] D'Annunzio, following Baudelaire, revives repetition with considerable effect to make up for lack of rimes in his *Elegie Romane.* See p. 69, "Villa Chigi."

[2] By R. B. Gent. (Barnfield?), London, 1594, a rare book. See Barnfield's own *Hellens Rape*, ed. by Grosart for the Roxburgh Club, 1876.

[3] A gentle shepherd born in Arcady,
Of gentlest race that ever shepherd bore.

No small influence in introducing this kind of repetition is due to the imitations of classic verse, and the struggles of the Areopagus to expel the tyrant Rime. Compare Spenser's own experiment: *Now doe I nightly waste*, quoted by Guest, *English Rhythms*, II. 270.

[4] A suspicion that R. B. is japing (see his *Amyntas: A-mint-Asse*, in the 4th of the fourteen "sonnets"), vanishes with careful reading of these highly interesting "experiments."

and it grows worse than tiresome in Gabriel Harvey's variation of the *ubi sunt* theme: —

> Ah, that Sir Humphrey Gilbert should be dead,
> Ah, that Sir Philip Sidney should be dead,
> Ah, that Sir William Sakevil should be dead,

which is not even humorous. Now it is clear that classical models play a part here. The pastorals of Vergil, the iteration of elegy imitated by Milton at the opening of *Lycidas*, are to be reckoned with; but not only was the throng behind all this, as shall be seen in a study of the *vocero*, not only are the charming iterations and incremental touches in Catullus,[1] —

> multi illum pueri, multae optauere puellae . . .
> nulli illum pueri, nullae optauere puellae . . .

along with store of ordinary repetition and a refrain, to be placed where they belong, in an alternating chorus of youths and maidens, with distinctly communal background; but there were cases in early English where the classical influence is slight, and the song of a swaying mass is clearly to be heard: [2] —

> Adam lay ibowndyn, bowndyn in a bond,
> Fowre thousand wynter thowt he not to long;
> And al was for an appil, an appil that he toke,
> As clerkes fyndyn wreten in here book.
> Ne hadde the appil take ben, the appil taken ben,
> Ne hadde neuer our lady aben heauene qwen.

In fact, early literature is full of repetition which suggests a recent transfer from the dancing and singing throng. So even the mediæval clerk[3] had not only Latin jingling in his

[1] *Carm.* lxii. 39 ff.

[2] Recorded as a fifteenth-century carol in the Sloane Ms.

[3] See, however, the caution uttered by M. Jeanroy against the idea that songs of the *Carmina Burana* represent popular poetry (*Origines de la Poësie Lyrique en France*, pp. 304 f.). Ingenious repetition, whether in refrains of the *triolet*

head, but also songs of the country folk buzzing in his ears; and it is no classical tone, despite the tongue, that sounds in his —

veni, veni, venias,
ne me mori facias,

while repetition takes a more artistic form in the vernacular:[1] —

Come, my darling, come to me!
I am waiting long for thee:
I am waiting long for thee,
Come, my darling, come to me!

Lips so sweet of red-rose grain,
Come and make me well again:
Come and make me well again,
Lips so sweet of red-rose grain!

Incremental repetition, then, as it is found in traditional ballads, lies midway between two extremes, one communal and one artistic. Behind it is the indefinite iteration, unchanged, of primitive song; before it is the repetition of artistic parallelism which is crossed by variation, mainspring

type, or in the Portuguese type represented by these verses, and in certain other poems of artificial construction (Jeanroy, p. 309): —

Per ribeira do rio
vy remar o navio;
et sabor ey da ribeyra!

Per ribeyra do alto
vy remar o barco;
et sabor, etc.

Vy remar o navio
hy vay o meu amigo;
et sabor, etc.

Vy remar o barco,
hy vay o meu amado;
et sabor, etc.

are probably no popular making. See, however, above, p. 139, the folksong of this type.

[1] "Chume, chume, geselle mîn." *Carmina Burana*, ed. Schmeller, pp. 208 f.

of the poetic dialect. Iteration is the spontaneous expression of emotion, and begins in the throng; it lies at the root of all rhythm, cadence, and consent; variation is the assertion of art, of progress, of the individual. These are the two great elements of poetry. Variation could take place in two ways. The communal singer had his stock of communal refrains and the like, derived from tradition of the singing and dancing throng; for communal purposes he could have added his own stanzas, just as Burns did in modern days. There was the chorus: —

Bonnie lassie, will ye go,
Will ye go, will ye go,
Bonnie lassie, will ye go
To the birks of Aberfeldy?

To this, and many a chorus like it, Burns added his own words.[1] But the early artists who worked out the scheme of national poetry went about their task by a different method. Their material was the unchanged repetition, probably in couplets corresponding to the forward-and-back of a dance, either in line, like some children's games now, or in a half circle, like that dance of the Botocudos. Out of this repetition they made the artistic parallelism found alike in Germanic epic and in Hebrew psalms, as well as the variation which Heinzel has so neatly compared for this same epic and for the Sanskrit hymn. As regards Germanic verse, Dr. R. M. Meyer[2] notes that repetition of words yielded to the necessity, imposed by rigid metrical law, to take a synonym which would rime with the principal word, thus ending in a mass of kennings or verbal variations. It is clear that the strophic ballad is based upon older conditions, as is proved

[1] See also R. H. Cromek, *Select Scottish Songs*, London, 1810, I. 14, —

Saw ye my Maggie?

[2] *Altgermanische Poesie*, pp. 228 f. See also Kluge, in Paul-Braune, *Beiträge*, IX. 462 f.

by preceding examples, and by the lack of variation in typical verses such as this, the opening of a pretty dance-song:[1] —

La rauschen, lieb, la rauschen!

The rigid structure of an alliterative verse calls for variation, not repetition, within its limits; variation in the ballads is incremental and close to actual repetition, being forced within a stanza only by the exigencies of rime: —

O where hae ye been, *Lord Randal, my son,*
O where hae ye been, *my handsome young man?*

The refrain, however, could hold to repetition pure and simple, leaving room for an increment of considerable effect at the climax; thus in the same ballad of *Lord Randal*, the refrain

For I'm weary wi' hunting and fain wad lie down,

turns at the end to —

For I'm sick at the heart and I fain wad lie down.[2]

Doubtless, too, variation began in the singing before it was evident in the record; that change of accent which editors claim for the well-known verses: —

Sigh nó more, ládies, sígh no móre . . .
Weep nó more, wóeful shépherds, wéep no móre

may have had its counterpart in far older and far ruder verse of the throng. If the earliest form of poetry was the

[1] Uhland, *Volkslieder*, I. 78.

[2] Variations may advance the sentence, or simply hold it; thus (*Barzaz-Breiz*):

Little Azénor the Pale is betrothed, but not to her lover,
Little Azénor the Pale is betrothed, not to her sweet "clerk;

no advance; otherwise in a refrain: —

Come hearken, hearken, O folk,
Come hearken, hearken to the song!

which suggests the syntactic structure of old English poetry due to alliterative variation.

iterated single verse, a statement of a fact, or, in the first instance, a fact stated not formally but by the repetition of words in a rhythmic period which was itself exactly repeated, it is clear that the progress of poesy may have begun by making a proposition of the single verse and then proceeding to add some new elements in the repetition of it. Artistic skill next fell upon the single verse,[1] fixed its cadence, curbed its repetition by syntactic relations, and, as in Germanic poetry, rang the changes on this law of variation. Now it is evident beyond all doubt how great a part incremental repetition must have played, and it is also evident that this can be studied best in a collocation of communal survivals, like the ballads, and primitive survivals, such as are found in savage songs. Let us look first at certain songs which belong between these two classes, then at a form of verse which is found in both, and finally at the ethnological or primitive material.

Radloff[2] collected an admirable series of songs and ballads in southern Siberia. Here are the homogeneous community, the oral and traditional verse, and the slow but sure ruin[3] of both due to importation of Mahometan learning, books and poets; here too are those fashions of making and keeping a song, half communal, half artistic, which yield to the conditions of written poetry. The gregarious song still lingers in chorus and in improvisations; while individual singers are

[1] A single sentence to the single verse is indicated in all primitive poetry, and is still the rule in Russian folksong: Bistrom, *Zeitschr. für Völkerpsy.*, V. 185. Progress lay both in intension and in extension, — regulation of the verse-parts, and combination of verses in a strophe. For example, an element like rime or assonance was used to bind verses now in couplets, now in a series like the old French *tirade*.

[2] *Proben der Volkslitteratur der türkischen Stämme Süd-Siberiens*, St. Petersburg, 1866 ff.

[3] *Ibid.*, III. xix. See above on the closed account. Exotic literature, and the *mullas*, learned poets, Radloff declares, are slowly driving out folksong of every sort.

working free from the throng, and are diverting the old broad current of repetition into channels and courses of art. But this individual artist[1] has a very short tether, and he is close to the community not only in fact but in the character of his work. Improvisation is the rule; composition of the deliberate modern sort is almost unknown. Festal throngs, not a poet's solitude, are the birthplace of poetry; and the folk, if they must listen and may not sing in chorus, choose a pair of singers to compete. "Some one present steps forward and challenges to a flyting. If no one appears in answer, the challenger sings improvised stanzas making fun of the people before him; but if a match is made up, then the two wage their duel in song until one fails to respond, loses the game, and gives a present to his conqueror." As with the Faroe islanders, so here on the Tartar steppes, and on the slopes of the Altai, if these rival songs show conspicuous merit, they are remembered, repeated, and sung as traditional ballads.[2] Radloff has several instances. A girl who enters such a flyting with a young man named Kosha, now flouts, now praises, and finally — another world-old trick of traditional song — falls into a series of riddles. What was first created, — who was so-and-so's father,[3] — when do the waters freeze? Kosha answers them all; the girl gives up, and presents him with a coat. Another pretty flyting[4] is also between youth and maid; the girl holds her own until the boy says he has wounded her brother, whereupon she sits down and weeps.

[1] For a study of the artistic side of this improvised song, see Chap. VIII. Here the communal conditions are to be emphasized, and the basis of unvaried repetition is to be inferred.

[2] Radloff, III. 34, note; 41.

[3] Compare Hildebrand in the older lay, bidding his son Hathubrand put him to the test of genealogies: —

> "ibu dû mî ênan sagês, ik mî dê ôdre uuêt,
> chind, in chunincrîche: chûd ist mî al irmindeot."

[4] Radloff, III. 48 f.

In all these, and in the solitary improvisations, there is constant repetition. Two verses of a challenge — all go by quatrains — are repeated in the answer; while in the continuous ballad, song oscillates, as Ten Brink says of this stage in the development of poetry, between memory and improvisation, production and reproduction. The singer has a mass of verses in his head, and puts his own thought only into the third and fourth lines of a quatrain,[1] the first and second coming from the common stock. That is the recurrent passage, the "ballad slang"; but actual repetition, in its incremental phase, is stronger here than in any poetry on record except that of the Finns. A fine example of this repetition and variation is in the *Kangsa Pi*, one of the historic songs;[2] mostly the stanzas are interlaced in pairs. Often the changes are mere emphasis, not progress; for example: —

If I had a white hawk,
  He would scream behind me;
If I had relatives on my father's side,
  They would follow behind me.

If I had a blue hawk,
  He would scream behind me;
If I had relatives on the Old One's side,
  They would follow behind me.

These changes of colour, variation on hard-and-fast lines, are very frequent and often inappropriate, as with a white horse and a blue horse;[3] one form of the change is not far remote from a Germanic kenning: —

[1] The so-called *Oelong*, with rime or assonance. *Ibid.*, III. xxii. The quatrain, as Usener points out in his *Altgriechischer Versbau*, seems to have been the favourite measure for popular verse.

[2] *Ibid.*, I. 218 ff.

[3] White and blue are the favourite variation. In a series, climax is often displaced by anticlimax, as in the quotation below: wife — betrothed; gold — silver; back — neck. For anticlimax with decreasing numbers, see Radloff, II. 670.

O Myrat mine, Myrat mine,
A *sea* is coming,—
How will you cross it?
On its *border* dwells a tribe,—
How will you come through it?

O Myrat mine, Myrat mine,
A *stretch of water* is coming,—
How will you cross it?
On its *banks* dwells a tribe,—
How will you come through it?

Thus a mother to her son; his answer is of the same kind; and so back and forth for nineteen stanzas, when the poem closes with two stanzas sung by the son happily returned from war. With this parallelism of form goes a parallelism of thought not unlike the implied simile in poetry of the schools; witness the hawk and the relatives, quoted just above, or these improvised verses:—

What has scattered the golden-seeming leaves?
Is it the white birch? It is indeed!
She whose hair streams down her back,
Is it my wife? It is indeed!

What has scattered the silver-seeming leaves?
Is it the blue birch? It is indeed!
She whose hair streams down her neck,
Is it my betrothed? It is indeed!

This is growing a bit too artistic for comfort; and presently in another song direct simile breaks out:—

As the meadow fire in spring,
  Warms this heart of mine;
As the bird that comes in spring,
  Implores this eye of mine.

As the fire that burns in autumn,
  Burns this heart of mine;
As the bird that comes in autumn,
  Mourns this eye of mine.

Improvised or not, these songs are not only of the individual lover, but of the artist, the bard, still close to his throng, to be sure, but with a clear notion of his dignity and a good care for his singing-robes. As one of these bards, though in another tribe,[1] prettily puts it: —

When the wind blows from the right hand,
Bends and bows the poplar;
When I sit and sing,
May there follow thirty songs!

When the wind blows from the left hand,
May the poplar move and quiver!
When I thus sit and sing,
May my own breast move and quiver!

Presently pen and paper will be found for the singer, and at last printer's ink to spread his songs; the days of communal chorus and communal repetition are numbered. One other effect of the old communal impulse, however, may be noted along with this trick of style. The rhapsode, singer, leader, where he is first seen detaching himself from the throng, has neither the individuality nor the artistic importance of what one now calls a poet. Every one knows the solicitude of Germanic singers to base their song upon tradition, to put their own invention into the background and appeal to the common stock: "we have heard tell of the Spear-Danes," — "I heard tell of Hildebrand and Hathubrand." This meant that the tale to be told had the communal stamp, and was worth hearing.[2] Egger[3] notes that the oldest Greek rhapsodes, like their songs, differed not one from the other in glory; the best song was simply the last which had been heard,[4] and there was no trace of rivalry among the bards, no

[1] Radloff, II. 669.
[2] See Vilmar, *Deutsche Altertümer im Hêliand*, Marburg, 1862, pp. 3 f.
[3] *Essai sur l'Histoire de la Critique chez les Grecs*, Paris, 3d ed., 1887, pp. 6 f.
[4] *Odyssey*, I. 352.

trace of partiality among the hearers. With the next age, the time of Hesiod, came the stress and struggle for a poet's crown; and since the crown was to be awarded to the best singer, judges were in demand, and so a rough criticism. It is easy to see that this stage would be reached in any growth of poetry when the bard began to talk of his thirty songs and of his quivering bosom; behind that stage lies the stage of the poets as deputies and mouthpieces of the throng; behind that, the throng itself.

We have now to look at a second class of material where primitive repetition, born of strong communal emotion, gets artistic control and so passes into new phases of development; this, confined to no one epoch of culture, must be sought in some universal human impulse. Birth, marriage, death, ought to give rise to such songs. Obviously, however, the first of these will be of the least value, and in point of fact songs of the sort were rarely recorded in early times, and perhaps rarely if ever made. Marriage and death, from the terms of the case, promise far better; and of the two, — for to treat them both would demand excessive space, — we shall take the songs of death, the *voceri*.[1] A brief glance at the marriage-songs, however, which are mainly sung in communal dance and procession, shows repetition everywhere, increasing with the older stages of culture. In German villages the whole community still has a share in the bridal;[2] while in Tyrol, if a girl goes outside the village for a husband, the youths mob her, tie her to a dung-cart, and lead her through the place, all singing derisive songs, until her father rescues her.[3]

[1] A study of marriage-songs must begin with choral sex-dances and songs of the great periodic excitement, the mating-time, still observed by Australian tribes, and work up through survivals of every sort to the festal "epithalamies" and their deputies in the poetry of art.

[2] E. H. Meyer, *Volkskunde*, p. 168.

[3] Perhaps a survival, but surely an exceptional case, valuable only for the communal feeling. See Pearson, who gives the facts, *Chances of Death*, II. 141.

Of course, the mobbing of unchaste women who marry is common enough; while in other cases of local indignation, crowds and derisive songs are always in order,[1] being represented under conditions of print by the "ballad," which can be used as a threat, like the modern reporter's interview or "exposure." Gretchen, in her terror, seems to hear these mocking songs. Poor Pamela hoped she would "not be the subject of their ballads and elegies," if she put an end to herself. But this is the other side of a joyous page. The later epithalamy was sung on private family occasions outside the bridal chamber and Puttenham gives a lively description of such festivities; but public and communal features are the older fact. In Greece[2] the bridal song comes from the festal crowd and accompanies the communal dance; the bride throws bits of food into the village fountain, about which the dances begin, — dances "which are regarded as the last act of the wedding ceremony." The songs for these dances, moreover, along with verses composed and danced at other stages of the affair, "form a considerable part of the national poetry."[3] In Albania[4] the bridal bread is baked on Thursday, and the kneading of it is begun with choral songs made for the occasion; on Sunday the marriage takes place, and from the procession of the groom and his friends down to the departure of the pair all is song and dance. The formal dance is opened by bride and groom, when a song is sung: "Raven

[1] *Old English Ballads*, pp. xxxii ff.

[2] Fauriel, *Chants Populaires de la Grèce Moderne*, Paris, I. 1824, II. 1825. See I. xxxvi. Roman literature gives hints of the same sort. The first epithalamium of Catullus (lxi) is "an imitation of the national custom": Teuffel, *Hist. Roman Lit.*, trans. Warr, p. 5.

[3] The older wedding in Greece was of the same kind. See *Iliad*, XVIII. 491 ff.; K. O. Müller, *Griech. Lit.*, p. 34. See too the burlesque at the end of Aristophanes's *Birds*, and H. W. Smythe, *Greek Melic Poets*, p. cxx.

[4] Hahn, *Albanesische Studien*, I. 144 ff.

stole a partridge. — Partridge? What will he do with the partridge? — Play with her, toy with her, and spend his life with her." English marriage customs, with communal dance and song, were of the same sort;[1] and "the poore Bryde" had to "kepe foote with al dauncers and refuse none, how scabbed, foule, droncken, rude and shamles soever he be," — an early puritan view of the case. Song and dance, communal rites throughout, were certainly characteristic of the Germanic wedding in its old estate, as is proved by divers names cited by Müllenhoff in his essay on our old choral verse,[2] and by the fact that a wedding was often called outright "the bridal song."[3] Neocorus,[4] too, tells of the customs in his time among the folk of the Cimbrian peninsula. In the East, again, down to this day, a wedding, like a funeral, is celebrated by the entire village for a full week; it was on communal epithalamies of the sort that one based the artistic bridal poem such as Budde[5] sees in Solomon's Song. The modern custom is said to keep many primitive traits. After a wedding,[6] which is usually in March, the pair are treated for seven days "as king and queen," and songs, now of communal victory and the like, now erotic, are sung by the folk; a great dance, moreover, is

[1] See the whole section in Brand's *Antiquities* under "Marriage Customs and Ceremonies." The quotation is from *The Christian State of Matrimony*, 1543.

[2] *De antiquissima Germanorum poesi chorica*, Kiel, 1847, pp. 23 f. — "carmina nuptialia, quorum varia erant nomina," etc. See also Kögel, *Geschichte der deutschen Lit.*, I. 44 f.

[3] Kögel, pp. 44 f.

[4] *Chronik*, ed. Dahlmann, I. 116 ff., 176. It is here that the good man breaks out in a lament for the "leffliche schone Gesenge" that have been lost. Bladé, *Poesies Pop. d. l. Gascogne*, I. xix ff., says the wedding songs are both traditional and improvised, taking the form of choral dialogues, where repetition is of course abundant.

[5] "Das Volkslied Israels im Munde der Propheten," in *Preussische Jahrbücher* LXXIII. (1893), 462.

[6] Wetzstein, "Die syrische Dreschtafel," in *Zeitschrift für Ethnologie*, V. (1873), 288 ff. See p. 297.

danced to the *wasf*, a song which praises the charms of bridegroom and bride. The chorus is naturally insistent and incessant, and a main characteristic of the songs is repetition.[1] But all folksong of the wedding tells this tale of dance and song, with repetition as the chief feature of the poetical style; and repetition is studied to even better advantage in that communal song of lamentation for the dead, which, for convenience, may pass by its Corsican name of *vocero*.

Mourners for the dead, now, save in the case of public characters, restricted to kin and friends, but once the whole community, are only mutes or audience to the act of burial; it is clear, however, that the priest and the service, or, as in France, the oration at the grave, along with the reticent group, are deputy for older and indeed still surviving songs of lament improvised and uttered by a near relative, and these again are but a development from the rhythmic wailings of a whole community or clan. Antiquity is no test whatever. A husband who advances to the coffin where his dead wife is lying and gives her a passionate farewell, after the manner of the French, while the funeral guests stand now in sympathetic silence, now with audible manifestations of grief, is doing precisely what Lucian describes as common in his day, barring the extravagance of the previous scene and the violent demonstrations made by Grecian women. Lucian thinks both demonstrations and oration ridiculous,[2] and he gives a kind of parody of the speech which a father makes over the body of his son. So too with the poetical lament, the elegy, mere antiquity goes for nothing; and the question is one of stages of evolution,

[1] The various German bridal songs printed by Firmenich, *Germaniens Völkerstimmen*, are mostly artificial things; and one which goes to a lively rhythm and is meant for a dance (I. 165) has fallen into mere barnyard filth.

[2] Lucian, *On Mourning*, 12 f. "A speech senseless and ridiculous," he says of the oration.

regardless of chronology, from the communal and choral wail up to the highly individualized and intellectualized monody of grief. The elegy of Simonides over the dead at Marathon was doubtless in its way as artistic as Tennyson's *Ode on Wellington;* and the same perspective must be kept in dealing with private outbursts of sorrow. Tennyson's own lines on the death of his brother are not a whit more modern in tone than the *Ave atque Vale* of Catullus which inspired them. The more primitive obligation was not to hear in respectful sympathy, not to read with intellectual approval, the oration or the poem, but to weep with them that weep and so to sing with them that sing. Uhland[1] cleverly notes the mythological projection of this older custom in that lament for Balder shared by all animate and inanimate creation. We are not, however, to think of the *vocero* as sprung from the ceremonies of a primitive funeral. Historians of literature are fond of such a process, and fix upon this or that religious rite as the source of some poem or song; Kögel,[2] for example, traces epic to a ceremonial rite as to its ultimate origin, and, for this particular case, insists that the *vocero* of a Germanic wife over her husband was a song of magic, a kind of incantation, asserting, wildly enough, that choral lament for the dead was unknown to the Germans of Tacitus, while magic songs had long been in vogue. This is distortion of facts and reversal of natural evolution. By the very terms of social organization, social consent must precede social institutions, and a ceremonial must usually be regarded not as the beginning but as the end of a social process. The prime factor in social expression was consent of rhythm; rhythmic cries at wedding[3] and at funeral do

[1] *Kl. Schrift.*, III. 445.

[2] See his *Gesch. d. d. Lit.*, I. 47, 51.

[3] Professor Smythe points out, *Greek Melic Poets*, p. cxiv, that Homer describes a hymeneal but "nowhere alludes to the religious element in the celebration of the rite."

not spring from the religious rites, although this or that wedding-song, this or that threnody, may have had such an origin; the rites are rather themselves an outcome, under priestly control and the hardening of custom into law, of this festal excitement, this communal grief. The priest, even the shaman, is deputy of that throng which was once active and is now passive; and when one considers the literature of death, one finds the earliest stages of funeral lament in that half chaotic chorus of repetition and tumultuous cries which cannot be derived from any ceremony, strictly so called, but is rather on the way to ceremony. At this literature we are now to look.

Homer has preserved in an artistic form echoes of primitive wailing, of primitive repetition and choral cries, when he describes the funeral of Hector.[1] "And the others . . . laid him on a fretted bed, and set beside him minstrels, leaders of the dirge, who wailed a mournful lay, while the women made moan with them." Andromache then leads the lamentation, "while in her hands she held the head of Hector, slayer of men. 'Husband, thou art gone young from life.' . . . Thus spake she wailing, and the women joined their moan." Then Hecuba; and again the line like a refrain, "Thus spake she wailing, and stirred unending moan." Lastly Helen; and again, "Thus spake she wailing, and therewith the great multitude of the people groaned." Wailings of the throng are echoed also in choruses of Greek tragedy;[2] but it is these epic passages and their details which carry one back into the communal realm, quite away from

[1] *Iliad*, XXIV, 719 ff., trans. Lang, Leaf, and Myers.

[2] See H. Koester, *de Cantilenis Popularibus Veterum Graecorum*, Berol., 1831, p. 15. Roman *neniae*, of course, are in point (see Sittl, *Gebärden der Griechen und Römer;* Cap. IV.); but the artificial element is very strong, and primitive survivals are few. Wordsworth, *Fragments and Specimens of Early Latin*, p. 562, says of the epitaphs on the Scipios, "Whether they were or were not fragments of *neniae* is quite uncertain."

the satire of Lucian,[1] however some of the features which he describes may seem to be repeated here. The song of lament, whether a domestic duty or a professional act, was mainly a matter for the women, and was originally improvised; at the funeral of Achilles,[2] it is his mother and "the deathless maidens of the waters" who wail about his pyre, and it is the muses themselves who raise the clear chant. So Hildeburh at the funeral pile, in that episode of the *Béowulf:*[3] —

> Sad at his shoulder sorrowed the woman,
> Moaned him in songs.

That a wailing chorus answered her wailing there can be no doubt, though nothing is said of it; that the song is not quoted, that the record of these rites is brief, can be explained easily enough, when one remembers the monk who set down this fine old epic with pagan delight in his heart but a crucifix before his eyes, and constant thunder of ecclesiastical denunciation in his ears. Those *neniae inhonestae*, the singing of diabolical songs and the dancing of diabolical dances[4] about

[1] Crude enough, to be sure, compared with Chaucer's humour in dealing with the funeral of Arcite: —

> "Why woldestow be deed," thise wommen crye,
> "And haddest gold ynough, and Emelye?"

For this is the conventional question, in whatever form, in the *vocero* of all places and ages: "Why did you die? You had enough to eat, you had clothes," etc. Old Egeus has the modern consolation, and philosophizes in no communal vein.

[2] *Odyssey*, XXIV. 59 ff.

[3] 1117 f. It has been noted that Kögel, *Gesch. d. d. Lit.*, I. 54, says, without good reason, that this was a magic song, a *spruch*. It was surely what it is called, a song of lament, a *vocero*, and doubtless asked the same old question.

[4] St. Augustine tells how such songs were sung at the tomb of St. Cyprian: "per totam noctem cantabantur hic nefaria, et *cantantibus saltabatur*." See also the well-known passage from Burchard of Worms: "cantasti ibi diabolica carmina et fecisti ibi saltationes" — *i.e.* at the "vigiliis cadaverum mortuorum." Müllenhoff, work quoted, pp. 26 ff., gives some of these protests of the church. On p. 30 he notes that the songs themselves were improvised: *extempore et subito facta*. The older the rite, the more choral and communal it grows. The names (*ibid.*, p. 25) are significant: *dâdsisas, leidsang, chlagasang*, etc., for older German; *lîcsang, lîcleôð* (*epicedium*), *byrgensang* (*epitaphium*), etc., for older English.

a corpse, all the "payens corsed olde rites," were denounced by bishops and councils of the church with a fervid iteration which at once accounts for the silence of the poets and testifies to the stubborn vogue of the ceremony. The dance is of course a survival of very primitive rites, as will be seen in the study of the actual *vocero*, and as can be learned from ethnology; for the epics it has been developed into funeral games, although in the *Béowulf* one finds an older stage of these ceremonies than in Homer. Besides Hrothgar's lament over Aeschere, a lament intensified by the absence of the dead body,[1] and the moanings of old Hrethel for his son,[2] there is the hero's own funeral, where, when all the clan, presumably, have mourned their lord, presumably in song, and when the wife has sung, like Hildeburh, her *giomorgyd*, her song of lamentation, at last the ashes are placed in the barrow, and twelve noble youths ride round it chanting the praises of the dead king. A close parallel to this ceremony is found far to the eastward. In what is now known to have been a Gothic rather than a Hunnish rite, warriors rode, "as in the games of the circus," round the body of Attila where he lay in state, and as they rode sang also a funeral song of praise; Jordanis[3] gives a Latin version of it, but as it stands in this guise, it has a very artistic and even artificial ring. The clan-grief and the clan-praise at Beowulf's funeral are nearer to the facts. As regards the riding, it is clear that this takes the

[1] *Béow.*, 1322, 2124 f.

[2] *Ibid.*, 2446 f., 2460. There is a sort of *vocero* echo here. Remarkable, too, in the story of the self-buried chief, is a *vocero* of that old man over himself, the last of the race burying his treasure as a kind of substitute: *ibid.*, 2233 ff. It is superfluous to point out how English lyric poetry, from the *Ruin* to the *Elegy*, and on to our own day, loves to linger by a grave. Traces of the *vocero* that led to the vendetta might be found in the countless stories of old Germanic feud.

[3] *De Orig. Act. Getarum*, ed. Holder, c. 49. A similar story is told (c. 41) of the funeral of King Theoderid of the Visigoths, killed in 451, and of the wild songs that were sung even on the field of battle as the warriors bore away the body of their king.

place of an older dance or march, just as the song takes the place of older wailings and cries. The processions of a whole community, at times of planting and of harvest, round the field, the barn, the village, to which we shall presently refer when considering the refrain, are matched by similar rites of marching with dance and song round hearth, grave, altar, in the ceremonies of wedding and burial. On the Isle of Man a wedding party goes three times round the church before it enters; and in many places the corpse is carried in the same way for a funeral. In the latter case, the solemn march is only a repetition of the dance round the corpse itself, the mourners going hand in hand, now slowly, now tumultuously, to the sound of their own wailing. Ethnological evidence, again, puts the songs and dances for the dead, as found among savage tribes throughout the world, in line with these survivals among the peasantry of Europe; no chain of evidence could be more complete. To this ethnological material we shall presently return; meanwhile it is in order to note the evidence in literature.

We have seen obvious cases of the *vocero* in oldest English, and it could be followed in other Germanic records. Probably many of the English and Scottish ballads began as a kind of *vocero*, something like the coronach of Highland clans: one thinks of *Bonny George Campbell*, with its repetition and refrain, and of *The Bonny Earl of Murray*, with its triad of incremental repetitions, ballads which follow close upon the death of their hero; of ballads less immediate but still memorial, like *The Baron of Brackley*, and perhaps *The Lowlands of Holland;* even of the widely spread ballads of a condemned criminal, the *Good Nights*, and such admirable precipitates of this kind as *Mary Hamilton*. For more direct evidence, the refrain line *Ohon for my son Leesome Brand!* [1] is promising; but it is only a line. One *vocero*, however, has come down

[1] Child, I. 182.

to us, although considerably changed from the normal and original pattern. In Aubrey's *Remains of Gentilisme and Judaisme*,[1] mention is made of "Irish howlings at Funeralls, *also in Yorkshire within these* 70 *yeares* (1688)"; and again, quoting the song, *This ean night*, Aubrey says it is from Mr. Mawtese, "in whose father's youth, sc. about sixty years since (now 1686), at country vulgar Funeralls was sung this song," by a woman like a *praefica*. Scott has a like account; it was sung a century ago[2] "by the lower ranks of Roman Catholics in some parts of the north of England. The tune is doleful and monotonous." The refrain, or, as Scott calls it, the chorus, is very insistent and belongs to genuine communal tradition; he quotes an account of Cleveland, Yorkshire, in the reign of Queen Elizabeth, which was found by Ritson in a manuscript of the Cotton library: "When any dieth, certaine women sing a song to the dead bodie, recyting the journey that the partye deceased must goe." The following stanzas will serve as specimens of this highly developed but interesting *vocero*: —

This ae nighte, this ae nighte,
Every night and alle;
Fire and sleete and candle-light,
And Christe receive thye saule.

When thou from hence away art paste,
Every night and alle,
To Whinny-muir thou comest at laste,
And Christe receive thye saule.

In Germany, the *vocero* lingered long, but is dying or dead; it was an improvised farewell in "free" rhythm.[3] A very interesting communal survival akin to the *vocero* was known

[1] *Folk-Lore Soc. Pub.*, IV. (1881), pp. 21, 31.

[2] Scott, *Minstrelsy*, 1812, II. 361 ff.

[3] Still found in remote places, — among Germans in North Hungary, and in Gottschee in Krain, speech-islands both. Meyer, *Volkskunde*, p. 272.

in Flanders down to the year 1840, — The Maids' Dance[1] at the funeral of a companion; it was sung and danced by the young girls of the parish. When the coffin had been lowered into the grave, all these girls, holding by one hand the cloth which had covered the corpse, went back to the church singing this "dance" with a force and a rhythmic accent which roused the hearer's surprise.[2] The two stanzas and the refrain are, of course, partly modern; but they show traces of the old dance and *vocero* noted below as surviving among the Corsicans: —

Up in heaven is a dance;
Alleluia.
There the maidens are dancing all.
Benedicamus Domino.
Alleluia, Alleluia.

It is for Amelia;
Alleluia,
We're dancing as the maidens dance.
Benedicamus Domino.
Alleluia, Alleluia.

But there is better material in the literature of other races. Nowhere, for example, is the wailing and chanting of women over the dead better attested than among the Hebrews of the Old Testament; Syrians of to-day hold to the same rites and sing a song of mourning strangely like that which Jeremiah heard twenty-five centuries ago.[3] The lament of David over Saul and Jonathan, known to be an actual *kîna*, with its personal touch of "my brother," and its communal refrain, *how*

[1] "Dans der Maegdekens," heard at Bailleul by Coussemaker. See his *Chants Populaires des Flamands de France*, Gand, 1856, pp. 100 f. Soon after 1840 it was forbidden, and the song is no more, save in the record. It goes back, says C., to the oldest times.

[2] *Ibid.*, p. 101.

[3] Budde, "Das hebräische Klagelied," *Zeitschr. f. alttestamentl. Wissensch.*, II. 26 f.; and Wetzstein, "Syrische Dreschtafel," as quoted above. See also same *Zeitsch.*, III. 299 ff. For the professional singing-women, the *praeficae* of Israel, see Jer. ix. 19.

are the mighty fallen, differs from the professional lamentation of the women, which was in a fixed rhythm,[1] while David's outburst is spontaneous and "free." In cases of this kind, to be sure, one must always reckon with the literary and artistic element; but David's *vocero* is close to the popular custom, and of more value to the student than the lament of tragedy old and new. Indeed, a kind of declamation over the dead relative is often found in tragedy, with some resemblance to the actual *vocero* both in matter and in style, but with an alien touch of rhetoric; so Hieronimo, showing the corpse of his son, has the repetition and play of words already noted among the early Elizabethans, and at far remove from that "O my son Absalom, my son, my son Absalom!" of the immediate lament:—

> Here lay my hope, and here my hope hath end;
> Here lay my heart, and here my heart was slain;
> Here lay my treasure, here my treasure lost,

and the rest. Hamlet and Laertes at the grave of Ophelia suggest further distortion, turning the lament into a kind of flyting. It is the actual *vocero*, and the communal conditions of it, from which one learns the course of poetry; and this actual *vocero*, even in its Homeric form, has two elements, the song of the relative and the answering wail of the throng. With later conditions the single song comes to be professional, as with Hebrews, Romans, and nearly all nations; or else the women move with sympathetic gestures now round the chief mourner, now round the corpse, singing and wailing as they go. Like modern Syria, modern Greece keeps the old custom; the myriologue has many features of the Homeric rite, particularly the primitive trait of improvisation. The song, says Fauriel,[2] is never composed in advance, but is

[1] Budde, "Die hebräische Leichenklage," *Zeitschr. d. deutsch. Palästina-Vereins*, VI. 181 f., 184 ff.

[2] Work quoted, p. cxxxiii.

always improvised in the very moment that it is delivered, and is always fitted to the person addressed. "It is always in verse; the verses are always in the metre of other popular songs; and they are always sung." Each village — and the communal trait is significant — has an air of its own for these lamentations, and sings them to no other air. Hahn's account[1] is worth quoting. When a man has died, the women of his family make a fearful cry,[2] which brings all the neighbouring women to the house, shrieking, howling, and gesticulating with the mourners. The actual relatives tear their hair, dash their heads against the wall, *call upon the dead by name*, and scream so loudly[3] and continuously that for a time they often lose their voices.[4] So the women; the men are more calm. The corpse is now washed and clad, whereupon the women seat themselves about it, and the real lament begins. "This is always rhythmic and generally consists of two verses sung by one voice and repeated by the whole chorus of women." Now it is traditional, now improvised. As fast as one woman is exhausted, another lifts her hand in signal and begins a new verse. On the way to burial they sing in the same fashion.

This song over the dead, which is found throughout the world, in Greenland, in Peru, in the Hebrides, among the Hottentots,[5] shows a course of development in which the detached or literary lament is the latest stage. Here it may be a great poem, pulsing with the grief of nations and close to

[1] J. G. Hahn, *Albanesische Studien*, I. 150 f.

[2] Precisely as among the Irish. See Miss Edgeworth's account, quoted by Brand, *Antiquities*, "Watching with the Dead."

[3] In a note, I. 198, Hahn notes that Plato forbade this wild cry (*Legg.* xxi), but allowed the song of lament. For calling on the dead, cf. Latin *inclamare*.

[4] One of the canons which condemned heathen customs at Christian funerals forbids not only song and dance, but also *illum ululatum excelsum*.

[5] The *vocero* sung by natives of Algiers has been noted as strongly resembling the Corsican. A specimen, quoted from Certeux and Carnoy, *L'Algérie Traditionelle*, is full of repetition and refrain.

the common heart, or a mere exercise made by rule; the gay science of Provence, like the school poetry of Germany and England, had minute directions for the making of a good *planch*.[1] "One may compose a song of lament in any melody," runs the Catalan rule, "save in the melody of a dance," — strange exception, when one comes to the dances which so often went with the real *vocero;* and Master Vinesauf,[2] in his *Poetria*, called out Chaucer's well-known gibe[3] by the recipe for a poem of grief. "When you wish to express grief," he advises, "say something like this;" and an appropriate sentiment follows. That is the literary stage, the detached lament; but behind the little artifice, as behind the great art, lies the real *vocero* with elements that need to be set in right perspective. We see the corpse, the wailing relatives, the singing relatives, the professional singing women, the whole clan in tumultuous grief, loud discordant cries, a choral wail which is rhythmic and articulate, chanted verses. Of all these the professional singing woman such as Jeremiah invoked, the *praefica* of Rome, the keener at an Irish funeral, is the nearest to literary lament, and connects the communal with the artistic. Behind her, and taking her place as one follows back the course of evolution, stands the "free" or natural mourner, now and then a man,[4] but usu-

[1] Springer, *Das altprovenzalische Klagelied*, Berlin, 1895, pp. 8 ff. It is this formal poem of grief which is in the mind of Crescimbeni, *Comentarj Intorno all' Istoria della Volgar Poesia*, 1731, I. 256, when he traces the Italian funeral song back to Latin and Greek.

[2] This English Boileau, who "flourished," in two senses, about 1200, is good reading. His *Poetria* begins at p. 862 of Polycarpi Leyseri . . . *Historia Poetarum et Poematum Medii Ævi*, Hal. Magd., MDCCXXI.

[3] *C. T.*, 4537 ff. The Latin:

Temporibus luctus, his verbis exprime luctum.

[4] Marcaggi, *Les Chants de la Mort et de la Vendetta de la Corse*, Paris, 1898, p. 193, gives a *vocero* said to have been made by a monk, who calls on the celestial powers to join the chorus and wail the death of his two friends: "Jesus, Joseph, Mary, Sacred Sacrament, and all of you here in chorus, sing this *lamento*." Bandits make a *vocero*, pp. 307 f.

ally wife or mother or sister of the dead. Behind these, again, stands the throng itself, the original mourners, clan or horde of a time when the bonds of mere community were stronger than any ties of kin, and when individual grief was hardly if at all lifted from the communal level; and with this stage one has come from elaborate verse, through choral lament, to mere iteration of clamorous grief, rhythmical by the consent of a throng and by the compulsion of dance, gesture, and spasmodic utterance. In this communal refrain, then, we reach the origin of all laments; here is surely one, at least, of the "beginnings of poetry"; and in the *vocero* of Corsica break forth even yet those cadenced interjections which were heard throughout the Orient, spread over Greece in the wailings for Adonis, and echo in the repeated denunciation of Jeremiah: "They shall not lament for him, saying, *Ah my brother!* or *Ah sister!* — They shall not lament for him, saying, *Ah Lord!* or *Ah his glory!* He shall be buried with the burial of an ass, drawn and cast forth beyond the gates of Jerusalem."[1] But these earliest cadenced cries are best approached by means of the second stage; and the song of grief can still be heard in Corsica from wife or mother of the dead, with all the force and naturalness of the *vocero* as it is described by Homer and in the *Béowulf*. Elsewhere, of course, and in Italy itself, one can find material of the sort. D'Annunzio describes, in terms said to be rigorously correct, a peasant mother's improvised *vocero* at sight of her drowned boy.[2] After a few moments of silence, broken only by wild outcries, she begins her spontaneous song in a short, panting rhythm, rising and falling with the palpitations of her

[1] Jer. xxii. 18. See below, on the Linos song.

[2] *Trionfo della Morte*, pp. 419 f. "Era l'antica monodia che da tempo immemorabile in terra d'Abruzzi le donne cantavano su le spoglie dei consanguinei." See another account of the Italian *vocero* in Guastella, *Canti Popolari del Circondario di Modica*, Modica, 1876, p. lxxix. He notes, moreover, that in Sicily the *prèfiche* are called *ripetitrici*.

heart; a characteristic noted also by writers on the Corsican *vocero*.

We turn, then, first to this Corsican lament.[1] *Voceri* they call the songs, as one might say "vociferations," a name doubtless due to the *gridatu* or inarticulate wailings of the throng, which precede the *vocero* proper; *lamenti* and *ballati* are terms sometimes used instead, the second, of course, referring to those dances which were once an inseparable part of the rite, but are now seldom seen. "Make wide the circle," runs one lament, "and dance the *caracolu;* for this sorrow is very sore."[2] As for the song itself, it is briefly but adequately defined[3] as an "improvised funeral song," sung by a near female relative of the dead man, in a strophe of six verses with four measures to the verse, that verse beloved everywhere of communal poetry; and since the same occasion begets them all, all *voceri* have considerable likeness one to another, with recurrence of word and phrase. The speech of Corsica is itself rudely poetic; and these improvisations, though full of traditional passages,—"sweeter than honey"; "better than bread,"—are direct in their diction, even to a point that seems at first sight to deny such a fundamental communal trait as repetition. Iteration, however, is there, insistently there, when one takes into account not only the refrain, always breaking down into sobs and re-

[1] Mérimée's *Columba* has made the *vocero* familiar to readers. See also Mar caggi, work quoted; Ortoli, *Les Voceri de l'Ile de Corse*, Paris, 1887; Paul de St. Victor, *Hommes et Dieux*, Paris, 1872, pp. 349–369, a reprinted article cannily decocted and pleasantly served in the English periodical *Once a Week*, 1867, pp. 437–442. St. Victor refers to the older collections of Tommaseo and of Fée.

[2] Marcaggi, p. 161. See above on the ride round the body of Beowulf and of Attila, and the older dance. The *caracolu* is "a sort of pantomime, a funeral dance done by the mourners round the corpse as they make gestures of grief." The *caracolu* is danced no more. And again, Marcaggi, p. 231, note: "*vocerare* ou *ballatrare* veut donc dire improviser un vocero,"—highly suggestive fact.

[3] *Ibid.*, p. 4; Ortoli, p. xxxiv. Of these two, Marcaggi prints mainly the older material, with a few new pieces of miscellaneous character, such as cradle-songs and serenades.

peated moans, but the evident suppression of repetition in the text. As to the refrain, the leader now bids all present join her in this wailing cry, and now bids them cease in order that she may be heard: —

> Di gratia, fate silenziu . . .
> Finitele ste gride . . .

and now, again, she takes the refrain bodily into her own song, beginning thus a new stanza. "*Di, di, dih!* Woe is me! Make one great cry of sorrow, brothers and sisters all," sings a wife over her husband; and this inarticulate bit of chorus, always sung, as Marcaggi says,[1] at the end of each stanza, by the women who surround the corpse, may be the imitation — echo would better hit the truth — of the old sobbing of the throng. As for the text, repetition is hardly to be expected in print, and the editors have doubtless done as Lyngbye did with Faroe ballads, though here and there occurs a line[2] like,—

> Chéta, chéta, chéta, o Sàgra,
> Chét' é nun piegna piu tantu.

They are keen to record the power of improvisation shown by their countrywomen; what use to print pages of iteration? A fine hint, however, can be found in Marcaggi's forewords, not only of the silly sooth but of the old time; he saw, he says, "one day a poor woman run shrieking from her house, her hair disordered, and coming to the public square, where the corpse of her sister-in-law lay, sing in a mournful and monotonous note, with grotesque leaps and bounds: —

> O commari Mari!
> O commari Mari!

People said," adds Marcaggi, "*that she was following the custom of a former age*, and that she lacked proper re-

[1] His philology is unnecessary, p. 85. Ortoli, too, should stick to his "espèce de sanglot," rather than follow his colleague's "racine de *titiare*" or contraction of *Oh Dio!*

[2] Ortoli, p. 248.

serve."[1] This is, indeed, the more primitive note; and the iterated cry, mere appeal to the dead, like those *cris d'enterrement* which Bladé heard at Gascon burials, was once sung by the swaying and dancing throng of mourners. Psychologically and physiologically this is quite in order; a kind of communal hysterics, intensely rhythmical, as with a badly frightened child, as with insanity, delirium, abnormal emotion of any kind, has the cadent and recurrent note at its utmost; and this woman, with her "lack of decorum," like that peasant on the beach by the drowned boy, is the modern survivor and deputy of panic emotion, a belated case in the pathology of epidemic grief. Between this mere iterated cry, as was said above, and the later professional song of lament,[2] lie the bulk of Corsican *voceri*, sung by sister or mother of the dead, and most characteristic when it is a violent death which they deplore and when they will stir to vengeance a group of male relatives standing sullenly by the corpse. For while a *vocero* in the case of some peace-parted soul, such as the village priest, is often a decorous and comforting office,[3] the passion of the thing is felt only over the bier of a man murdered in feud. St. Victor, whom all the others quote on this point, describes the scene. At first, in the chamber of death, rises a great wail of lament, through which oaths of vengeance flash like lightning; men draw their daggers, and dash their guns upon the stone floor; women dip their handkerchiefs in the blood still oozing from the wounds;[4] some-

[1] *Manquait de tenue*, M., pp. 24 f.

[2] See Marcaggi, pp. 157, 231, for a *vocératrice célèbre*. "La vocératrice marche toujours à la tête des pleureuses,"—in going to the funeral.

[3] Such is No. X. in Marcaggi, a "*vocero* sung by a woman in the square of Canonica in the midst of a great crowd of women, priests, doctors, and magistrates come from neighbour villages."

[4] A child who does this, and makes a *vocero*, declares that he will bind the kerchief about his neck whenever he feels moved to laugh,—a grim bit which throws into the shade that "child on the nourice's knee" of English ballads, who vows revenge if he shall live to be man.

times they are moved to a frenzy that vents itself in dancing round the corpse amid loud cries, until silence is demanded and the dead man's mother, wife, sister, moves to the bier and begins her *vocero*. There is no art in it; "the excuse for its violence is in its explosive force, . . . it sings through the mouth of a wound." It begins, however, in a plaintive way, calls tenderly upon the dead, then tells the story of his taking off; now the gently cadenced movements of the singer grow more violent, and presently she breaks into a storm of imprecations and into wild appeals for the vendetta.[1] One after another of these singers improvises such a lament, and for every stanza a chorus of sobs and cries and moans, often, one gathers, of articulate words, rises from the throng. The passion, too, is real; readers who come of northern blood must banish certain associations of the cardboard castle, the cloak and sword, loud baritone confidences, and stage moonlight. These *voceri* of vengeance are not rated as rant by the law, which often and vainly tries to put them down. Thus among the Basques, a race, as George Borrow declared, not of poets but of singers, laws were passed against the old fashion of the funeral;[2] it was forbidden "to make lamentations, to tear one's hair, to bruise the flesh, to wound one's head, to chant death-songs." A Basque chorus of lament is described by Michel. "All the women join in it with deep sighs and cries of grief, addressed now to the dead and now to themselves; they begin with high tones, then fall into a deep note, and pronounce from time to time *ayené*, a Basque word which means *Alas!*" It is quite clear that in these repeated words of the chorus one finds the origin of the *vocero*, the "cry" of

[1] On the vendetta in Italy during the renaissance, see Burckhardt, *Cult. d. Ren.*,[6] II. 179 ff.

[2] J. F. Bladé, *Dissertation sur les Chants Historiques des Basques*, Paris, 1866, pp. 6 ff.; Borrow, *The Bible in Spain*, 1843, II. 394; F. Michel, *Le Pays Basque*, 1857, pp. 277 f.

communal grief; and a study of such cries at the actual burial, as they are still heard in Gascon funerals,[1] shows to what beginnings one must refer the more elaborate *voceri* of the Corsicans. As early as 1340 a law was passed at Tarbes against "cries and lamentations at the return from a burial." According to Bladé, the Gascon burial cries are a kind of recitative, lacking rime and even what modern ears demand in the way of rhythm, for they are now divorced from the dance, and at best are timed to the steps of the procession. They begin when a funeral procession starts from the church to the cemetery, and are a series of "distinct exclamations combined into irregular stanzas"; mostly they begin "in a high note, falling slowly, to rise again at the end." The iteration of these cries is insistent; Bladé quotes a long *cri* of the sort:[2]—

Ah!
Ah! Ah! Ah!
Ah! Pauvre!
Ah! Pauvre!
Ah! Pauvre!
Mon Dieu!
Mon Dieu! Mon Dieu!

Ah!
Pauvre Père!
Pauvre Père! Pauvre Père!
Vous êtes mort, pauvre Père!
Pauvre Père, vous êtes mort!
Vous êtes mort!
Vous ne reviendrez jamais!
Jamais! Jamais!

Then the first stanza is repeated. The choral possibilities of this cry are clear enough, and sung to the dance

[1] "They have not utterly disappeared from my country," says Bladé, *Poésies Populaires de la Gascogne*, introduction to Vol. I. p. xi; and he prints a collection of them, pp. 212–231.

[2] This is Bladé's French rendering, pp. 212 ff. Beaurepaire, work quoted, pp. 24 f., says these cries are no longer heard in Normandy.

about a corpse, as was undoubtedly the primitive case, its rhythm would have been exact and no "recitative." A further step is taken when individual and artistic touches make themselves felt in a pretty little *cri* which is sung by a mother[1] over her child:—

Pauvret!
Ah!
Tu seras bien seulet
Au cimitière
Cette nuit,
Et moi
Je te pleurerai
A la maison.
Mon Dieu!
Ah!

Repetition is the original rhythm, the original poem; then comes improvisation by the individual, begetting the increment and founding a "text," while variation plays upon the repeated words. Such is the course of poetry, and in particular of the *vocero;* repetition lies at the heart of it. Wetzstein,[2] describing the Syrian song of lament sung by the women, lays stress upon the constant iteration in it, and upon the chorus which consists mainly of a single word,—"woe!" "alas!"—counterpart of the chorus in Corsican and Pasque *voceri*. Indeed, the *vocero* is not only inscribed with woe, but was once nothing else; and fragments of this or that "cry" of burial and of death found their way into the mythology and the recorded poetry of Phœnicians, of Egyptians, and of Greeks. Brugsch,[3] in his study of the songs about Adonis and Linos, makes it clear that Linos was simply a personification of these Phœnician cries of lament, *ai lenu*, the choral "alas!" or "woe to us!" The

[1] "The men, old and young, take no part," Bladé, I. xiii.

[2] "Die syrische Dreschtafel," *Zeitschr. f. Ethnologie*, V. (1873), 295 f.

[3] *Die Adonisklage und das Linoslied*, Berlin, 1852, pp. 16 ff.

refrain or repeated cry of grief sung by mourners about their dead finds thus both mythical and ritual projection and the immortality insured by great artistic song. This *ai, ai,* seems to be one of the oldest choral funeral cries, common, as Brugsch puts it, "to the whole Orient as well as Egypt"; and he follows it down to the exquisite elegy of Bion. Linos, in the vintage songs, was made a personification of this cry,[1] became a Greek, was said to be buried in Argos, and was worshipped on Helicon amid lamentations of matron and maid gathered at the yearly festival. One remembers Ezekiel's wrath over the women who, in the gate of the Lord's house, were weeping for Tammuz. In the Egyptian lament of Isis for Osiris, the opening words, "Come back," are repeated, as in the choral cry from which it sprang, and are in accord not only with the *vocero* of Europe, but with the refrain of a dirge in India:[2] —

> We never scolded you; never wronged you;
> *Come to us back! . . .*
> *Come home, come home, come to us again!*

The Egyptian *vocero*, the *ai en Ise*, is worth quoting in full:[3] "Come back, come back, God Panu, come back! For they which were against thee are no more. Ah, fair helper, come back to see me, thy sister, that love thee; and drawest thou not nigh to me? Ah, fair youth, come back, come back! I see thee not, my heart is sore for thee, my eyes seek thee. I wander about for thee, to see thee in the form of Nai, to see thee, to see thee, fair lord, in the form of Nai, to see thee, the fair one, — to see thee, to see thee, God Panu, the fair one! Come to thy darling, blessed Ounophris, come to thy sister, come to thy wife, come to thy wife, God Urtuhet,

[1] K. O. Müller, *Gesch. d. Griech. Lit.*, I. 28, makes Linos the personification of the soft spring slain by heats of summer.

[2] Quoted by Tylor, *Primitive Culture*, II. 32.

[3] Taken from the German rendering of Brugsch.

come to thy spouse! I am thy sister, I am thy mother, and thou comest not to me; the face of gods and of men is turned to thee, while they weep thee, seeing me that weep for thy sake, that weep and cry to heaven that thou hear my prayer, — for I am thy sister that loved thee on earth. Never lovedst thou another than me, thy sister! Never lovedst thou another than me, thy sister!" Like the companion lament of Nephthys, this is distinctly a *vocero* of the sister over the brother; and the repeated *mââ-ne-hra*, "come home," the refrain of the piece, gave rise to the name Maneros, fabled to be a prince of Egypt, a fact which reminded Herodotus of the similar song of Linos in Greece. In his chapter on the Lityerses song, Mannhardt[1] notes that this name, too, with that of Bormos, both supposed to be sons of a king, like Maneros, Linos, Mannerius, was developed out of an old refrain. The Greeks, singing a lay which corresponded to the Maneros, went with choral cries and music to seek the vanished Bormos. So, too, with Hylas; a Bithynian festival is on record, where sacrifice is made at the scene of his capture by the nymphs; and the festal throng thereupon wander over the hills and about the Hylas Lake, crying incessantly upon his name. It is needless to follow all these myths and the ritual connected with them; nor can we turn aside and study the memorial festivals of the dead, like that old Germanic feast in November, now surviving in All Souls' Day, where masses said for the repose of Christian dead, and flowers laid upon their tombs, took the place of older sacrifice, dance, and song.[2] What one sees beyond question is the origin of funeral songs in the communal chorus, and what one infers with great probability is that death, and the resulting expression of com-

[1] *Mythologische Forschungen*, pp. 16, 55. Herodotus, II. 79, distinctly says that the Maneros song was of the people.

[2] For the general custom, see Tylor, *Primitive Culture*, II. 36 ff.; for Germanic relations, Pfannenschmidt, *Germanische Erntefeste*, pp. 165 ff.

munal grief in choral song and dance, had much more to do with earliest forms of poetry than even the erotic impulse. Sociology now declares that primitive feeling for children, relatives, clan, was far keener in its emotional expression than the sense of sexual desire.[1] The importance of the love-lyric, now overwhelming, and mainly an individual outburst, yields in primitive life to the importance of the choral *vocero* over a dead clansman; so that, using the terms in a modern way, one must reverse that saying of the preacher: it was death that was stronger than love. Coming back to modern survivals, one finds this *vocero* common, both in its individual and in its choral form, among the Celts. Leaving the Ossianic lament alone in its gloom, one may take the honest and homely prose of Pennant,[2] who made a tour through Scotland in the year 1769, and saw a lyke-wake[3]— he calls it a "late-wake"—in the Highlands. "The evening after the death of any person, the relatives and friends of the deceased meet at the house, attended by bagpipe and fiddle; the nearest of kin, be it wife, son, or daughter, opens a melancholy ball, dancing and greeting, *i.e.* crying violently, at the same time; and this continues till daylight, but with such gambols and frolics among the younger part of the company that the loss which occasioned them is often more than supplied by the consequences of that night." This is eighteenth-century humour, and an eighteenth-century reason to explain the hilarity is quoted from Olaus Magnus. Unfortunately Pennant did not hear what he calls the "Coranich";

[1] Grosse, *Anfänge der Kunst*, p. 234.

[2] *A Tour in Scotland*, 3d. ed., Warrington, 1774, p. 99.

[3] Chaucer, who puts several home touches not known to Boccaccio or Statius into his account of the funeral of Arcite in the "Knight's Tale," speaks of the *lyche-wake* as well as of the *wake-pleyes*, — the latter, of course, funeral games. Pennant, by the way, in his *Second Tour in Scotland* (Pinkerton, III. 288), speaking of Islay and its antiquities, says "the late-wakes or funerals . . . were attended *with sports and dramatic entertainments*. . . . The subject of the drama was historical *and preserved by memory*." (No italics in the original.)

but he learned that such a song is generally in praise of the dead, a recital of his deeds or the deeds of his forbears. Questions, too, were addressed to the corpse, why, for example, he chose to die — a common trait of the *vocero*, already put to use by Chaucerian humour,[1] and noted by old Camden; Pennant remarks that the mother of Euryalus makes the same query.[2] But Pennant had heard such songs in the south of Ireland; and this feature of an Irish wake is still accessible to the curious. On its native soil it has been often studied and described.[3] When the corpse has been laid out, "the women of the household range themselves at either side, and the keen (*caoine*) at once commences. They rise with one accord, and moving their bodies with a slow motion to and fro, their arms apart, they . . . keep up a heart-rending cry. This cry is interrupted for a while to give the *ban caointhe*, the leading keener, an opportunity of commencing. At the close of every stanza of the dirge the cry is repeated." The authors give the air to which keens are chanted. "The keen usually consists in an address to the corpse, asking him, 'Why did he die?' — or a description of his person, qualifications, riches; it is altogether extemporaneous." A note attributes the ease of improvisation to the fact that assonance, "vocal rime," is enough to satisfy the needs of Irish verse. The keener is often a professional and paid; sometimes a volunteer and a member of the family. "Any one present, however, who has the gift, may put in his or her verse; and this sometimes occurs. . . . Besides *caoines*,

[1] See above, p. 222.

[2] *Æn.*, X. 473 ff.

[3] Perhaps best in Mr. and Mrs. S. C. Hall's *Ireland: its Scenery, Character*, etc., 3 vols., London, 1841–1843. See I. 222 ff. The authors mention the women who wept over Hector, with the odd explanation that the Greeks were once in Ireland. Other accounts of Irish funerals are quoted in Brand-Ellis, *Popular Antiquities*, as of "the men, women, and children" who go before the corpse and "set up a most hideous *Holoo, loo, loo*, which may be heard two or three miles round the country."

extempore compositions over the dead, *thirrios*, or written elegies, deserve mention. They are composed almost exclusively by men, as the *caoines* are by women." One thinks of Marcaggi's poetical bandits and their written effusions as compared with the improvised songs of the *voceratrice* over her dead. It is odd to see how the zeal of certain antiquarians would reverse the law of nature, and make this improvised keen a degenerate form of older and carefully composed elegies of Irish "bards." O'Conor thought the old keen to be "debased by extemporaneous composition";[1] and a Mr. Blanford[2] describes the degradation in detail. The keen, he says, was once an antiphonal affair prepared beforehand, and sung by bards with the aid of a chorus, — elaborate in every way. On the decline of these bards, "the Caoinan fell into the hands of women, and became an extemporaneous performance." Like the degeneration theory of ballads, this account of the keen goes to pieces under the test of comparative and historical studies. Spenser, to be sure, speaks of these bards, and not without respect;[3] but it is clear that the ancestral line of the keen among Irishmen runs back to "the lamentations at theyr burialls, with dispayrefull outcryes and immoderate wailings,"[4] which he mentions in his argument to prove that the Irish are descended from the Scythians. Would that Spenser had not cut short his tale

[1] Quoted by J. C. Walker, *Historical Memoirs of the Irish Bards*, London, 1786, pp. 20 f. The keening of women who follow the hearse, dressed sometimes in white and sometimes in black, "singing as they slowly proceed . . . extempore odes," is sufficiently like the march of the *praeficae* at a Roman funeral; and in neither case has one the primitive form of the rite.

[2] *Transact. Royal Irish Academy*, IV., "Antiquities," pp. 41 ff., read December, 1791.

[3] "Present State of Ireland," *Works*, ed. Morris, pp. 625 f. Camden, about the same time, *Britannia*, trans., ed. 1722, p. xix, speaks of the bards as men who "besides . . . their poetic functions do apply themselves particularly to the study of genealogies." See also Evan Evans, *Specimens of the Poetry of the Antient Welsh Bards*, . . . London, 1764, p. 91. This is not primitive song.

[4] Spenser, p. 633.

"of theyr old maner of marrying, of burying, of dauncyng, of singing, of feasting, of cursing, *though Christians have wiped out the most part of them*," — best reason for telling in detail of all the Christians had left!

Wailings, cries now articulate and now inarticulate, but wrought by repetition, by the cadence of rocking bodies, or of measured steps, by the spasmodic utterance of extreme emotion, into a choral consent which is not harmony, perhaps, to modern ears, but which has a rhythm of its own, — these are the raw material of the poetry of grief. Like the "cries" at a Gascon burial, like the Irish keen, is the *rauda* of Russian Lithuania, which Bartsch[1] significantly calls "a preliminary stage of actual folksong." This *rauda* or *daina* is sung by women; it lacks what one calls melody and verse; and it is sung mostly on the way to the burial or at the grave. Prætorius, at the end of the seventeenth century, describes the Lithuanian *vocero* as a mingled song and sob, with the usual questions to the corpse, so familiar in the Irish keen — why did the man die, had he not enough to eat and drink, had he not clothes and shoes?[2] Brand, who made his tour in 1673, tells the same story; relatives and friends, however, are here seated round the corpse, shrieking and howling, to be sure, but in words of a more lyric tone: "Why hast thou

[1] "Totenklagen in der litauischen Volksdichtung," *Zst. f. vgl. Litteraturgesch.*, N. F., II. 81 ff.

[2] A similar series of questions, with interesting details of the ceremony, is given in the *Itinera Constantinopolitanum et Amasianum* ab Angerio Gislenio Busbequij . . . Antverpiæ, 1681, p. 28: "deuertimus in pagum Semianorum Iagodnam: ubi ejus gentis ritus funebres vidimus multum à nostris abhorrentes. Erat cadauer in templo positum detecta facie: iuxtà erant apposita edulia, panis et caro et vini cantharus: adstabant coniunx et filia melioribus ornata vestibus, filiae galerius erat ex plumis pavonis. Supremum munus, quo maritum jam conclamatum uxor donauit, pileolum fuit purpureum, cuius modi virgines nubiles illic gestare solent. Inde lessum audiuimus et naeniam lamentabilesque voces; quibus mortuum percunctabantur *quid de eo tantum meruissent, quae res, quod obsequium, quod solatium ei defuisset; cur se solas et miseras relinqueret: et hujus generis alia.*"

left us? Whither art thou gone? I shall go to thee, but thou wilt not come to me."[1]

Enough has been said to show the origins of the *vocero* in Europe. Among the Tartar folk of Siberia, songs of lament, although nearly always improvised, have more the character of an elegy, and are sung by the relatives of the dead during a full year after the funeral.[2] If the husband dies, it is his wife who makes the song; if son or daughter dies, it is the mother; while a dead mother is sung by her daughter or a near female relative. Men sing these songs only when a rich or powerful person dies, and then only at the funeral:[3] one thinks of David over Jonathan and Saul, and of that old king in the *Béowulf*. Among the Eskimo,[4] however, occurs a *vocero* precisely like the type which has been found common to the primitive customs of Europe, — a song by the near relative, with chorus of moans, sobs, and cries from the women who stand about. Coming to the distinctly savage state, one finds material enough to fill a book, all going to prove that a choral cry and not an individual composition must be taken as starting-point of the *vocero*. "Of the Tasmanians, Mr. Davis relates[5] that 'during the whole of the first night[6]

[1] Compare the pathetic word of David about his dead child: 2 Sam., xii. 23.

[2] Spencer, *Sociology*, I. § 142, quotes Bancroft, of the Indians of the West, that for a long time after a death, relatives repair daily at sunrise and sunset to the vicinity of the grave, to sing songs of mourning and praise. Hahn tells the same thing of his Albanians, *Alb. Stud.*, I. 151 f.

[3] Radloff, III. 22.

[4] Often quoted from Kranz, *Grönländische Reise*. See also Boas, "The Central Eskimo," in *Report Bur. Ethn.*, 1884-1885, Washington, 1888, p. 614.

[5] Quoted Spencer, *Soc.*, III. § 126.

[6] There was also a lament sung hard upon the death of a warrior in battle. As the Goths bore away their dead king, singing a song of woe in the midst of flying weapons, so with many savages. In a skirmish which followed the murder of Captain Cook, a young islander was killed, and the Englishmen next morning saw "some men carrying him off on their shoulders, and could hear them singing, as they marched, a mournful song." Cook's Last Voyage, in Pinkerton, *Voyages and Travels*, XI. 723.

after the death of one of their tribe they will sit round the body, using rapidly a low, continuous recitative, to prevent the evil spirit from taking it away.'" Naturally the artist comes early upon the scene; dirges, eulogies, elegies of every sort, are built on this choral foundation; and that communal magic, if it was anything more than a Tasmanian *vocero*, is soon replaced by the magic of the individual shaman. To put him in the van of funeral lament, however, to say that he preceded communal and choral wailings for the dead, is ignoring the facts of primitive life and the instincts of human nature. Comparetti makes the magic songs of the Finns precede their heroic and legendary verse, and this may well be true; but the communal lament is older than both, for, as was seen in the case of the Botocudos, primitive folk have no legend, no history, and as for the magic, while the sayings of a shaman would get the earliest record, they demand a communal background. For it is the unavoidable condition of all recorded literature that what is of the moment and of the mass dies with its occasion; while only individual skill, the hand of a single performer, is moved to keep the record of his doing on purpose to a life beyond life. Even the humblest shaman, too, learns his art and his rude ritual from an older artist in magic,[1] and so his making becomes a tradition and his verses flit from mouth to mouth. But the history of religion has taught us to look elsewhere than to the temple and the priest and the Deus Optimus Maximus of civilized worship, if we would find the beginnings of cult and the earliest divinity. As we go back to a horde of homogeneous men, so we go back to a horde of homogeneous spirits; as one spirit rises above the rest, so the shaman is deputed, with his superior powers,[2] to cope

[1] On *neniae* as incantations, see Grimm, *Mythologie*,[4] p. 1027.

[2] The phrase for a capable person in incantation is found for Germanic usage in the Merseburg Charm, here said of Wodan himself, — *sô hê unola conda;* in

with the superior god. It was the "we" of the horde, in the new sense of coherence and social being, which started that communal thinking and made that communal belief in the "they" of a surrounding and potent host of spirits; and it is not unreasonable to suppose that communal appeal, sheer cries and leaps in some wild consent of rhythm, must have begun those magic rites which are perhaps to be surmised in no very advanced stage in the songs of Mr. Davis's Tasmanians. Actual incantations that come down to us are full of repetition, and frequently have a chorus or refrain;[1] elements that point back to a communal source. Among American Indians the necromantic songs abound in a chorus which is nearly all repetition, like[2] —

Na ha, Yaw ne;
Na ha, Yaw ne.

But it is the *vocero* which we are now to study among savage tribes. A case or so from Africa and Asia will do for that side of the world — evidence is more than abundant — and then America may tell its tale at a time when borrowing is out of the question. M. Adanson, a correspondent of the Royal Academy of Sciences, travelled in Senegal about 1750;

Anglo-Saxon the same phrase is used for a skilled poet: *se þe cuðe*, *Béow.*, 90; and in Old Saxon for a wise man: *ên gifrôdôt man the sô filo konsta wisaro wordo*, *Hêliand*, 208.

[1] For example, in mere invocation, the *Erce, Erce, Erce, eorðan modor* of an Anglo-Saxon charm (Grein-Wülker, I. 314), and the actual spell against stitch in the side (*ibid.*, p. 318): —

Wert thou shot in the fell, or wert shot in the flesh,
Or wert shot in the blood [or wert shot in the bone],
Or wert shot in the limb . . .

with more of the sort, and the solemn, —

This to heal shot of gods, this to heal shot of elves,

and so on, with a refrain in the epic part, —

Out, little spear, if it in here be!

[2] Schoolcraft, *Indian Tribes*, I. 367 ff.

his account[1] of *vocero* and dance is fairly representative of the case. One night in a village he was awakened by a "horrid shrieking," and found that a young woman had just died. What follows is interesting for comparison with the custom in modern Greece. "The first shriek was made," says M. Adanson, "according to custom, by one of the female relations of the deceased before her door. At this signal, all the women in the village came out and set up a most terrible howl, so that one would have thought they were all related to the deceased;" the traveller forgets that in certain levels of culture the clan, even the horde, is above kin. The noise lasted till break of day; relatives then went into the dead woman's cottage, took her hand, and asked her questions, — the common trait of the *vocero* everywhere. When she was buried, the lamentations ceased; but for three nights the young people danced a memorial dance. At this the performers sang a song, "the burden of which was repeated by all the spectators." Then follows the description of certain erotic features of the dance, and the usual testimony to that exactness of time observed in song and movement and gesture. The *vocero* itself is mainly a lament; Mungo Park speaks of "the loud and dismal howlings," another of "leaping and dancing"; while in Loango relatives "weep, sing, and dance" about the corpse.[2] In Korea, after a night of merriment the body is carried to its tomb; "the bearers sing and keep time as they go, whilst the kindred and friends . . . make the air ring with their cries." [3]

Interesting are the accounts of American Indians in the days of discovery. Jean de Lery, a Frenchman who went to Brazil with the Protestant emigrants in the sixteenth century,

[1] Translated from the French in Pinkerton's *Voyages and Travels*, XVI. 598 ff. See pp. 623 f.

[2] *Ibid.*, XVI. 877, 685, 596.

[3] *Ibid.*, VII. 534.

and wrote an account of his journey,[1] was struck by the likeness between the funeral laments made by savages, and the *voceri* of the women of Béarn singing over their dead husbands. He quotes one, a good document. "'La mi amou, La mi amou: Cara rident, œil de splendou: Cama lengé, bet dansadou: Lo mé balen, Lo m'esburbat: Matî depes: fort tard au lheit.' That is to say, 'my love, my love, laughing face, fine eye, light limb, brave dancer, valiant mien, lovely mien, early up and late to bed.'" So too the Gascon women: "'Yere, yere, o le bet renegadou, o le bet iougadou qu 'here': that is to say, 'O the brave Protestant, O the brave player that he was!' And so do our poor American women, who, besides a refrain for each stanza,[2] always throw in a 'He is dead, he is dead, for whom we now are mourning,' whereupon the men respond and say: 'Alas, it is true; we shall never see him more until we are behind the mountains, where, as our Caribs tell us, we shall dance with him'—and other things of the sort, which they add in their response." Lescarbot,[3] quoting Lery about the Brazilians, remarks the agreement in songs of lament between them and the Canadians "fifteen hundred leagues away." Such a song ran—

Hé hé hé hé hé hé hé hé hé hé,

a monotonous performance on paper, with the notes *fa fa sol fa fa sol sol sol sol sol*, not too elaborate music; but bodily graces made up for this, since they then "shrieked and cried in fearful wise the space of a quarter-hour, and the women leaped into the air with such violence as to foam at the mouth." Then once more the tuneful mood began, and they

[1] *Histoire d'un Voyage fait en la Terre de Bresil autrement dite Amerique* . . . a la Rochelle, MDLXXVII. pp. 336 f.

[2] "Au surplus au refrein de chacune pose."

[3] *Histoire de la nouvelle France*, Paris, MDCIX. See pp. 691 ff. On the title-page he declares himself "témoin oculaire d'une partie des choses ici recitées."

sang, "Heu heüraüre heüra heüraüre heüra heüra onech." In this song they are mourning for their dead parents. As with Lery and Lescarbot, so the spirit of comparison is astir in Lafitau,[1] who, however, has less to tell of folklore at home, and a great deal to say of the ancients, as may be gathered from the title of his book; the laments for the dead he calls *nénies,* and speaks of the "matron" who plays the part of *praefica.* He tells, however, a plain story of the savage customs. When a corpse has been dressed and laid in state, tears and lamentations, restrained up to that time, begin to break forth, but in order and cadence. The "matron" leads the other women, who "follow in the same measure, *but use different words, according to the relation which they bear to the deceased,*" — second stage of the *vocero,* with a survival of the chorus, however, far more pronounced than in Corsica. Men, too, mourn their dead, but in a nobler way, singing the death-song and dancing the hereditary dance;[2] but these *voceri* of the women are of great interest. Grosse[3] quotes from Grey the Australian *vocero* for a young man, where "the young women sing — 'My young brother,' — the old women sing — 'My young son,' — and all in chorus sing — 'Never shall I see thee again, Never shall I see thee again.'"

In Schoolcraft's[4] time things had undergone no great change; for "every person aggrieved makes his own com-

[1] *Mœurs des Sauvages Ameriquians, Comparées aux Mœurs des Premières Temps,* . . . 2 vols., 4to, Paris, 1724. See II. 321. Lafitau spent five years in a mission in Canada, and also got information from a brother Jesuit of sixty years' experience in the new world (I. 2). It was this book which moved Dr. John Brown, a century and a half ago, to write his essay on the history of poetry and music, and to use so effectively the comparative method in literature.

[2] *Ibid.,* II. 395.

[3] *Anf. d. K.,* p. 229.

[4] *Indian Tribes,* IV. 71, question 254 (see I. 556): "Is it the custom to call on certain persons for these laments? Are the laments themselves of a poetic character?" Answered by Mr. Fletcher for the Winnebago Indians.

plaint, and it is pitiful to see a married person commence wailing and singing *kitchina takah,* then wailing again *kitchina,* — 'men's friend.' These are all the words," — a significant fact. "The same way in other deaths the deceased is bewailed." Here is the single *vocero;* but it is a faint affair in comparison with the volume and sound of the funeral chorus. Schoolcraft's evidence all runs this way. "Choruses," says Mr. Fletcher,[1] "are about all the Indians sing." Carver,[2] to be sure, like the other travellers, tells of a mother who seemed to improvise a song of lament over her dead child at the time when it was laid among the branches; but he is emphatic about the chorus, and calls it "a not unpleasing but savage harmony." A recent writer,[3] noting the monotonous choral songs at funerals, thinks "these chants may no doubt occasionally have been simply wailing or mourning ejaculation." As one comes to lower levels of culture, among the Patagonians, for example, and the interior tribes of Africa, mere choral iteration of monotonous sounds and beating the ground with the feet — perhaps not so much "to keep off the evil one"[4] as to find the communal consent — are the prevailing characteristics of the *vocero.* The funeral dance of the Latuka, which Baker saw,[5] really comes to this; while the feathers, the bells, the horns, are easily recognized as lendings of an incipient culture, and teach the plain lesson that the state of the African savage is not to be transferred outright to primitive man. Indeed, it is quite evident that such perfect consent of communal voice and step as was shown by the Botocudos may be confused and broken in what one must call higher stages of culture, — for example,

[1] *Ibid.*, answer to question 253.

[2] *Three Years' Travel through the Interior Parts of North America* (1766–1768), Philadelphia, 1796. See p. 179.

[3] *Rep. Bureau Ethnol.*, I. 194 f.

[4] Wallaschek, *Prim. Mus.*, p. 54.

[5] *Ibid.*, p. 198.

that dance of the Latuka. In Nubia Miss Edwards[1] saw a ceremony, mainly dance, at the grave of a member of the tribe, which seemed to her artificial in the extreme. "The lamentation itself is a definite musical phrase executed by women who, beginning on a high note, proceed down the scale in third-tones to the lower octave or even the twelfth. It is taught, like the *zaghareet*, or cry of joy, by mothers to their young daughters in their earliest years." It is only when the historian looks at all this evidence of savage dance and cry, of feminine song and choral response, of refrain passing into rite and myth, of detached and artistic lament, and when he applies to it the evolutionary test, the comparative and historical test, that it lies in true perspective and allows him to draw some definite conclusion about one at least of the beginnings of poetry. The *vocero* began as communal wailing, horde or clan or house mourning the brother and inmate in rhythmic cries to the cadence of the dance; with new domestic ties of blood, in which of course the mother and sister are supreme,[2] these two stand out as singers of the solitary *vocero* to which the crowd makes answer in refrain. The inevitable sundering of individual and chorus now makes headway, the former passing into literature, the latter, dropping its concomitant dance and surviving as refrain, dies slowly out in all save a few isolated communities, and in all recorded verse except here and there a chanted dirge. But in each of these diverging fortunes, as in the earliest, so in the last estate of the *vocero*, in elegy, threnody, ode, one common trait abides; and everywhere it echoes the insistent

[1] Wallaschek, *Prim. Mus.*, p. 199. It is needless to insist on the custom of dancing at funerals, and, in memorial rites, over the graves of the dead; mediæval councils were full of warning against this habit. The "dance of death," of course, became symbolic and artistic.

[2] Denied as a literal fact, as an affair of government and authority, the matriarchate, so called, is sufficiently proved as the early form of family life.

voice of repetition.[1] As an example of this repetition, as well as of the *vocero* in its earlier stage, we may conclude with an iterated verse sung by a negro woman, once a slave, who still lived with her master's family in the South.[2] She had just buried her husband, but went about her tasks as usual and waited upon the children of the house. Suddenly, however, in their presence, and to their great fright, she burst out with these words, —

O dem ropes dat let him down!

and continued to sing them without ceasing, in a strange crooning way, the better part of an hour, and at intervals during some days. It were to consider too curiously, perhaps, if one should compare this crude case of "vision" with certain forms of poetry that bear a similar relation to the original song of grief.

So much for the *vocero*. It has led us from the ballads back to that ethnological evidence making so strongly, in diction as in rhythm, for the primitive note of iteration, for the fundamental element which marks the communal origin of poetry, precisely as variation has marked its individual and artistic course. Repetition of sounds, when joined with act of labour, with march or dance, with strong emotion of a festal or communal kind, made possible the perception of consent, or, to speak with Professor Baldwin Brown, of order. It begets this sense of order in other arts; repetition of a certain kind of line on a jar made a

[1] As the clan or horde had its song of triumph, and this is echoed and prolonged in "national" songs like the *Marseillaise*, or, better, the *Ça ira*, so the clan grief can expand into a national lament. Something of this sort is found in that wail over the downfall of their power sung by the Moors in Spain and so potent to stir the heart that it was forbidden by government; its refrain, *Woe is me, Alhama*, has all the iterated passion of grief that one finds in the primitive *vocero*. Then there is the song or psalm of the captives in Babylon, — and the list could be extended indefinitely.

[2] The story is at first hand.

rhythm of decoration, just as a series of similar groups of words, of steps, made poetry and dance. How important repetition must have been in early poetry, and in any unrecorded verse, is clear when one reflects that the invention of writing turned poetry from an art wholly of time and succession to an art half plastic; we see the line, the stanza, nowadays, and repetition is an impertinence in poetry, because hearing has become a secondary and imagined process. The æsthetic value of repetition in primitive verse gets a new aspect when one considers

> Wie das Wort so wichtig dort war,
> Weil es ein gesprochen Wort war;

although that other protest is right enough for one who has only modern poetry in view: —

> Im Anfang war das Wort? . . .
> Ich kann das Wort so hoch unmöglich schätzen.

For repetition as the main element in savage poetry it is useless to spread out evidence; no one denies the fact, and ethnology is full of it. From surviving incremental repetition, as in the *Kalevala* and in the ballads, one passes back, with the increment steadily diminishing, to outright and unrelieved iteration. The Africans have songs, some of them known as "national," which consist of a single word, arranged in rude rhythmic groups, repeated for hours; and they get as much satisfaction from it as presumably those Ephesians got out of their own vehement and repeated cry. Lery and Lescarbot heard these songs of an iterated word. Lafitau[1] says that Father Marquette saw Indians dance the calumet dance, and was surprised "that the slave in singing said nothing but the single word *Alleluia,*" — of course an accidental coincidence of sounds, — "pronouncing the *u* after the Italian fashion, and dividing the word into two parts."

[1] Work quoted, II. 324.

The iterated word in primitive song has its meaning somewhere, but often shades back into an inarticulate sound, and shades forward into a traditional and unintelligible cry, mere relief of emotion. Perhaps words of this sort went with the "detestable air" which Mary Shelley heard at the *festas* near her house in Italy.[1] The countryfolk, "like wild savages, . . . in different bands, the sexes always separate, pass the whole night in dancing on the sands close to our door, running into the sea, then back again, all the time yelling one detestable air at the top of their voices, — the most detestable air in the world." The favourite song of the Botocudos, their lyric mainstay, was just *Kălăuī ahâ*, repeated indefinitely. The chorus of Indian war-songs, in North America, "consists for the most part of traditionary monosyllables which appear to admit often of transposition, and the utterance of which, at least, is so managed as to permit the words to be sung in strains to suit the music and dance."[2] Dr. Brinton, in a summary of the characteristics of American aboriginal poetry,[3] — which was always sung, — noting that repetition is the groundwork, says that this element of iteration has two forms: a verse is sung repeatedly, which of course makes some statement, or there is a repeated refrain; but this refrain is wholly interjectional and meaningless. The Fuegians often sing not so much as a word, but only a syllable repeated forever. Progress is in the text, and by the individual; communal reminiscence is in the refrain: it is clear, then, that the refrain is the

[1] Account of Shelley's last days, quoted in *Harper's Magazine*, April, 1892, p. 786.

[2] Schoolcraft, III. 326, "Poetic Development of the Indian Mind." For a good collection of facts about iterated words as song, see the sixth chapter of Wallaschek's *Primitive Music*. For example, p. 173, "The Macusi Indians in Guiana amuse themselves for hours with singing a monotonous song, whose words, *hai-a*, *hai-a*, have no further significance." See also pp. 54, 56 f.

[3] *Report Proceed. Numism. and Antiquar. Soc., Philadelphia*, 1887, pp. 18 f. (Printed 1891.)

original "poem," and to the refrain one must look for an idea of beginnings. A. W. Schlegel[1] conjectured that the earliest forms of lyric poetry were due to an "effort of the human heart to express a feeling or mood and to give it permanence by tone and rhythm," this effort resulting at first "in simple words and interjections often repeated." These are kept in the chorus or refrain; incremental repetition, as was shown above, works its way in the text. The chorus, to be sure, rises soon to the dignity of a coherent sentence; but its communal and retrograde force still is strong, and it insists on naked repetition, while individual singers cherish the increment. Miss Kingsley[2] heard the Bubis sing in chorus over and over for hours this verse and nothing more, —

The shark bites the Bubi's hand.

A more advanced stage is seen in the cautious but distinct incremental repetition of a singer among the North American Indians; we quote from Schoolcraft:[3] —

Ningah peendegay aindahyaig:
We he heway . . .[4]

That is, "I will walk into somebody's home." The following words proceed very cautiously. "The composer appears to commence with delicacy . . . singing that he would walk into some indefinite home. The next line implies that he will walk into his or her home. In the third line . . . he

[1] Lectures, as quoted, II. 117, speaking of poetry before Homer. On the origin of poetry in unintelligible sounds, see Ragusa-Moleti, *Poesie dei Popoli Selvaggi*, Torino-Palermo, 1891, pp. vi ff., and Jacobowski, *Anfänge der Poesie*, p. 66, who assumes that early man held fast to those tones and gestures which expressed an original sensation or emotion. On the repetition of mere sounds to express emotion, see Alice C. Fletcher, *Journal American Folklore*, April–June, 1898, p. 87.

[2] *Travels in West Africa*, pp. 66 f.

[3] V. 559 ff. "Original Words of Indian Songs literally translated."

[4] "Choral chant, four times repeated." All Schoolcraft's examples here are full of repetition.

will walk into her home during some night. He then informs her that he will walk into her dwelling during the winter. In the fifth line" — it is really a stanza, with that eternal chorus — "he becomes decisive and bold, and says he will walk into her lodge this night." So, too, the warrior sings:[1] —

I will kill, I will kill,
The Americans I will kill!

But the repeated air of that "cereal chorus,"[2] when a girl gets a crooked ear at the husking, has the stricter note: —

Wagemin, wagemin,
Paimosaid:
Wagemin, wagemin,
Paimosaid.

The work of developing poetry from a rhythmic chaos of wild and repeated cries up to a chorus of this kind was a communal achievement; art is responsible for increment and variation. Communal consent in rhythm caused the repetition of more or less articulate sounds, and so developed that most important element in primitive speech now known as emphasis. Repetition, which is modern emphasis in sections, marks the event or sensation which it records as something out of the common, holds it in the ear and before the mind as something to note and to keep noting, and so makes for memory, not idly called the mother of the muses, while it heightens the actual emotional state. Just as certain early efforts of plastic art expressed great wisdom by several heads, great strength by a number of hands, great fecundity by many breasts, so early man by the iteration of a word gave it poetic force; a better art seeks perfection of the single feature, and fitness of the single word. It has been shown already how poetry made a gain when repetition of a

[1] *Ibid.*, III. 328.

[2] *Ibid.*, V. 563 f. See below, p. 310.

certain number of sounds gave ease to the instinct for harmony, and a yet greater gain when the regular recurrence of a louder sound or a longer sound satisfied the craving for finer distinctions;[1] it has been shown how the mere zeal of repetition was crossed by increment and variation, until the oldest element of poetry was made superfluous in the plainer form and was almost utterly driven out of diction, with no refuge but rhythm and certain forms of lyric sacred and profane. In this plain and outright form of repeated words, however, it lingered long in ballads, in festal rites, and of course among the savages; it is in the refrain, therefore, that one can still find some hints of the actual beginnings of poetry. The refrain has been touched incidentally in the treatment of repetition; it is now to be considered for itself.[2] Important as it is in ballads, the refrain has even weightier meanings when studied in what may be called the occasional poetry of the people.

The refrain, which in its communal function survives as

[1] See above on Rhythm. In addition to the references given there, see some sensible remarks in Emerson's "Poetry and Imagination"; for scientific discussion of repetition as basis of rhythm, see Gurney, *Power of Sound*, pp. 455 f., and Masing, *über Ursprung u. Verbreitung des Reims*, pp. 9 f. J. Grimm pointed out that alliteration is really a form of repetition, *Kl. Schr.*, VI. 161 f. Adam Smith, *Essays*, pp. 154 f., has some curious remarks on repetition as possible in music, but impossible in poetry.

[2] W. von Biedermann, in two articles, — "Zur vergleichenden Geschichte der poetischen Formen," *Zeitschr. f. Vergl. Litteraturgesch.*, N. F., II. 415 ff.; IV. 224 ff., and "Die Wiederholung als Urform der Dichtung bei Goethe," *ibid.*, IV. 267 ff., — traces the development of poetical style from this fundamental fact of repetition. First, simple words were repeated, then only part of the words in a sentence: such is the case in old Chinese, in Zend, in Accadian. Then came parallelism; then the repetition of similar sounds; *and finally metre or rhythm* (*Versmass*). Where were the dancing throngs in this interesting stretch of development, with rhythm as an afterclap of rime? As later in his review of Bücher's *Arbeit und Rhythmus*, so here, Biedermann denies that rhythm came into poetry through music and the dance. He fails, however, to make good this assertion by any show of proof (see above, p. 75); but his references are useful for the student of repetition. For another scheme of repetition in poetry, see R. M. Meyer, *Altgermanische Poesie*, pp. 12 f.

repetition pure and simple practised by the throng, and in its artistic function has come to be the means of marking off a strophe or stanza, is really the discredited and impoverished heir of that choral song which by general consent stands at the beginning of all poetry. This choral song, under the influence of art and the reflecting, remembering, individual mind, was developed into such forms of epic, drama, lyric, as meet us, more or less divested of communal traits and conditions, on the threshold of every national literature. Greek tragedy is a well-known case in point. The refrain, however, is not a development but a survival,[1] so far, at least, as communal conditions are involved; and even in ballads what is called the refrain or the burden is a slowly yielding communal element fighting hopelessly against invading elements of art. In other words, as the ballad recedes into primitive conditions, the refrain grows more and more insistent, so that for the earliest form of the ballad, now nowhere to be found, but easy to reconstruct by the help of an evident evolutionary curve, one must assume not the refrain as such, but rather choral song outright. Different altogether from this communal survival is the artistic use of the refrain. The extreme of art and often of artifice is reached in those forms of verse which were developed out of the older minstrelsy of France, and are known as *ballade*, *rondel*, *triolet*, *chant royal*, with a refrain as their distinguishing feature; it is conceded, however, that in the first instance this refrain was everywhere taken from popular song.[2]

[1] Hence the inadequate character of its treatment, say for Old Norse, by Vigfusson and Powell, *Corp. Poet. Bor.*, I. 451 ff. R. M. Meyer, *Altgerm. Poesie*, p. 341, takes a more excellent way, but he lays too much stress on the ancient refrain, and not enough on the ancient choral and the primitive communal conditions of song. Much more to the point is the admirable though incomplete chapter on "Early Choral Song" in Posnett's *Comparative Literature:* see especially pp. 127 ff.

[2] Wolf, *Lais*, pp. 23 f. The refrain was insistent in all poetry of the troubadours and trouvères, and so leads back to refrains as the prevalent characteristic

Learned poetry of the Middle Ages,[1] to be sure, imitated not the vernacular refrain, but the refrain of classical verse; this, however, in its turn had been taken from the poetry of the people, and, whether one considers the *Hymen, O Hymenaee* of Catullus,[2] or the later *Cras amet qui nunquam amavit,* which trips so featly through the *Pervigilium Veneris*[3] and keeps such true step with the popular rhythm of its stanzas, is at no great remove from communal song.

But refrains of artistic poetry are of subordinate interest for our study of primitive verse; and it is clear that all investigations which neglect the older and more popular phases, which neglect the primitive choral song and the primitive communal conditions, can lead to no valid conclusions about the refrain. It is something, of course, when Bujeaud explains this or that refrain of a modern song as imitated from sounds of some musical instrument, or taken from the *argot* of the streets;[4] but when Rosières[5] undertakes to tell the whole

of all songs in the vernacular. See Wolf's references, pp. 22 ff., and notes, pp. 184 ff. For a modern study of this development of artistic forms of the refrain, see the third chapter of the third part of Jeanroy's excellent *Origines de la Poésie Lyrique en France au Moyen Age,* Paris, 1889.

[1] Ebert, *Lit. d. Mittelalters,* II. 63 f., 64 note.

[2] See lxi, lxii. The Hymen cry, taken from the Greek, was there a lending of communal wedding songs: see Smythe, *Greek Melic Poets,* p. 496. More artistic refrains are the

Currite ducentes subtegmina, currite, fusi,

of Catullus, lxiv. 323 ff., and the recurrent lines in Spenser's *Prothalamion* and *Epithalamium,* which, of course, are on the same artistic plane with that marriage-song of Peleus and Thetis.

[3] Walter Pater's pleasant account of the making of this song (*Marius the Epicurean,* p. 73) is not improbable, in spirit at least; and it must be borne in mind that this was the metre of marching songs of Roman soldiers and other popular verse. See Du Meril, *Poésies Populaires Latines,* Paris, 1843, pp. 106–117, including the *Pervigilium Veneris.*

[4] Bujeaud, "Refrains des Chansons Populaires," in *Le Courier Littéraire,* 25 Mai, 1877, pp. 256 ff. For reference to this article, the present writer is indebted to Boynton's dissertation, named and quoted below.

[5] "Le Refrain dans la Littérature du Moyen Age," in *Revue des Traditions Populaires,* III. 1 ff.; 82 ff.

story of the refrain, and settle its origins beyond doubt, saying now that it "springs from the periodic return of full sounds," now that it is a *tra-la-la* to take the place of musical instruments, now that it is "a little poem stuck in all the fissures of a big poem," and now, with a passing recognition of communal conditions, but with sufficient vagueness, that it voices popular song, then, indeed, one feels the vanity of dogmatizing to the full.[1] The need of comparative, historical, and genetic study is also evident in a similar essay on the refrain in Middle High German. Freericks[2] regards the original refrain not as repetition of the words of a singer but as an expression of sentiment which they evoke, coming back in cries of sorrow or of joy. "When utterances of this sort continually interrupt the song, there is the refrain in its simplest form." So too Minor,[3] in his book on German metres, calls the refrain "the original cry of the throng in answer to the song of the singer." Against all this, Dr. R. M. Meyer, in two essays,[4] makes emphatic and successful protest. With an eye on conditions and not on theory, Meyer shows the refrain to belong to the oldest poetry of man, — inarticulate cries at first, in rhythmic sequence, to express fear, wonder, grief, affection. The refrain, for example, is the original part of a threnody, as we have seen very plainly in our study of the *vocero;* in short, so far from being an aftergrowth of communal song, this refrain is declared by Dr. Meyer to be the very root of the matter. With more attention to choral

[1] J. Darmesteter, *Chants Pop. des Afghans*, Paris, 1888–1890, p. cxcvi, calls the strophe "abstraction faite du refrain," — a more excellent way than these theorists take with their "little poem stuck in the cracks of a big poem," and such clever nonsense.

[2] "Der Kehrreim in der mhd. Dichtung," *Jahresber. d. Königl. Gymnas. zu Paderborn*, 1890.

[3] *Neuhochdeutsche Metrik*, p. 392. See R. M. Meyer, below.

[4] *Zeitschr. f. vergleich. Lit.*, I. 34 ff.; *Euphorion, Zeitschr. f. Litteraturgesch.*, V. (1898), 1 ff. He points out that nobody heeded his view of the case, but that the works of Grosse, Groos, and Bücher all brought confirmation to it.

song in the horde or clan, Posnett has come closer to the facts than Meyer, who failed to appreciate all the communal conditions of such early verse; for while Meyer referred to inarticulate cries as a beginning of the refrain, it is evident that these immediately formed the chorus, and that the refrain is rather survival and deputy of this old chorus than the chorus outright. The refrain, in other words, allows one to feel one's way back to the choral song of the horde,[1] but is not to be transferred to those primitive times even in its unintelligible and inarticulate forms. To make this clear, we must study the refrain in its various communal survivals.

Records of early literature and early religion show the refrain in its original guise as a part of the choral song, and it echoes audibly the steps of the dance. Nowhere is this echo more insistent than in that hymn of the Arval brothers, sung, of course, with a dance that was confined to the priests, and already come a long way from the shouting and leaping throng of primitive time; nevertheless, as a hymn used in processions about the fields, it is to be connected with the survivals of similar rites and the songs still heard from European peasants at the harvest-home. In the inscription which preserves it, each verse, except the last, is given thrice.[2] A free translation[3] follows: —

Help us, O Lares, help us, Lares, help us!
And thou, O Marmar, suffer not
Fell plague and ruin's rot
Our folk to devastate.

[1] All early accounts of dances among savages, South Sea islanders, and the like, assert this priority of chorus over refrain. There are no spectators, no audience, or "public"; all sing and all dance. See Wallaschek in his first chapter, and Yrjö Hirn, *Förstudier till en Konstfilosofi*, Helsingfors, 1896, p. 148.

[2] Zell, *Ferienschriften*, II. 111 f., notes that this sort of repetition is found in old Etruscan prayers as well as in the liturgy of the Roman church.

[3] By Wordsworth, work quoted; see, too, F. D. Allen, *Remnants of Early Latin*, p. 74, with interesting remarks on the fragments of the *Carmina Saliaria*, the *axamenta*.

Be satiate, O fierce Mars, be satiate!
  Leap o'er the threshold! Halt! now beat the ground!
Be satiate, O fierce Mars, be satiate!
  Leap o'er the threshold! Halt! now beat the ground!
Be satiate, O fierce Mars, be satiate!
  Leap o'er the threshold! Halt! now beat the ground!
Call to your aid the heroes all, call in alternate strain;
    Call, call the heroes all.
Call to your aid the heroes all, call in alternate strain.
Help us, O Marmar, help us, Marmar, help us!
Bound high in solemn measure, bound and bound again,
  Bound high and bound again! [1]

Refrain and iteration are here in thrall to religious ceremony, and the priest has laid hands upon the rough material of the throng; but the throng is present, takes part, — even if, in later time, by deputies, — and invention is at a minimum, appearing only in its regulative, and not in its originating force. It is easy to see how question and answer, strophe and antistrophe, are simply a development and division out of the crowd with one voice, as in the Greek chorus. So, too, in an Assyrian hymn: [2] —

Who is sublime in the skies?
  Thou alone, thou art sublime.
Who is sublime upon earth?
  Thou alone, thou art sublime.

The Hebrew psalms [3] show very clearly a more or less artistic use of the refrain sung under congregational and therefore

[1] Kögel, *Gesch. d. d. Lit.*, I. 31, 34 f., points out the close resemblance of the conditions and circumstances of this hymn with those of the old German hymns, of which we have no example; he therefore infers for the latter the same repeated cries to the god, and finds confirmation for this inference in the dancing, the repetitions and the cries of a Gothic Christmas play, written in Latin, in Greek characters, but with a Gothic original peeping through. Müller's attempt to restore this Latin-Gothic hymn is highly interesting.

[2] Westphal, *Allgem. Metrik*, p. 37.

[3] Also dramatic poetry, as in Job; for example, the refrain in the speeches of the messengers who tell Job of his calamity, "And I only am escaped alone to tell thee." See Moulton's arrangement in his edition of Job, pp. 10 f.

to some extent communal conditions.[1] These communal conditions can be guessed in their older and simpler form from such an account as is given of David and his dancing before the ark, when he "and all the house of Israel brought up the ark of the Lord with shouting and with the sound of the trumpet";[2] the personal song detached itself from the rhythmic shouts of the dancing or marching multitude precisely as the song of the wife and sister over their dead came out clearer and clearer from the wailings of the clan. So, if D. H. Müller be right, following in the path marked by Lowth, the form of Hebrew prophecy was at first choral, then was divided into strophe and antistrophe, yielding in time to an impassioned solo of the prophet himself. In any case, this single prophet, in historical perspective, lapses into the throng, into those "prophetic hordes" which Budde compares with modern Dervishes, "raving bands" now forgotten or dimly seen in the background of a stage where noble individuals like Amos, still in close touch with the people, play the chief part, and hold the conspicuous place.[3] As Amos and his brother prophets yield to the later guild whose prophecies were written, so one goes behind Amos to the "bands," to communal prophecy, to the repeated shouts and choral exhortation, and so to the festal horde of all early religious rites. The backward course would be from a prophecy writ-

[1] For these refrains see Driver, *Introd. to the Lit. of the Old Test.*, p. 366 (original ed., p. 344). They are sometimes exactly repeated, sometimes varied. For the poetry due to the Hebrews in general, see Renan, *Mélanges*, p. 12.

[2] 2 Sam. vi, 14 f.

[3] Lowth, *de sacra Poesi Hebr.*, ed. Rosenmüller, p. 205, citing "Nehem. xii, 24, 31, 38, 40, et titulum Ps. lxxxviii." D. H. Müller, *Die Propheten in ihrer ursprünglichen Form*, Vienna, 1896, I. 246 f., — a somewhat discredited work with regard to the theory of Hellenic and Hebrew relations, but seemingly sound in these facts. Budde, *Religion of Israel to the Exile*, pp. 97, 100. The "prophets" who came to England from the Cevennes make another modern instance; and there are many more in the great development of religious enthusiasm in the seventeenth century.

ten to be read, to the chanted blessing or imprecation of the seer; thence to a singing and shouting band under the leadership of one man, with constant refrain; and at last to the shouting and dancing of purely communal excitement, the real chorus. Moses and the children of Israel "sang a song unto the Lord, saying, I[1] will sing unto the Lord. . . . And Miriam the prophetess . . . took a timbrel in her hand, and all the women went out after her with timbrels and with dances. And Miriam *answered* them, Sing ye to the Lord." Here is certainly no premeditated verse; and it must be borne in mind that refrains, except where they have a sacred tradition behind them and are kept up by the priests, as in the Arval "minutes," easily drop from the record. Oral tradition, on the other hand, is fain to hold fast to all these vain repetitions; they are the salt of the thing. Now and then an unmistakable refrain is preserved. "And it came to pass as they came, when David returned from the slaughter of the Philistines, that the women came out of all the cities of Israel, *singing and dancing*, to meet King Saul, with timbrels, with joy, and with instruments of music. *And the women sang one to another in their play*, and said:—

> "Saul hath slain his thousands,
> And David his tens of thousands."[2]

That women in all nations and at certain stages of culture make songs of triumph like this, as they dance and sing, is known to the most careless reader; one or two chorals,

[1] Exod. xv. 1. 20 f. Clearly the whole tribe: see above, p. 186.

[2] 1 Sam., xviii. 1 ff. Lowth says of the *one to another*: "hoc est, alternis choris carmen amoebaeum canebant; alteris enim praecinentibus 'Percussit Saulus millia sua,' alterae subjiciebant 'et David suas myriadas.'" Perhaps. *Amant alterna Camenæ*. But it was rude amœbean, then, a tumultuous chorus, just as in the Fescennine songs of old Italy, and in the songs of Roman soldiers, a roughly divided pair of choruses sang alternately: see Zell, *Ferienschriften*, II. 149. On the choral nature of old Hebrew poetry see this whole passage in Lowth, pp. 205 f.

strangely similar to these songs of the Hebrew women, may be noted from mediæval Europe. Now it is the singing of Gothic songs of welcome by those maidens who come from their village, as the women of Israel from their cities, to meet and greet Attila,[1] dancing as they sing. So the daughter of Jephtha greeted her sire with the singing and dancing maidens; and so in Cashmere a stranger is still met by the women and girls of a village, who form a half circle at the first house where he comes, join their arms, and sing eulogies of him, dancing to the tune of the verse. Malays and even Africans do the same.[2] Again, it is in the seventh century, and an obscure saint, Faro by name, has won the gratitude of a community; straightway a song is made and sung "by the women as they dance and clap their hands."[3] It was not often that a saint's name lent grace to these songs of the women and saved them from clerical wrath; the decrees of councils, the letters of bishops, refer

[1] In the year 446. The story is often quoted from Priscus, 188, 189.

[2] Böckel, work quoted, p. cviii.

[3] "Ex qua victoria carmen publicum juxta rusticitatem per omnium ora ita canentium, feminaeque choros inde plaudendo componebant." Mabillon, *Acta Sanctorum ordinis S. Benedicti*, Venetis, 1733, II. 590. This clapping of hands as one dances and sings is often found in communal records, and is common among savages, negroes, and the like. Among tribes on the White Nile, where no musical instruments were to be had, girls clapped their hands to the song and dance: Wallaschek, p. 87, and also cf. p. 102, the account of women seen by Captain Cook to snap their fingers in marking time for their song. The practice is common elsewhere; for Polynesia generally, see Waitz-Gerland, *Anthropol.*, VI. 78 f. Sidonius Apollinaris speaks of it, I. 9: —

> Castalidumque choros vario modulamine plausit
> Carminibus, cannis, pollice, voce, pede;

while a dance to this hand-clapping is represented on an Assyrian monument: see Herrig's *Archiv*, XXIV. 168, quoted by Böckel in the introduction to his Hessian ballads. — That actual songs were made by these women is clear; see the passage from Guillaume de Dôle, quoted by Jeanroy, *Origines*, p. 309: —

> que firent puceles de France
> a l'ormel devant Tremilli
> on l'en a maint bon plet basti.

perpetually to the wicked verses and diabolical dances in which maids and even matrons indulged at the very doors of the church. Sometimes, however, national glory covered the shame. In the chronicle of Fabyan,[1] who is here telling no lies, it is said that after Bannockburn songs were made and sung with a refrain "in daunces, in the carols of the maidens and minstrels of Scotland, to the reproofe and disdaine of Englishmen"; and Barbour,[2] mentioning a fight in Eskdale where fifty Scots defeated three hundred English under Sir Andrew Harcla, says he will not go into details, seeing that any one who likes may hear —

> Young wemen, quhen thai will play,
> Syng it emang thame ilke day.

One is even fain to believe that Layamon[3] was thinking of the women when he said that after a treaty of peace,

> Tha weoren in thissen lande blisfulle songes.

That the record of these refrains is so meagre and baffling need cause no surprise. The histories of national literature are disappointing to the student of beginnings, for the reason that they almost invariably[4] study these beginnings as conditioned by the habits of authorship in modern times; they are always looking for original composition, for expres-

[1] London, 1811, p. 420. See also Ritson, *Scottish Song*, I. xxvi, f.

> Maydens of Englande, sore may you mourne
> For your lemmans ye have lost at Bannockisburne!
> *With heve a lowe.*
> What, weeneth the King of England
> So soone to have won Scotland!
> *With rumbylowe.*

This refrain, as will be seen, is a kind of water-chorus.

[2] *Bruce*, ed. Skeat, E. E. T. S., p. 399.

[3] *Brut*, ed. Madden, 9538 f.

[4] A notable exception is K. O. Müller, who studied early Greek song in connection with early Greek life, an example — as Posnett notes in some excellent remarks, *Compar. Lit.*, p. 104 — which subsequent historians have neglected to their own harm.

sion of individual feeling, for a story, and therefore turn aside from these stretched metres of an antique song. But the story, and the expression of personal emotion, are precisely what one seldom if ever finds at the beginning of a literature; one finds there, when one finds anything, the chorus or its deputy the refrain. The refrain was a constant element in early Greek song, "an essential mint-mark";[1] not only the early melic verse, but a study of the chorus[2] in dramatic survival, proves this beyond doubt, and one is amazed to find Rosières, in the essay quoted above, saying that the ancients, particularly the Greeks, had no need of the refrain, and hardly used it at all. How important, on the contrary, this refrain must have been, how it works back through the alternate strains of chorus and solo to the throng of communal singers and dancers, could be shown for classical poetry, and can be proved by mediæval and modern refrains, some already noted under the *vocero*, and others presently to be considered in songs of labour and of the harvest. True, the records are scanty; and the unwary historian of English poetry in the early stage, reviewing his material, announces that, with the exception of some insignificant charms, there is just one poem with a refrain, the "Consolation" of Deor, the king's minstrel out of place, — taking, that is, a lyric of individual and artistic reflection as the only example of that part of poetry which above all belongs to the communal and spontaneous expression of the throng. Recorded poetry has here a poor tale to tell, and even that is usually marred in the telling. Where, then, is the old refrain of the English folk, and where was the chorus? Had they no dances, no ballads, no communal singing? If the evidence of ethnology from tribes and communities of men in

[1] Smythe, *Melic Poets*, p. 490.

[2] For reference to the older literature of this subject, see Blankenburg, *Litterar. Zusätze*, I. 235 ff.

every degree of culture is to be accepted, it is certain that Englishmen of that early day had dance, ballad, chorus, and refrain. We know that their old heathen hymns went with the dance; and the dance means a strophic arrangement. What, then, has become of this refrain? So far as the old English poetry has found record at the hands of the monk, it is in a fixed alliterative metre, without strophes,[1] suited to epic and narrative purposes, suited to recitation and a sort of chant, but not, in its literary shape, suited to refrain and chorus.[2] One does not dance an epic, or sing it; it is chanted or recited; and even Anglo-Saxon lyric, barring that little song of Déor, is elegiac and highly reflective. The refrain, says Dr. R. M. Meyer,[3] is to be assumed for oldest Germanic poetry, although it was thrown out by the recited alliterative verse, only to come again into recorded literature with the introduction of rime; but no one supposes that Englishmen ceased in that interval to dance and sing. It is a defect of the record. The chorals and refrains, even the ballads of which William of Malmesbury speaks as crumbling to pieces with the lapse of time, were simply deemed useless if not harmful, and had no claim whatever to the life beyond life. Nor is this chorus, this refrain, simply assumed for oldest Germanic poetry; it is proved, and nowhere proved so well as in Müllenhoff's essay.[4] Many conclusions of this sturdy and often too intolerant scholar have been rejected by later investigation;

[1] Déor's song, of course, is divided into strophes or stanzas by means of this refrain.

[2] See above, p. 86, on the dispute between Sievers and Möller, and their agreement regarding this change from song to recitation.

[3] *Altgerm. Poesie*, pp. 341, 345.

[4] *De Antiquissima Germanorum Poesi Chorica* . . . Kiel, 1847. "Antiquissimum enim omnium poesis genus haud dubie illud est, quod choricum dicitur." See p. 5: "Carmina vero haec sacra . . . ex communi populorum usu, *non a rhapsodis recitata neque a singulis, sed semper a choro sive pluribus simul et cantata et acta sunt.*"

but his assertion in regard to choral poetry as the foundation of every literature remains an article of faith among those who deal at first hand with the material involved, and writers since his day who have undertaken to describe the different kinds of Germanic choral song have done little more than follow in his steps.[1] There is no need, then, to rehearse this proof of the existence of refrain and chorus as main form[2] of poetry among the ancient Germans; it is in order simply to trace these and other choral songs in the later fragments and the surviving refrains, whether sung at the solemn procession round the fields, or sung to the festal dance at harvest-home, or in whatever survivals they may be found, and to compare them with kindred refrains and kindred customs elsewhere. From this point of view, even the blackness of thick darkness which broods over Anglo-Saxon communal song, that darkness of superstitious fear felt by monks who knew these customs and these songs to be of the devil himself, and would not write them down, is lifted a little. We look, then, at refrains of labour, refrains of actual work, too trivial usually for record, and at those refrains and chorals of the harvest feasts, of plantings, sowings, reapings, which had the taint of heathendom upon them, and so were either left in silence or coaxed into a harmless formula; we look, too, at refrains and chorus of the dance, the sunnier side of life, and still more provocative than labour as an occasion of communal song. For the refrains of war, and even for the choral raised by a whole army as it marched

[1] The best recent summary is that of Kögel in the first volume of his *Geschichte der deutschen Litteratur*.

[2] See p. 6 of Müllenhoff: "Actionum autem choricarum triplex est genus: pompa, saltatio, ludus; quorum et simplicissimum est pompa et quasi primitivum." He treats only the first of these three; but a valuable paper on the sword-dance ("Ueber den Schwerttanz," in the *Festgabe für G. Homeyer*, 1871), the essay *De Carmine Wessofontano*, and many hints in his introduction to the *Sagen, Märchen u. Lieder d. Herzogth. Schleswig-Holstein u. Lauenburg*, 1845, make up the omission.

to battle, an occasion which Müllenhoff calls the supreme moment of all Germanic life, the fierce and clamorous words needing no leader,[1] and the wild rhythm asking no aid from trumpet or drum, there is ample evidence; and indeed these war chorals might be connected by easy stages with the ridiculous marching songs already noted above. From the *barditus* to "ma poule a fait un poulet" were a pretty journey; but we will keep to the ways of peace, and the *saure wochen, frohe feste* of everyday life will yield material enough in regard to this communal refrain.

Songs of labour are found everywhere; but there is a great chasm between the actual refrains, the survivals of communal or even solitary song which come from the real scene of labour and from the real labourers, and those songs which are made for the labourer. Nowhere is the difference between *volkspoesie* and *volksthümliche poesie* so evident; and we have here no concern with poetry, however successful, which has been written for the edification of "honest toil."[2] It is the song of actual labour to which we now turn, as it has abounded in all the activities of life, and which, like the ballad, is fast vanishing from the scene. Sometimes the labour was solitary, and the song was a plaintive little lyric when it was made by the lonely maiden grinding at her hand-mill:

Alone I ground, alone I sang,
Alone I turned the mill. . . .[3]

[1] Kögel, work quoted, p. 18. See his references, p. 17, for these refrains and songs of war.

[2] Well meant but ludicrous compilations, designed to offer songs of solace and cheer to all sorts of labourers, and to drive out the idle rimes which they are wont to sing, are cleverly noted in Hoffmann von Fallersleben's *Unsere Volksthümlichen Lieder*, Leipzig, 3d ed., 1869; the specimens he gives in his introduction are highly amusing, and are taken from Becker's *Mildheimisches Lieder-Buch*, 1799, which provides special songs for the butcher, the chimney-sweep, the scissors-grinder, and all the rest. See Hoffmann, pp. vii ff.

[3] A Lithuanian mill-song: see Bücher, p. 39. See also Porthan, work quoted

but often even this grinding of the mill was social, as in Poland, where it was the manner of the women to repeat a word in chorus.[1] Plutarch has preserved an old Greek "song of the millstone,"[2] which he heard a woman sing; from the older Scandinavian literature[3] comes a lay, sung by two maidens, Menja and Fenja, as they grind out King Frodi's fortune, which may hold bits of the actual refrain of labour, and has, too, its touch of folklore, explaining "how the sea became salt"; but the real and primitive choral of such labour is sufficiently attested by those women in Poland, and by a similar case among the Basuto tribe,[4] where, as Cassilis says, to relieve the fatigue of solitary grinding, "the women come together and grind in unison, by singing an air which blends perfectly with the cadenced clinking of the rings upon their arms." There is plenty of evidence for this choral of the grinding women in places and times so widely sundered as to forbid all idea of borrowing, and to leave the conditions of communal labour and communal consent as the only explana-

above, p. 198. He gives a pretty little song of a Finnish woman who calls for her absent husband in no recondite terms, ending: —

Liki, liki, linduiseni,
Kuki, kuki, kuldaiseni! —

that is, "prope, prope, deliciae meae; juxta, juxta, corculum meum."

[1] "Agrestum quendam concentum edere solent . . . hocque verbum ad cantilenae similitudinem repetunt." Pistorius, *Polon. Hist. Corp.*, I. 46, quoted by Bezzenberger, *Zeitsch. f. vgl. Lit.*, N. F., I. 269.

[2] Smythe, *Greek Melic Poets*, pp. 160, 510 f. — Bücher, p. 38, notes that this song, like many a lost refrain of the same kind, disregards the rules of classical metre, and follows the movement of the millstone. — Pennant (*Second Tour in Scotland*), Pinkerton, III. 314, compares the singing at the mill of the island women with Aristophanes' *Clouds*, Act V. scene 11.

[3] *Pros. Edda*, ed. Wilken, "Skáldskaparmál," xliii. pp. 123–134; cf. 4: —

sungu ok slungu
snúðga steini . . .

[4] Böckel, work quoted, lxiii f., where there are other references of the sort. So in pounding wheat, women in North Africa sang a national song in chorus, always pounding in time with the music, Wallaschek, p. 220.

tion. Originally there was a spontaneous chorus or refrain[1] — in the strictly choral sense, that is, and not in the technical meaning presently to be considered — suggested by the movements, cadence, and sounds of the work itself; improvisation added words at will, until at last art seized upon the material and gave now a song like that of Fenja and Menja, now even a jolly refrain such as one finds in an audacious song of Beaumont and Fletcher's *Maid of the Mill.*[2] Everywhere labour had its refrain and song, and even the scanty remains of Hellenic communal poetry tell of songs for reaper, thresher, miller, for the vintage, spinning, weaving, for the drawers of water, oarsmen, rope-makers, watchmen, shepherds, and for the common labourers marching out to their work. Rome itself, in the old silent period, has something of this song for the attentive ear;[3] and allusions scattered throughout the Bible show that the Hebrews sang at their work in house and in field. A few echoes of such singing come from Egypt; while darker and darkest Africa, along with savage tribes over the world, shows yet more elementary, and hence more insistent and necessary[4] connection between work and song. With the breaking up of communal conditions, with the advance of individual and initiative art, these songs of labour, like the ballad, like all communal poetry, tend to disappear or yield to alien verse. Often the individual works in silence, when his labour demands intelligent thought, but where labour is automatic or monotonous, where-

[1] Bücher, p. 60, is emphatic on this point, that the refrain is to be regarded as the oldest part of all songs of labour.

[2] Act V.

[3] Zell, *Ferienschriften*, II. 99 ff., "Ueber die Volkslieder der alten Römer," is still the best piece of information on the subject, although it was published in 1829.

[4] In carrying loads, in cutting, and the like tasks, the Lhoosai in southeast India "clear the lungs with a continuous *hau! hau! uttered in measured time by all;* without making this sound they say they would be unable to work." Lewin quoted by Böckel, p. lx.

ever it is collective, the labourer sings, and always will do so; the important fact is that he now ceases to sing the old refrain or song of the labour itself, born, as Bücher[1] shows so plainly, of the very movements and sounds which it called forth. For good reason, *andere zeiten, andere lieder.* Neus[2] noted that the Esthonians, a century ago, sang their own songs, and sang always as they worked in the fields or came together for festal occasions; now, — and "now" is fifty years ago — he says that either the song is silent, or else it is changed for an imported German ditty. All the more need, then, to collect and study such survivals of the refrains of labour as can be found. Speaking of the decline of folk-song in Germany, not only of the making but even of the singing, Professor E. H. Meyer[3] remarks that collective labour still has some power here and there to stir the old instinct into a fitful activity. Now it is in the spinning-room, — where Böckel[4] a few years ago could hear Hessian folk-songs in the making — now at the berry-picking in Nassau, at the flax-breaking, and elsewhere in cases where companies of peasants still ply the monotonous tasks of their forefathers. And in all these cases, as in the beginning, so in the end, women are the mainstay of communal song.[5]

Of particular trades and callings, perhaps sailors, oarsmen, and watermen generally, would furnish more refrains than

[1] *Arbeit u. Rhythmus*, pp. 30 ff. This chapter, quoted above, pp. 107 ff., gives ample references for the subject.

[2] *Ehstnische Volkslieder*, 1850, p. 1.

[3] *Deutsche Volkskunde*, 1898, pp. 331 f.

[4] Work quoted, p. cxxiii. The spinning-room for winter, and in summer the *rundgänge*, when youths and maidens arm in arm go by long rows singing songs to their march, are still a refuge for actual poetry of the people. But, as he says, it is dying fast.

[5] Böckel, work quoted, p. clii, notes that the three classes who spread and sing songs of the folk are women, soldiers, shepherds. Blind minstrels, of course, are to be added for the chanting and reciting guild, and in Russia the tailors. But women, soldiers, and shepherds best keep the old clan instincts.

could be found in any one industry of the land. Sailors' chanteys are still heard in every ship;[1] but they are now apt to echo those songs of the street and the dance-hall which have been picked up at port, and they have seldom a traditional interest. Here and there, however, the genuine refrain is clear enough, and attests itself by its power to withstand the *discrimina rerum* and the changes of time; it is said that modern Greek sailors, when reefing sails, have nearly the same melodious calls as those preserved in a play of Aristophanes.[2] Negro roustabouts on the Mississippi sing interminable refrains, while a capable leader improvises stanzas on the work in hand or on current events; a process which is matched by refrains and songs of manual labour in every part of the world. A well-known passage in the *Complaynt of Scotland*[3] gives the cries and songs both of weighing anchor, — where a leader sings and the rest answer "as it had bene ecco in an hou heuch," like the echo in a hollow ravine, mainly in repetitions, — and of hoisting sail, with iteration of short running phrases such as: —

> Grit and smal, grit and smal,
> Ane and al, ane and al, —

and not stopping here, undertakes to set down the "chorus" of guns heavy and light as a spirited sea-fight begins. In

[1] Laura Alexandrine Smith, *Music of the Waters*, London, 1888; John Ashton, *Real Sailor Songs*, London, 1891. Boatmen's songs changing or dying out: Bücher, pp. 128 f. Bücher's little group of boatmen's songs, pp. 118 ff., 66 ff., is far more valuable than these long and random collections. See his comments, pp. 68 ff. For example, the boat-song of North American Indians, taken from Baker, is foolishness to the Greeks who make collections for popular use, but is full of instruction for the student of poetry; it runs, without the musical notes: —

> Ah yah, ah yah, ah ya ya ya,
> Ah ya ya ya, ah ya ya ya,
> Ya ya ya ya ya ya.

[2] Böckel, p. lx. Roman oarsmen had not only the *celeusma* to time their strokes, but often a song of their own: Zell, II. 208.

[3] Ed. Murray, E. E. T. S., pp. 40 ff.

the old play *Common Conditions* occurs a pirates' song, the stanzas in quatrains, with a jolly refrain or chorus: —

> Lustely, lustely, lustely let us saile forthe,
> The wind trim doth serve us, it blows from the north.

Hoisting, pulling, however, and work of the sort on shipboard, yield in importance, so far as refrains are concerned, to the regular cadence of the oar, where voices have kept tune and oars have kept time from earliest days. Not only in the classical period, where actual song and music came to take the place of the refrain,[1] but with Egyptians, Africans, Tonga Islanders, wherever rowing is practised, these refrains are known; the Maoris, for example, "row in time with a melody which is sung by a chorus sitting in canoes." The same thing is told of the Indians of Alaska.[2] A refrain already noted seems to have served in England both for hoisting and for rowing; Skelton mentions it:—

> Holde up the helme, loke up, and lete god stere,
> I wolde be mery, what wynde that ever blowe,
> *Heve and how, rombelow, row the bote, Norman, rowe!*

and D'Israeli says that sailors at Newcastle in heaving anchor still have their *Heave and ho, rumbelow;* while it is recorded that in 1453, Norman, Lord Mayor of London, chose to row rather than ride to Westminster, and the watermen made this roundel or song: —

> Rowe the bote, Norman,
> Rowe to thy Lemman, —[3]

so that two refrains are confused in the laureate's account, and the exquisite reason, with a Lord Mayor in the case, is no

[1] Bücher, p. 68.

[2] Wallaschek, pp. 41, 47. See, too, p. 166: "Mr. Reade observed that his people" — Africans — "always began to sing when he compelled them to overcome their natural laziness and to continue rowing."

[3] Chappell, *Pop. Music Olden Time*, pp. 482, 783; Skelton, *Bowge of Court.*

more probable than such stories of origins are wont to be. For example, Cnut is credited[1] with a little song, which he is said to have composed as he rowed by Ely and heard the chanting of the monks; "ordering the rowers to pull gently, and calling his retinue about him, he asked them to join him . . . in singing a ballad which he composed in English and which begins in this way: —

"Merie sungen the muneches binnen Ely,
Tha Cnut ching rew ther by.

"Roweth, cnihtës, noer the land,
And herë we thes muneches sang."

Several things here are noteworthy; both Grundtvig and Rosenberg have pointed out[2] that this song is composed in a two-line ballad strophe of four accents to the verse, the kind afterward so common in Scandinavia and in England; and whatever Cnut's share in the making of it, it is at least of the eleventh century, and is the first recorded piece of verse to break away from the regular stichic metre of our oldest poetry. Moreover, it is said that Cnut improvised the song, and that he called on the others to join him; the lines quoted then, so Grundtvig infers, are the burden or chorus of the song itself; and it is interesting to know that in the days of the chronicler, say about the middle of the twelfth century, this refrain as well as the song was sung in the choral dances of the English folk. Doubtless it was sung to the oar itself; and that may have been the first of it, with royalty as an afterthought.[3]

[1] "Cantilenam his verbis Anglice composuit;" see *Historia Eliensis*, II. 27, in Gale, *Hist. Script.*, I. 505; it gives the account here quoted, then the verses, adding "et caetera, quae sequuntur, *quae usque hodie in choris publice cantantur*." . . .

[2] *Danmarks Gamle Folkeviser*, III. x f.; *Nordboernes Aandsliv*, II. 408.

[3] Refrains of rowing are found in many Danish ballads, mostly irrelevant, as these refrains so often are, but unmistakable. See Steenstrup, *Vore Folkeviser*, p. 77, for several examples.

Coming to land, one would think that the blacksmith, rhythmic as his work may be, must have little breath to spare for song; and, indeed, Bücher could find but one specimen which seemed to hold the genuine rhythm of the anvil. Had he looked to the English, however, he would have met more; an old "Satire on the Blacksmiths"[1] preserves a refrain probably sung to the work itself, or, at worst, imitated from its cadence:—

Thei gnaven and gnacchen, thei gronys togydere. . . .
Stark strokes thei stryken on a stelyd stokke,
Lus! bus! Las! das! rowten be rowe,
Swych dolful a dreme the devyl it todryve!
The mayster longith a lityll, and lascheth a lesse,
Twineth him tweyn and towcheth a treble,
Tik! tak! hic! hac! tiket! taket! tyk! tak!
Lus! bus! Las! das! swych lyf thei ledyn.

St. Clement is the patron of blacksmiths, and while Brand's account of the festivities gives no refrain, but only poor doggerel and mimicry, it is clear that processions, songs, and dances were a feature of the saint's day,[2] once regarded as the beginning of winter; so that communal origins may even lurk in the traditional anvil song, quoted by Dickens,[3] "that

[1] In Wright-Halliwell, *Reliquiae Antiquae*, I. 240: it belongs to the fourteenth century. Some rimes for St. Clement's day are printed by G. F. Northall, *English Folk-Rhymes*, 1892, mostly begging verses (pp. 222 ff.): although there is a ceremony at Woolwich connected with blacksmiths, song, however, yielding to formal speech.

[2] 23 November. See Hampson, *Medii Aevi Kalendarium*, I. 61; and Brand-Ellis, *Antiquities*, same date. The Germanic year has been recently studied by Dr. A. Tille, *Yule and Christmas*, London, 1899; he corrects in some particulars the current ideas set forth by Weinhold, according to which the seasons were regulated by natural signs,—solstice and the like. Dr. Tille contends that this was rather done by economic conditions. Before the German had a settled agricultural life, Michaelmas superseded Martinmas, the oldest Germanic festival. Actual harvest festivals are comparatively late. While Dr. Tille's idea of borrowing and of Christian influence goes entirely too far, his emphasis on economic conditions must be noted and approved.

[3] *Great Expectations*, Chap. XII.

imitated the measure of beating upon iron, and was a mere lyrical excuse for the introduction of Old Clem's respected name":—

> Hammer, boys, round — Old Clem,
> With a thump and a sound — Old Clem.

Again, there is the tinker with his catches, which moved Overbury[1] to a theory of origins; "from his art was music first invented, and therefore is he alwaies furnished with a song," to which his hammer keeps time. Of course, the only point of interest in these songs of the trades is the survival of a refrain which carries the sound and cadence of the work itself. Thus in the old play of *Tom Tiler and his Wife*, it is probable that an actual refrain has crept into the lively song of which Dame Strife sings the first staff, with its

> Tom Tiler, Tom Tiler,
> More morter for Tom Tiler, . . .

clearly an echo from the roof. But there is more of the communal strain in spinning-songs;[2] for here is the home of balladry, a city of refuge even to this day,[3] and here the women make as well as sing the song. Echoes of the wheel itself[4] are not infrequent; perhaps they are too close to art in that pretty song of sewing, knitting, and spinning, sung by three women in the first act of *Roister Doister*:—

[1] Or rather Mr. J. Cocke; see note to *Works*, ed. Rimbault, p. 288, and p. 89. See also the tinker as "master of music" and chief singer of catches, in Chappell, pp. 187, 353.

[2] Among the Romans, too; see Tibullus, Eleg. II. 1:—

> Atque aliqua assiduae textis operata Minervae
> Cantat, et applauso tela sonat latere.

[3] See letter in *Evening Post*, quoted above, p. 168; Böckel, work quoted; and the preface written by "Carmen Sylva" for the Countess Martinengo's *Bard of the Dimbovitzka*, London, 1892.

[4] It is almost superfluous to mention Gretchen and the recurrent echo of her wheel in the stanza *Meine Ruh' ist hin*. But this, of course, is art.

Pipe mery Annot, *etc.*
Trilla, trilla, trillarie,
Worke Tibet, knitte Annot, spinne Margerie :[1]
Let us see who shall winne the victorie. . . .

although, what with incremental repetition in other stanzas, and the audible whir of the wheel, this is like the songs which still move women to emulation under like circumstances in the spinning-rooms of Europe. "In Northamptonshire, when girls are knitting in company, they say" — surely sing? —

"Needle to needle, and stitch to stitch,
Pull the old woman out of the ditch;
If you ain't out by the time I'm in,
I'll rap your knuckles with my knitting-pin.

The 'old woman,' 'out,' and 'in' are the arrangements of the wool over and under the knitting-pins."[2] The same authority gives other rimes of this sort, more or less suggested by the movements of the work; for instance, a song of Cumberland wool-carders: —

Tāary woo', tāary woo', tāary woo' is ill to spin,
Card it well, card it well, card it well ere you begin.

Slightly different is the song of Peterborough workhouse girls in procession, where the refrain is quite primitive in form:[3] —

And a-spinning we will go, will go, will go,
And a-spinning we will go.

[1] A version of "The Cruel Brother" (Child, I. 147), from Forfarshire, has along with the common refrain two lines at the end of the stanza which partly echo the refrain of labour: —

Sing Annet, and Marret, and fair Maisrie,
An' the dew hangs i' the wood, gay ladie.

[2] Northall, *English Folk-Rhymes*, p. 322. See the interesting notes from Southey's *Doctor*, xxiv, about Betty Yewdale and the song she and her sister had to sing while learning to knit socks. The song kept time with the work, *and had to bring in the names of all the folk in the dale.* See on cumulative song above, p. 200.

[3] Dyer, *British Popular Customs*, p. 42.

Bell[1] records what seems to be a real refrain of the spinning-wheel in the Greenside Wakes Song:—

> Tread the wheel, tread the wheel, dan, don, dell O.

The flyting that goes with this refrain is negligible,—a man and a woman on horseback with spinning-wheels before them, singing alternate stanzas in the midst of the fair, with its dancing and merriment, a sort of side-show; but the refrain may well be old.

Songs of the crafts, however, are less likely to hold the festal, gregarious, communal note than those old refrains which took their cadence from the movements of workers in the field. An agricultural community, whether in its rudest stages, a horde that lives in fertile river bottoms as distinguished from the nomadic, predatory bands of the plain, or in the civilization of feudal Europe, always tends to homogeneous conditions and always fosters communal song. Where these conditions survive, this song in some degree survives with them. Corsican labourers in the field, says Ortoli,[2] still sing so at their work; the Styrian threshers, eight together, make their flails chorus thus:—

> Hiwer, hawer, hawerhaggl,
> Hiwer, hawer, hawerhaggl,

while Silesians, with two, three, four, five, six, hear as many different refrains made by the strokes of the flail;[3] and Bladé[4] prints a song of Gascon peasants which seems to give again all the stages in the culture of the vine,—a stanza or two may follow for example of the repetition and the refrain:—

[1] *Ancient Poems, Ballads and Songs*, London, 1857, pp. 187 f. Greenside is near Manchester.

[2] *Voceri*, pp. 244 f., with a specimen song taken from Viale.

[3] E. H. Meyer, *Volkskunde*, p. 236.

[4] *Poes. Pop. Gasc.*, II. 224 ff. See his references for this interesting subject.

Plante qui plante,
Voici la belle plante ;
Plante qui plante,
Voici la belle plante
    Plantons, *plantin*,
    Plantons le bon vin.
Voici la belle plante en vin,
Voici la belle plante en vin.

De plante en taille,
Voici la belle taille;
De plante en taille,
Voici la belle taille.
    Taillons, *taillin*,
    Taillons le bon vin.
Taillons la belle taille en vin.
Taillons la belle taille en vin.[1]

Early English drama was evidently fond of songs not unlike this, and in *Summer's Last Will and Testament* Nash brings harvesters on the scene singing what appears to be a song of harvest-home, if one may judge by the refrain of *Hooky, Hooky*, said by a Dodsley editor[2] to be heard still in some parts of the kingdom. " Enter Harvest," run the directions, "with a scythe on his neck, and all his reapers with sickles, and a

[1] Coussemaker in his section of songs for the dance, work quoted, pp. 338 f., gives a "ronde" sung during the fête at Bailleul: —

Now the salad must be sowed,
Now the salad must be sowed,
Salad, salad, salad, salad, salad,
Now the salad must be sowed.

Now the salad must be cut, —

then plucked, washed, dried, and so on. The list of these songs could be extended indefinitely; the fact that this of the salad is sung at a quite alien festivity simply proves the vogue of the thing. One must refer, however, to the dances of Catalonian peasants and children, the songs for which are little more than repetition and refrain descriptive of country toil, as quoted by Wolf, pp. 34 f., of his *Proben Portugiesischer und Catalanischer Volksromanzen*, Wien, 1856.

[2] Ed. 1825, IX. 41. The phrase "to town" at which our editor boggles, ignorant of its real meaning, is a further proof of the traditional character of this song.

great black bowl with a posset in it, come before him; they come in singing: —

> Merry, merry, merry, cheary, cheary, cheary,
> Trowl the black bowl to me;
> Hey, derry, derry, with a poup and a lerry,
> I'll trowl it again to thee.
> *Hooky, hooky,*[1] *we have shorn,*
> *And we have bound,*
> *And we have brought Harvest*
> *Home to town.*

The tendency to put popular and traditional songs into a play was common everywhere. Hans Sachs[2] used a May-song for the ring-dance which is clearly made in its turn out of a lusty old refrain: —

> Der Mei, der Mei,
> Der bringt uns blümlein vil.

Best of all, however, George Peele, who in his *Old Wives' Tale* gives tryst to countless waifs of folklore and popular stories, makes room there for a pretty song of harvesters. "Ten to one," cries Madge, when they first enter upon the stage, "they sing a song of mowing," but they are sowing, it seems; and once again they come in, this time with a song of harvest. The present writer has ventured[3] to change the first song so as to make it agree with the second, not an auda-

[1] "Is your throat clear for *hooky hooky?*" asks Harvest; and the reapers sing the refrain again. Later he speaks of weeping out "a lamentable *hooky hooky.*" Drake connected *hooky* with *hockey*, the hock or harvest cart sung by Herrick. But perhaps "hooky" is to be kept without any such change. Leyden, see *Complaynte of Scotland*, p. xciii, speaking of ring dances at the *kirn* or feast of cutting down the grain, says that reapers who first finished the work danced on an eminence, in view of other reapers, and began the dance "with three loud shouts of triumph, and *thrice tossing up their hooks in the air.*" Cf. the Oxford Dict., s.v. *hook*, the common word for reaping scythe or sickle from Anglo-Saxon down.

[2] In his *Neydhardt mit dem Feyhel*, 1562. See Uhland, *Volkslieder*, I. 58, and notes, *Schriften*, III. 24. Böhme follows the song back to the fourteenth century. In the play it is sung by the duchess and repeated by the chorus, as in popular dances of the day.

[3] In his edition of the play for Macmillan's *English Comedies.*

cious feat when one considers the case. The songs, with an interval between, would then run as follows: —

Lo, here we come a-sowing, a-sowing,
  And sow sweet fruits of love.
All that lovers be, pray you for me, —
  In your sweethearts well may it prove.

Lo, here[1] we come a-reaping, a-reaping,
  To reap our harvest fruit;
And thus we pass the year so long,
  And never be we mute.

The refrain is easy to detach from the rest; and it is clear, too, that actual imitation of sowing, reaping, binding, often went with the song, probably in this case a combination of gesture and word known still in games of modern children.

These songs, particularly the Gascon vintage chorus, are simply a festal recapitulation of the rustic year, with more or less echo of actual refrain sung to the labour in its various stages. From the moment when communal labour began to sow the seed — in Japan[2] the peasants still plant their rice in cadence with a chorus, and in Cashmere[3] the onions are sown with accompaniment of "a long-drawn, melancholy song," — through process after process, down to the picking,[4] reaping, harvesting, and so to the festal imitations just noted, even to the ritual of priestly thanksgiving, every stage is marked by communal singing, except that in the function last named the

[1] The reapers now appear "with women in their hands."

[2] Described to the writer by a Japanese gentleman.

[3] Bücher, p. 49.

[4] Twelve centuries before Christ, Chinese women gathered plantain with a song that is particularly rich in repetition and refrain; Bücher quotes the translation of Strauss, of which a stanza runs thus: —

Pflücket, pflücket Wegerich,
  Eija zu und pflücket ihn!
Pflücket, pflücket Wegerich,
  Eija zu, ihr rücket ihn.

The whole song minutely follows the process of picking.

community turns passive, the guild replaces the throng, and art has begun its course. Hence it is that most of the survivals of song and refrain come down to our day with more or less magic in the case. Rites are performed by the head of a family, and are even transferred from the field to the home; as when[1] at flax-planting a German wife springs about the hearth and cries, "Heads as big as my head, leaves as big as my apron, and stalks as thick as my leg!" In Silesia,[2] again, husband and wife sing together a song with the refrain, —

Om Floxe, om Floxe, om Floxe!

Even in the field itself, song is mingled with these symbolical and even religious rites; incantations, such as that Anglo-Saxon charm[3] for making barren or bewitched land bear again, are strongly tinged with clerical lore, and in this case involve a visit to the church altar. The Romans, too, had spells and charms for restoring fields to fertility when other spells and charms had bewitched them; harmful rites of this sort were forbidden in the laws of the twelve tables.[4] Cor-

[1] Grimm, *Mythologie*,[4] pp. 1036 f. He notes the frequency of this shouting, leaping, and singing at the planting of crops. It all goes back, of course, to communal rites.

[2] E. H. Meyer, *Volkskunde*, p. 225.

[3] Grein-Wülker, *Bibliothek*, I. 312 ff. To describe the whole ceremony in this case as original, is highly absurd.

[4] Zell, *Ferienschriften*, II. 118, 212; see Plin. *Nat. Hist.*, XXVIII. 2: "qui fruges excantasset." Standard works for the investigation of these relics of ancient cult are Mannhardt, *Wald-und Feldkulte*, 2 vols., 1875–1877; the same author's *Mythologische Forschungen*, already quoted; Pfannenschmid, *Germanische Erntefeste*, Hannover, 1878; and, pioneer of them all, Tylor's admirable work on *Primitive Culture*. For children's games, as last refuge of many of these rites, see F. M. Böhme, *Deutsches Kinderlied u. Kinderspiel*, Leipzig, 1897, which could be enlarged by a judicious use of Firmenich, *Germaniens Völkerstimmen*, in four volumes. Böhme says the *Ringelreihen* of these games are "uralte Reste chorischer Aufführungen bei den Jahres-und Gottesfesten unserer heidnischen Vorfahren," and gives cases which support his statement. Processional songs of the old cult survive in the *Ansingelieder*, *Umzugslieder*, and so forth, of the children, now mainly begging-rimes like the wren-song in Ireland and England, parallel to the swallow-song in Rhodes. Again, children have games which imitate sounds

ruption is rife in these things; but in a charm[1] for the old English peasant to get back his strayed or stolen cattle, amid the hocus-pocus of Herod and Judas and the holy rood and scraps of Latin, a few lines echo the old repetition, but have no refrain: —

> find the fee[2] and drive the fee,
> and have the fee and hold the fee,
> and drive home the fee.

A thousand things of the sort survive, but seldom touch the refrain; perhaps the charm to make butter come from the churn, common in 1655,[3] had a choral element: —

> Come, butter, come!
> Come, butter, come!
> Peter stands at the gate
> Waiting for a butter'd cake, —
> Come, butter, come!

We turn back to the actual labour of the fields, and the songs and refrains that went with it. A refrain[4] has come down to us from the harvesters of ancient Hellas, — "Sing the sheaf-song, the sheaf-song, the song of the sheaf," which is not unlike the type just considered in George Peele's "Lo, here we come a-reaping"; while that waif of Germanic myth,[5] the story of Scéaf, where the "sheaf" is made the

and movements of labour; Böhme gives a few. See also G. F. Northall, *English Folk-Rhymes*, pp. 360 ff. Halliwell, of course, includes some of these in his nursery-rimes. See also W. W. Newell, *Games and Songs of American Children*, N. Y., 1883. These songs of the children would lead us too far a-field, and we shall cling to the scanty survivals of the songs and refrains of labour itself.

[1] Grein-Wülker, I. 323 f., especially version C.

[2] Cattle.

[3] Halliwell, *Nursery-Rhymes*, p. 129.

[4] Mannhardt, *Mythol. Forsch.*, pp. 228 ff., J. Grimm, *Kl. Schr.*, VII. 229, in a paper on the "Nothhalm," with account of harvest rites.

[5] This child of destiny, asleep on a sheaf of grain, is wafted to the kingless land in a boat, — the Lohengrin parallel. For all the enticing material see Grimm, *Mythologie*,[4] III. 399 ff.; Müllenhoff, in *Zeitschr. f. deutsch. Alth.*, VII. 410 ff., and in his *Beowulf*, pp. 5 ff., with strongly established probability that the myth celebrates the beginnings of agriculture among Germans by the North and Baltic seas.

name of an agricultural god, or culture-hero, as one will, reminds us of Phrygian countryfolk who at their reaping sang "in mournful wise" the song of Lityerses, itself said to be the outcome of an old refrain, lapsing into a *vocero* for the hero's death. Burlesque laid unholy hands upon the custom and the myth; the story growing out of the song passed into a tradition which coldly furnished forth the satire and comedy of a later day; since any song of the harvest-field or the threshing-floor came to be called a Lityerses,[1] the name was seized upon for certain comic features, and grew to be a symbol of an insatiable eater. Yet dramatic allusions and uses of more serious nature, like the song recorded by Peele, were doubtless common in Greece and throughout the Orient. It has been said already, in speaking of the *vocero*, that the song of Maneros was sung by Egyptian reapers, just as they sang on the threshing-floor the song of the oxen treading out the corn; while at the harvest-home Greek husbandmen, if Mannhardt's surmise[2] is right, sang a variant of the Maneros; and Homer is witness for the singing of the Linos at the time of vintage.[3] If, now, one seeks for similar songs in the fields of modern Europe, one finds, to be sure, hints in plenty, descriptions by this and that traveller, and fragments of actual verse; but conditions of religious ceremonial have broken up the old refrains and barred any handing down of a Germanic Linos or Lityerses. Customs, too,

[1] Mannhardt, *Myth. Forsch.*, pp. 15 ff. That the Greeks sang at reaping, as at planting (Smythe, *Melic Poets*, p. 498, girls sing a sowers' song), is beyond question. See Mannhardt's note and references, as above, p. 2. He remarks that the Lityerses song in Theocritus (Id. X.) is an imitation of a real Greek folksong of labour, not, however, of the original Lityerses. Mr. Lang notes the resemblance of this situation to the famous scene in Molière's *Misanthrope*.

[2] Work quoted, p. 17. See his *Wald-u. Feldkulte*, p. 262.

[3] That the Romans had these refrains of harvest and vintage, as well as their Fescennine flytings and improvised satire, is beyond dispute (Zell, II. 122 ff.), but nothing of it all has come down to us. Fortune has been kinder with regard to the songs and refrains sung in processions about the Roman field.

have changed; and few are the places where folk at harvest-home do as their forbears did, when "the whole family sat down at the same table, and conversed, danced, and sang together during the entire night without difference or distinction of any kind" as between master and man, mistress and maid.[1] Add to the case that great transfer of vital interests upon which economists lay such stress, from open-air life to home-life, from the throng with its indiscriminate dance and merriment, often, too, its indiscriminate morals, its communal habit of thought and expression, to the individual responsibility, the sober pleasures and the stricter morals of the fireside, from the delight in movement, noise, cadence of many voices, to lamplight and the printed page and meditation: add this to the account, and one sees how ill it must have fared with the communal refrain of work, feast, and ceremonial rite. Reactions come, of course, and no one denies a constant market for cakes and ale; but what is a church fair, even a camp-meeting, to the old vigil? The wife of Bath is still with us, but she has to make shift with an afternoon tea. Disintegration, due to the lapse of communal feeling, has either broken up the traditional refrains, leaving only *Hooky, hooky*,[2] and unmeaning things of the kind, or else has favoured the making of doggerel which may or may not mean something, and which in any case threatens the student with perils of a too curious interpre-

[1] Chappell, II. 580. See his quotation from Tusser. Even here, in the Eastern states of America, middle-aged men have watched the passing of the "wealthy farmer," who now exists only in newspapers, and even there is kept at long range, — "of Indiana," "of Texas." Yet we knew him in our boyhood. The communal farmer occurs in old English novels, and in some new ones; but he is passing rapidly into tradition. See a paper on "England's Peasantry," by the Rev. Dr. Jessopp, in the *Nineteenth Century and After*, January, 1901; he tells of the communal conditions which once prevailed, of the change to the present, and is "inclined to doubt seriously whether before another century has ended there will be any such thing as an agricultural labourer to know."

[2] On the modern corruption of old refrains, see Pfannenschmid, pp. 207 ff., 468 ff.

tation of chops and tomato-sauce. Even where there is neither corruption nor distortion, there is unblushing if often innocent substitution of modern mawkishness. Precisely as one boggles, when reading Herd's *Scottish Songs*, to find under the title "I wish my Love were in a Myre" the familiar translation of Sappho's "Blest as the Immortal Gods,"— so, in coming to the "Cornish Midsummer Bonfire Song," in Bell's collection, a title to make any student of communal poetry get out a fresh pen, and in reading, too, that here "fishermen and others dance about the fire and sing appropriate songs," one pulls up with a rude shock at—

> Hail! lovely nymphs, be not too coy,
> But freely yield your charms,[1]

which, while appropriate in sentiment, has not the note of simplicity that one expects from Cornish fishermen dancing round the bonfire of heathen tradition. True, this is a very bad counterfeit; but many a verse quite as alien at heart, if not on the face, has been foisted upon communal and traditional song.

The best survivals come from the harvest field, and mingle refrain with improvisation. Very common in old times and in new is the note of ridicule, particularly for the wayfaring man, converted temporarily into a fool, who passes by the labourers; such a man even now gets rude handling as well as rude rimes, and this was the case in Hellas.[2] In an often-quoted Idyll of Ausonius there is reference to the exchange

[1] Compare the song sung on this occasion in Bavaria as the peasants dance about the fire and leap over it for good luck (Firmenich, II. 703):—

> Haliga Sankt Veit,
> Schick uns a Scheit;
> Haliga Sankt Wendl,
> Schick uns an Bengl;
> Haliga Sankt Florio,
> Kent uns des Fuiar O!

Kent = kindle.

[2] Mannhardt, *M. F.*, pp. 32 ff., 51.

of abusive lyric compliments between workers in the field and the boatmen on the Moselle; while any one can note how this instinct for a flyting between labourers in a band and the *spectator ab extra*, alone or in company, holds always and everywhere, while, on the other hand, the solitary labourer and the solitary wanderer are wont to pass the time of day with full courtesy and often with an inexplicably kindly feeling. German peasants breaking flax in the fields still sing to the rhythm of their strokes; as in the old days, a stranger who passes by them is sure to be hailed in improvised verses not of a complimentary kind. Particularly if the stranger be a young gentleman, a possible suitor for one of the daughters at the great house, sarcastic song greets him from twenty or thirty throats, mainly a refrain, and that partly of an imitative character, with derisive lines like: —

Too fat is he quite,
And he isn't polite,

with the refrain for conclusion, —

Hurrah, let him go![1]

All this, of course, to the exact time of the work in hand. When no stranger offers, mutual flytings will serve. Near Soest all the young people shout and sing throughout the entire process of preparing flax, — "unsung flax," they say, "is good for nothing," — and songs are improvised in satire of one another, with a refrain *rummel dumm dum* or *rem sen jo jo*. Travelling in Wales, by the bye, had once these chances of

[1] Quoted by Reifferscheid, *Westf. Volksl.*, Nos. 49, 50, 51. See the note, p. 188, and variants. The habit is widespread through Westphalia and the Rhinelands. A refrain printed by Firmenich, *German. Völkerstimmen*, III. 175, keeps time with the work (near Iserlohn): —

Dai Klinge dai klank,
Dai Hüppe dai sprank,
Wuol üöwer de Bank,
Wuol niäwen den Pal.

satire, and Aubrey tells about them, thinking doubtless of his favourite time "before the civil warres." For in Wales there were not only "rymers . . . that upon any subject given would versify extempore halfe an hour together," but "the vulgar sort of people . . . have a humour of singing extempore upon occasion: *e.g.* a certain gentleman coming to ——, the woemen that were washing at ye river fell all a singing in Welsh, w^{h} was a description of ye men and their horses."[1] How facile the black fellows of Australia, Africans, and savages everywhere, can be with this improvised ridicule, mainly practised on the march, or at some sort of labour, all travellers testify. Samoans sing instead of talking "as they walk along the road, or paddle the canoe, or do any other piece of work. These songs often contain sarcastic remarks, and in passing the house or village of parties with whom they are displeased, they strike up a chant embodying some offensive ideas."[2]

We must keep to the harvest fields. Wordsworth's solitary reaper called forth an exquisite lyric; but there is material more attractive for the student of refrains, however it lack poetic merit, in Boswell's and Johnson's stories of a Highland harvest, and one would be glad indeed if the doctor, who had all of Wordsworth's curiosity on this point, could have made the reapers tell him what they sang.[3] He was coming close to Rasay in a boat, while, as Boswell says, the boatmen "sang with great spirit," and Johnson remarked that "naval music was very ancient";[4] then the

[1] Aubrey, *Remains of Gentilisme.* Folk-Lore Soc., IV. (1881), pp. 81 f., under "Rymers." On p. 169 he says, "when I was a boy, every gentleman almost kept a harper; and some of them could versifie."

[2] Wallaschek, p. 179.

[3] He too heard a girl "singing an Erse song," as she span; and he had his jest, "I warrant you, one of the songs of Ossian." Hill's Boswell, V. 133 f.

[4] Before this he had been in a boat and heard one Malcolm sing "an Erse song, the chorus of which was 'Hatyin foam foam eri,' *with words of his own.* . . . The boatmen and Mr. M'Queen chorused, and all went well." *Ibid.*, V. 185.

men were silent, and from the near fields was heard the song of reapers, "*who seemed to shout as much as to sing*, while they worked with a *bounding activity*." Johnson's own account[1] of reaping on Rasay may refer to this or to another occasion. "I saw," he says, "the harvest of a small field. The women reaped the corn, and the men bound up the sheaves. The strokes of the sickle were timed by the modulations of the harvest-song in which all their voices were united. They accompany in the Highlands every action which can be done in equal time with an appropriate strain, which has, they say, not much meaning;[2] but its effects are regularity and cheerfulness." These hints from the Highlands are of peculiar importance because of the undoubted homogeneous conditions of life in the clans, keeping songs of this sort in an almost primitive state. Significant is the rhythm of shouts, significant the preponderance of the refrain. Lady Rasay showed Johnson "the operation of *wawking* cloth. Here it is performed by women who kneel upon the ground and rub it with both their hands, singing an Erse song all the time." Boswell speaks of their "loud and wild howl"; and Dr. Hill[3] quotes Lockhart that women at this work screamed "all the while in a sort of chorus. At a distance the sound was wild and sweet enough, but rather discordant" at close quarters.

The Lowlands of Scotland, too, had their *kirn*,[4] and the English harvest-home, practically the same thing, had merry songs and refrains down to living memory. What must

[1] *A Journey to the Western Islands*, Dublin, 1775, p. 97.

[2] The doctor complaining that he never could get an Erse song explained, was told "the chorus was generally unmeaning," which, of course, would point to a predominance of the refrain; Johnson himself slyly quoted an unintelligible refrain from an old English ballad. Hill's Boswell, V. 274.

[3] V. 203; Lockhart's *Life of Scott*, IV. 307. Pennant tells the same story in his *Tour in Scotland*.

[4] See above, p. 281, quotation from Leyden. See also for Scottish custom, Chambers, *Book of Days*, II. 376 ff.

these songs have been, when, if Professor Skeat[1] is right in his estimate and inference, on one estate of two hundred acres in Suffolk no less than five hundred and fifty-three persons were assembled for harvest? At almost any period of English country life one finds the rural philosopher looking back, like the Rev. Dr. Jessopp now,[2] to kindlier and more communal times, greater harvests, keener jollity, a wider and deeper social sense; so Overbury's franklin felt that he held a brief for the *tempus actum*. "He allows of honest pastime, and thinkes not the bones of the dead anything bruised, or the worse for it, though the country lasses dance in the churchyard after even-song. Rocke Monday, and the wake in summer, shrovings, the wakefull ketches on Christmas eve, the hoky or seed-cake, these he yearly keepes." Of this festal round harvest-home was culmination, since it knitted the bond between labour and rest, and was the pledge of plenty, the high tide of the agricultural year. Three elements may be noted in this harvest-home so far as the refrain is concerned; first, the shouting, the choral cries and songs of the labourers in the field as the last sheaf is cut and bound; secondly, the march homeward with the hock-cart to the cadence of loud refrains and songs, with the thrice-repeated procession about barn and yard; and thirdly, the more elaborate ceremonial of those gatherings which marked the safe accomplishment of harvest. Moreover, in any of these cases a progress may be noted from the rude but cadenced shouts, the refrains and chorals, through definite songs of harvest, up to all manner of offshoots and distortions, — fixed rites, speeches, sermons, pantomime, beggings, what not; but even in the last and worse estate of the communal harvest-song there is everywhere echo of the refrain, everywhere echo of the dance.

[1] Note to Passus, IX. 104, ed. of *Piers Plowman*, version C.

[2] Above, p. 286.

The breaking up of communal labour has left mainly the songs and cries of working folk on any given farm or estate; but the songs of a common festival for harvested crops still linger in customs of the village, — now a traditional march of the elder folk, now some half-understood dance and walk of the maidens, such as Hardy describes in his *Tess*, and now a mere song of village children coming in a band from the search for berries, as in the Black Forest: —

> Holla, holla, reera,
> Mer kumme us d'Beere.[1]

Lithuanians coming back from the field, or in any communal gathering, when they have sung through their traditional stock of songs, call for a new ditty; amid jest and jollity some one strikes up a *daina* of his own, composing as he sings; the rest repeat in chorus, correct the words, add to them, — and so a new song is made, and, if it finds favour, is handed down, and even passed to the neighbour villages. This custom, however, is fast going out of date.[2]

In some places the day when harvest begins is still a time of communal and ritual importance; Würtemberg reapers, men and women, gather in the early dawn and sing a choral for blessing on their work.[3] As they go to the field, the throng still sing choruses, improvised verses, and traditional ballads; and when they march home at dusk to their village, they sing songs, often modern enough, but, as

[1] E. H. Meyer, p. 133.

[2] Kurschat, *Litth. Gram.*, p. 445, quoted by Böckel, p. cxx.

[3] Pfannenschmid, p. 392. The song, "Die Ernt' ist da, es winkt der Halm," is clearly an outgrowth of the older refrain. See also p. 92. An actual refrain at the work is printed by Firmenich, III. 631: —

> Ei Hober, Hober, zeitige Hober!
> Ei Mädl, kom und schneid den Hober!
> Ei dirre Hober, dirre Hober!
> Ei Knechtl, kom und benn den Hober!

Pfannenschmid points out, substitutes for older and doubtless far more communal singing, which indeed lingers in the unintelligible refrain. In many places, however, chorus, refrain and song, whether communal or alien, to be sung at harvest and threshing, are dying out or dead; in Normandy, says Beaurepaire,[1] at the *fête de la gerbe*, when the last of the wheat is threshed, no song of any sort is heard, though elsewhere the festival is loud with chorus. A scrap of the refrain sung in another part of France —

> Ho! batteux, battons la gerbe,
> Battons-la joyeusement, . . .

Beaurepaire heard, to be sure, here and there in Normandy; but it was no longer a refrain of labour, and was attached to a love-song.[2]

The main ceremony, of course, is at the end of harvest. In many places a custom still prevails, that when the last sheaf is to be cut, a portion of grain is left standing, and the reapers now dance about it with repeated cries, sometimes of vague mythological tradition like "Wold, Wold, Wold," and with songs; now bare their heads, and pour food and drink upon the spot; now let the "bonniest lass" cut this remnant, dress it, and bring it home as the "corn-baby"; now throw their

[1] *Étude*, pp. 24 f.

[2] In this dying of communal song, its heart, the refrain, beats strong to the end, despite the other failing powers. See Beaurepaire's valuable testimony to this fact, *Étude*, pp. 39 ff., 48 f. "Deux lignes au plus composent le couplet. Le refrain est vraiment la partie importante, il supplie à la pauvreté ou à l'absence de la rime. . . . Au reste, il ne faudrait pas s'y tromper, la longueur du refrain, et son retour continuel, que nous serions tenté de considerer comme un défaut, forme précisement un des plus sûrs moyens du succès de la Chanson de Filasse. Elle exige, en effet, peu d'efforts de mémoire, elle permet à tous les laboureurs de prendre part fréquemment au chant; et avec son allure monotone, elle s'adapte merveilleusement à la marche lente et reguliere de travaux de la campagne. Aussi croyons-nous que c'est en partie à la predominance du refrain, que la chanson cuellissoire doit sa vogue et sa popularité." He gives another song with a refrain of planting.

sickles at it to see who can cut it down;[1] and so on, in variety of form, but all to the same purpose. In Flanders they sing, when the last load is taken from the field,

> Keriole, keriole, al in!
> 't loaste voer goat in.
> Keriole, Keriole, al in![2]

There is every reason to think that some rite of this sort, accompanied with communal refrain and song, was once universal in agricultural life.[3] The corn-baby just described as decked in silk and ribbons and brought home with singing, is also known as the kirn-baby, the ivy-girl, and the maiden; so that harvest-home is here and there called the maiden-feast.[4] The songs belong primarily on the field and with the homeward faring cart; but customs change. In Suffolk at harvest suppers some one is crowned with a pillow and the folk all sing *I am the Duke of Norfolk*,[5] though elsewhere in the country the old note remains. Still farther from the field, Hertfordshire countrymen sing *The Barley Mow* in alehouses after their day's labour; but in another part of Suffolk this is a festal song chanted at the harvest-supper "when the stack, rick, or mow of barley is finished." It is a song of repetitions, and holds an old refrain.[6] For this song at the harvest-home supper, its variations, corruptions,

[1] Pfannenschmid (on the cries and songs) pp. 404 ff.; Mannhardt, *M. F.*, pp. 167 ff., for the religious significance; J. Grimm, *Kl. Schr.*, VII. 225 f.; *Book of Days*, II. 377 f. Other instances are presently to be recounted.

[2] Firmenich, IV. (*Anhang*), 687. A longer version on p. 693. Keriole = *Kyrie eleison*,— substituted for an older heathen cry.

[3] See Mannhardt's chapter on "Demeter," work quoted; also pp. 20 ff.

[4] For all this English material, see Brand-Ellis, "Harvest Home," in the *Antiquities*.

[5] Chappell, I. 120.

[6] *Ibid.*, II. 745, one version. See for variants, and similar songs, J. H. Dixon, *Ancient Poems, Ballads, and Songs of the Peasantry of England*, *e.g.* pp. 175 ff., London, Percy Soc., 1846; Broadwood and Maitland, *English Country Songs*, pp. 150 ff., London, 1893.

survivals, its refrains, and its choruses, one would need a book; a description or two of recent doings must suffice. "At the harvest suppers up to some twenty years ago," say Broadwood and Maitland, "while the other guests were still seated at the table, a labourer carrying a jug or can of beer or cider filled a horn for every two men, one on each side of the table; as they drank, this old harvest-song was sung and the chorus repeated, until the man with the beer had reached the end of the long table, involving sometimes thirty repetitions of the first verse. After this, the second verse was sung in the same manner." The chorus — from Wiltshire — ran thus: —

So drink, boys, drink, and see that you do not spill,
For if you do, you shall drink two, for 'tis our master's will.

What is left here of communal song is the fact of the chorus and the infinite repetition; the song has a poor mixture of the bucolic with the buckish. The older collection of Dixon gives a better song: —

Our oats they are howed and our barley's reaped,
Our hay is mowed and our hovels heaped,
Harvest Home! Harvest Home!
We'll merrily roar out Harvest Home!
Harvest Home! Harvest Home!
We'll . . .

with another repetition of the line.[1] The men who sang this chorus were still in thrall to an old custom at the barley

[1] In the fifth act of Dryden's opera, *King Arthur*, is a harvest-song with this chorus: —

Come, boys, come! Come, boys, come!
And merrily roar out Harvest Home!

and the directions are that the actors shall sing this as they dance, a good communal trait. The words of this song grew popular, were varied, and became a ballad; it is in order for some one to show that harvest-home songs, like other popular verse, come from operas, plays, concerts, and the like.

harvest. On putting up the last sheaf, which is called the craw, or crow sheaf, the man who has it cries out, —

> I have it, I have it, I have it!

Another asks, —

> What hav'ee, what hav'ee, what hav'ee?

And the answer comes, —

> A craw, a craw, a craw!

Then wild cheering, and off they go to the supper, where they sing a well-known cumulative song about the brown bowl, the quarter-pint, the half-pint, and so on.

These repeated cries, however, take us back to the field. In Devon, as Brand relates, they still cried "the neck"; a little bundle was made from the best ears of the sheaves, and when the last field was reaped, all gathered about the person who had this neck, who first stooped and held it near the ground. All the men doffed their hats and held them likewise and then cried, in a very prolonged and harmonious tone, *The Neck*, at the same time raising themselves upright, and elevating arms and hats above their heads, the holder of the neck doing likewise. This was done thrice; after which they changed their cry to *wee yen,*[1] *way yen*, prolonged as before, and also sounded thrice; then boisterous laughter, amidst which they break up and hurry to the farmhouse, — a maimed rite, indeed, but of interest when compared with kindred doings. For the words are surely wreckage of an old refrain, full of repetitions, like that song Montanus rescued from the rites of midsummer-eve along the Rhine. Under the "crown," boys, girls, and their elders dance in a ring and sing as they dance a sort of refrain which is made of incremental repeti-

[1] Perhaps "we end," as Brand suggests; but perhaps and probably not. At another place in Devonshire they cry "the knack," and a rime is repeated: —

> Well cut, well bound,
> Well shocked, well saved from the ground.

tions into a description of the game they are playing; meantime one person stands in the midst of the ring until he has played his part to the choral suggestion, a common element in other games of children. In these and kindred ceremonies it is clear that a concerted shouting was the main feature, but the shouts were rhythmical and went with the communal dance, not with a disintegrated, howling mob. At Hitchin farmers drove furiously home with the last load of harvest, while the people rushed madly after, shouting and dashing bowls of water on the corn; but this is chaotic, for old Tusser[1] knew a better way:—

> Come home lord singing,
> Come home corn bringing.

In Germany the last load of grain is brought home with throwing of water and singing of traditional songs and shouts for the master. So too in English "youling," when cider is thrown on the apple trees, at each cup "the company sets up a shout."[2] Doubtless the elaborate chorus of the Arval brothers had once its wild but cadenced shout of the whole festal throng, as they "beat the ground" in communal consent of voice and step; and this primitive shout recurs in all folk-song, not only in the *schnaderhüpfl*, in the *jodel* which ends a stanza, but in those cries at the dance which have crept into the ballad itself. But the cadenced shout, the refrain, the infinite repetition of a traditional song, pass with the dance that timed them, and decorous reapers may now depute one of their number to act as spokesman; hence, as in

[1] *Five Hundred Points of Husbandry*, Eng. Dial. Soc., 1878, p. 126, under August. Hentzner noted the shouting of the people *in the cart*. See Furnivall's Harrison, *Descrip. Eng.*, p. lxxxiv. A curious custom of the largess-shilling in Suffolk is described by Major Moor, note to Tusser, p. 294. The reapers answer their leader's "Holla Lar! Holla Lar! Holla Lar!—jees," with "o-o-o-o-," head inclined, and then, throwing the head up, vociferate "a-a-a-ah." This is thrice done by harvesters for a shilling.

[2] Brand-Ellis, "Twelfth Day."

Mecklenburg, the recited poem, or the little speech, or even, as in Hanover, a figure made of the stalks is furnished with a letter to be read aloud for the behoof of neighbours; and there are other infamies of the sort. So passes the old Harvest-home.

Of vast importance for agricultural life, and resonant with refrain and song, were those processions about the field, about parish boundaries, to sacred wells,[1] to woods and groves to bring in the May, and for a hundred other purposes to a hundred other resorts. The solemn procession of a community, along with the festal dance, forms the oldest known source of poetry; and Kögel points out that in German even now the proper word for celebrating a festal occasion is *begehen*, while the corresponding noun is used in a mediæval gloss for *ritus* and *cultus*. The song of the Arval brothers had its origin in such a procession about the fields; and Vergil's advice[2] to the farmer shows that this rite was no monopoly of priests, or even of the man skilled in incantations, but a communal affair,—marching round the young crops, and dance and song at harvest:—

. . . thrice for luck
Around the young corn let the victim go,
And all the choir, a joyful company,
Attend it, and with shouts bid Ceres come
To be their house-mate; and let no man dare
Put sickle to the ripened ears until,
With woven oak his temples chapleted,
He foot the rugged dance and chant the lay.[3]

[1] See Uhland, *Kl. Schr.*, III. 389 f., and note, with references, 467 f., for the "bornfart," "bronnefart," with "dantzen, rennen, springen, jagen," closely connected with the May feasts. On the whole subject of processions, see Pfannenschmid's second chapter along with his notes, pp. 342 ff.

[2] *Georg.*, I. 343 ff.

[3] Translation of J. Rhoades. The last line—'det motus incompositos et carmina dicat'—is suggestive: "spontaneous gestures and steps, with song," emphasize a purely communal dance as compared with the ritual of the Brothers.

There can be no question of borrowing in these songs and dances, even in the simpler forms of ritual, which are found wherever rudest agriculture has begun. Doubtless only a change of religion deprives us of those songs, or some echo of them, which were sung in the famous procession of Nerthus,[1] the *terra mater*, goddess of fertility and peace among the Germanic tribes who lived by the northern oceans two thousand years ago. These people, so Tacitus[2] records the rite, "believe that she enters into human activity, and travels among them." Drawn by cows, she is accompanied in her mysterious wagon by a priest; "those are joyful times and places which the goddess honours with her presence, and her visit makes holiday."[3]

Tacitus was interested in the mysteries of the rite; would that he had heard and transmitted the songs that rang out in honour of this German Demeter, and had described the dances of the folk about their fields![4] For, as Kögel points out, the later procession to bless crops and to ban all things hostile to

Tibullus, by the way, has the Lares, not Ceres, in mind for the dance and song of his rustics: *Eleg.*, I. 1, 23 f.

> Agna cadet vobis, quam circum rustica pubes
> Clamet: *Io! Messes et bona vina date!*

[1] A "queen," accompanied by a guard of brothers and young folk generally, goes on Whitsuntide in Servia from farm to farm; at each she stops and her companions form a circle (*kolo*) and sing their songs. Each line is thrice repeated, and then follows the refrain *Leljo!* Then the dancers hold one another by the belt and dance in a half-circle, led by an exarch. Between the songs any ready young man cries out a lusty phrase or two, or makes a verse, after the fashion of the German *schnaderhüpfl.* See A. W. Grube, *Deutsche Volkslieder*, Iserlohn, 1866, pp. 132 f.

[2] *Germania*, xl.

[3] The procession of the Phrygian goddess, the *magna deum mater materque ferarum et nostri genetrix*, described by Lucretius in often-quoted lines, *Rer. Nat.*, II. 598 ff., with its Dionysian features, cannot be discussed here; Germanic and modern examples must suffice.

[4] It is a commonplace in sociology that agricultural communities worship female deities as representatives of fertility, while the god like Tiw or Woden springs from warlike and nomadic conditions.

their thriving, a custom still common in certain parts of Europe, is only a repetition of this old progress. Half-way between the time of Nerthus and the present occurs that Anglo-Saxon charm for making barren or bewitched land bear fruit; amid its excrescences of ritual, and under the alien matter, still lingers a hint of the old communal procession, the old communal song and dance; and perhaps Nerthus is dimly remembered in the cries of, —

> Erce, Erce, Erce, earth's mother,

which has a repetition familiar from many survivals,[1] and in the lines: —

> Hail to thee, Earth, all men's mother,
> Be thou growing in God's protection,
> Filled with food for feeding of men!

Again, one has the extremes of shouts, communal cadenced cries, and songs which are often quite irrelevant; thus in Brandenburg on Easter Monday girls march by long rows, hand in hand, over the young corn of each field, singing Easter songs, while the young men ring the church bells;[2] but one learns that Wends of the fifteenth century greeted the early corn as they ran round it in wild procession, and hailed it "with loud shouting."[3]

About the year 1133, and along the lower Rhine, a procession was in vogue which may have been a survival of the

[1] For example, the rain-song in Servia, an interesting ceremony, full of cries and with a refrain sung by dancing maidens. The *dodola*, a girl otherwise naked, but entirely covered with grass, weeds, and flowers, goes with a retinue of maidens from house to house; before each house the girls form a dancing ring with the *dodola* in the middle. The woman of the house pours water over the *dodola*, while she dances and turns about; the other maidens now sing the song for rain, each line ending with the refrain, *oj dodo oj dodo le!* See Grimm, *Mythologie*[4], p. 494. Similar customs prevail in Greece; the song is here full of repetitions. See Grimm, *Kl. Schr.*, II. 447. In the *Athenæum*, No. 2857 (1882), G. L. Gomme has some interesting notes on a survival of these processional rites.

[2] E. H. Meyer, p. 223.

[3] Grimm, *Mythol.*,[4] I. 52.

worship of that goddess recorded by Tacitus and called Isis because her symbol was a ship; for in the mediæval rite such a ship was placed on wheels and carried about the country, followed by shouting bands and hailed at every halt with song and dance.[1] The songs, *turpia cantica et religioni Christianae indigna concinentium*, were condemned by clericals,[2] and the dances of scantily clad women, not unlike the festal dances of savage women in many places at this season of the year, were doubtless not only intrinsically objectionable, but pointed back to the heathen doings from which our Germanic folk were so slowly converted. A glimpse at this older worship is given by Gregory in his often-quoted story of the Langobards who offered a goat's head to their "devil," running about in a circle and singing impious songs.[3] A survival of some such heathen rite, with ridiculous perversion of Christian legend, is the feast of the ass, the festival of fools, on Christmas or on St. Stephen's day, when during mass the priest brays thrice and the congregation respond in kind; here and there, as in France, a hymn is sung, with refrain from the throng:[4]—

Hez, Sir Ane, hez!—

and ending in what Hampson oddly calls "an imitation of the noisy Bacchanalian cry of *Evohe!*"—

[1] References *ibid.*, I. 214 ff., with similar cases. See also III. 86 f.

[2] William of Malmesbury tells a story to show that the church could do better than condemn. In 1012 fifteen young men and women were dancing and singing in a churchyard and disturbed Robert the priest. He prayed at them, and for a whole year they had to dance and sing without ceasing until they sank to the middle in the earth.

[3] Gregor. M. *Dial.*, III. 28, quoted by W. Müller, *Geschichte und System der altdeutschen Religion*, Göttingen, 1844, pp. 74 f. The first book of this excellent treatise is even now the best summary of old Germanic rites,—clear, compact, and with all necessary references. For the boar's head and the famous Latin song, at Oxford, see Grimm, *Mythol.*[4], p. 178; for the vows, Grimm, *Rechtsalterthümer*, pp. 900 f.

[4] From Du Cange, s.v. *Kalendae.* See too Hampson, *Med. Æv. Kal.*, I. 140 ff.

Hez va! Hez va! Hez-va-he!
Bialz, Sire Asnes, carallez
Belle bouche car chantez, —

a very far cry, indeed. After service, crowds marched through the streets, sang Fescennine songs, danced, and ended by "dashing pails of water over the precentor's head." It is needless to follow this degenerate choral over Europe, as it blends thus with rites of the church, passes into the song of the waits, and lingers in degraded form with the beggars or children who parade the countryside at Martinmas or in Christmas week, singing refrains that echo older and better song and doggerel that echoes nothing.

A soule-cake, a soule-cake,

was the refrain which Aubrey heard; but in modern Cheshire it is —

A soul! A soul! A soul-cake!
Please good Missis, a soul-cake![1]

printed here with full apologies to all outraged friends of the immensities and the eternities, who sought nobler stuff in a book on the beginnings of poetry. On Palm Sunday, near Bielefeld in Germany, the children go about with branches of willow and sing "all day long" —

Palm'n, Palm'n, Påsken,
Låt't den Kukkuk kråsken,
Låt't dei Viögel singen,
Låt't den Kukkuk springen![2]

Most stubborn, of course, is this converted or Christian survival, and almost as stubborn the custom of the village and

[1] Broadwood and Maitland, p. 30. Survivals of procession song (*Ansingelieder*) are printed by Böhme, *Kinderlied*, pp. 331 ff. The refrain has some body in a song "'t Godsdeel of den Rommelpot," printed by Coussemaker, *Chants Pop. des Flamands*, p. 95, and also found in different parts of Germany. The begging songs for Martinmas Eve, found in Flanders, are widespread in Germany; Firmenich, work quoted, prints a good dozen and more from different places. The steps of dance and march are best heard in his version from Oldenburg, I. 231.

[2] Firmenich, I. 281.

of remote agricultural communities; such a procession as Coussemaker[1] describes, popular throughout Flanders and Brabant, with a fixed refrain, held its place even in the cities. Occasionally Church and State were opposed;[2] a proclamation of Henry VIII forbade processions "with songes and dances from house to house," and even carols were forbidden by act of Parliament in Scotland. Wakes[3] were either abolished, or else passed into that curious communal revival, the love-feast and the watch-meeting of Methodists. But the communal song and procession are fast dying out, and the new century will hear little of them; although early in the old century the Christmas days[4] heard many a shouting throng, now with cries of *au guy*, now *gut heil*, now *hogmenay trololay, give us your white bread and none of your gray!*

[1] *Reuzelied*, pp. 139 ff.: —

> Als de groote Klokke luyd
> De Reuze komt uyt.
> *Keere u e's om, de Reuze, de Reuze,*
> *Keere u e's om,*
> *Reuzekom.*

That is, "When the big bell sounds, Reuze (giant?) comes out. *Turn back, Reuze, Reuze, turn back, good Reuze.*" The text is corrupt, and Reuze is not easy to explain; but one need not appeal with Coussemaker to the Scandinavians to establish the antiquity of this procession and this refrain.

[2] Hampson, I. 61.

[3] For a good description of wakes, see Brand-Ellis, and Song 27 of Drayton's *Polyolbion*, where such cheering is recorded of the villages —

> That one high hill was heard to tell it to his brother,
> That instantly again to tell it to some other.

[4] Besides T. Wright's *Songs and Carols*, Percy Soc., 1847, see W. Sandy's *Christmas Carols, Ancient and Modern*, London, 1833, with a long introduction, and the same editor's *Festive Songs*, Percy Soc., 1848. Sandys (*Carols*) gives the cries or refrains of many Christmas songs: —

> Nowell, nowell, nowell, nowell, —
> No — el, el, el, el, el, el, el, el, el, el, —
> Noel, Noel —

à moult granz cris, the familiar refrain in France.

and whatever other etymological puzzles the scanty records can show. These fragments of festal song are too far gone in corruption for profitable use. Aubrey[1] felt the lapse, and made such *memoranda* as these: "get the Christmas caroll and the wasselling song;" "get the song which is sung in the ox-house when they wassell the oxen," that is, with echo of an old refrain, where they drink "to the ox with the crumpled horne that treads out the corne"; and he has noted a few of these songs. The civil wars, he thinks, made an end of these old customs; "warres doe not only extinguish Religion and Lawes, but Superstition; and no suffimen is a greater fugator of Phantosmes than gunpowder." But peace has its victories of this sort. Not long ago the procession about village and parish boundaries was common enough; the whole community took part in this festal affair, and all sense as of an individual purpose or individual ownership was laid aside. Shout, dance, song, banquet, even directly ceremonial acts, were the concern of a homogeneous throng, "our village" in strictest communal sense. On the march — for example, the boundary march at Hamelin, in the late autumn, — rose traditional songs, varied by noise of every sort; and at the feast which followed, gentle and simple joined hands in the dance, until, with recent innovations, the gentry withdrew, became mere onlookers, and at last left the old rite to fall, like most communal traditions, into a shabby, vulgar, discredited uproar of the lower classes, a thing common and unclean. A quite similar case of degeneration is quoted by Brand from the *Gentleman's Magazine* for June,

[1] *Remaines Gentil.*, pp. 9, 21, 23, 26, 31, 36, 40, 161, 180. "Little children," he says here, "have a custome when it raines to sing or charme away the Raine; thus they all joine in a Chorus, and sing thus, viz.: —

Raine, raine, goe away,
Come againe a Saterday.

I have a conceit that this childish custome is of great antiquity."

1790, as going on at Helstone in Cornwall.[1] But where the prosperity of crop and barn is in question, the rites are more stubborn and hold their ground. This Helstone song welcomes summer; but before that was sung, processions of all kinds were wont to go about the fields, and in 1868 what the *Times* newspaper called a "ritualistic revival" came off in Lancashire, priest and choir making a progress through the fields with cross and banners, and singing as they went. Rogation week is still known as gang-week.[2] In older times the community itself was priest and choir; the cases are plentiful and may be read in Brand's account of "parochial perambulations." Then there is the song of bringing home the May,[3] the dance and song about the Maypole, with material and survival beyond one's compass; enough to let them echo in the verses put by Nash into his chaotic but pretty play, where the clowns and maids sing as they dance: —

> Trip and goe, heave and hoe,
> Up and down, to and fro;
> From the town to the grove
> Two and two let us rove.
> A-maying, a-playing :
> Love hath no gainsaying ;
> So merrily trip and go.[4]

[1] See the Helstone Furry-Day Song, Bell, *Ancient Poems*, pp. 167 f., with a refrain of some value.

[2] Also cross-week and grass-week. See Dyer, *British Popular Customs*, pp. 204 ff., for a sympathetic account of the customs still lingering in England.

[3] The standard description of English May-games, of course hostile, is that of Stubbes in his *Anatomie of Abuses*, ed. New Shaks. Soc., p. 149. See also the diatribe in John Northbrooke's *Treatise wherein Dicing, Dancing . . . are Reprooved*. London, 1579. He leans to Chrysostom's view (that is, Age takes this side against Youth, in the dialogue) that dancing "came firste from the Diuell"; and p. 68 b (only one page of the leaf is numbered) he describes the May.

[4] Compare the chorus of the Maypole song in *Actæon and Diana*, in Chappell, I. 126: —

> Then to the Maypole come away,
> For it is now a holiday.

The voices of the real maying folk are here, and the steps, lightly touched by art in the transfer to the play; in that Furry-Day Song at Helstone, with its opening about Robin Hood and Little John, there is a rougher but less effective refrain: —

With ha-lau-tow, rumble O!
For we were up as soon as any day O!
And for to fetch the summer home,[1]
The summer and the May O!
For summer is a-come O!
And winter is a-gone O!

What the poet can do with a fragment of communal song, with a heart full of communal sympathy, and with that final touch of art and individual reflection, may be felt by any one who will read in the echo of this rough old chorus those exquisite verses of Herrick to Corinna.

Songs that may pass as communal drama hold something of this old refrain of labour; so, for example, in the flytings of winter with summer or with spring,[2] which seem to go back in England to times before the conquest. A refrain, with change of "summer" to "winter" in alternate stanzas, runs through a ballad printed by Uhland:[3] —

"Trip and go" was "one of the favourite Morris-dances," and the words seem to have become a proverbial expression. See Chappell, I. 126, 302. It was on the basis of some refrain of this sort that the first part-song in English, the famous Cuckoo Song, was built up. Ten Brink is surely right in giving it a communal origin, though not communal making.

[1] "We have brought the summer home," is the spirit of all the May refrains, as the young folk come back with flowers and boughs. See Brand, "Maypoles."

[2] Still in vogue in some parts of Germany. See E. H. Meyer, p. 256.

[3] *Volkslieder*, I. 23. For the whole subject, see Uhland's *Abhandlung über die deutschen Volkslieder*, pp. 17 ff. Suspicion has been expressed that these flytings are a late echo of the Vergilian eclogue through such a transmitting element as the mediæval *Conflictus Veris et Hiemis* and the song to the cuckoo: —

Salve, dulce decus cuculus per saecula, salve!

Comparison of the fragments, however, shows this suspicion to be groundless, and it is thoroughly discredited by Uhland, *Kl. Schr.*, III. 24. See also Ebert, *Christ. Lat. Lit.*, II. 69.

Alle ir herren mein,
Der Sommer ist fein!

Another refrain is sung "by all the youth," when a mock fight between the two is ended, and winter lies at jocund summer's feet:—

Stab aus, stab aus,
Stecht dem Winter die Augen aus!

In the strife by deputy,[1] owl appearing for Hiems, and cuckoo for Ver, there is the call of the bird for refrain; or else it is holly for summer and ivy for winter, a chorus,[2] said to have been written down in Henry VI's time, running—

Nay, Ivy, nay,
Hyt shal not be, iwys;
Let Holy hafe the maystry
As the maner ys.[3]

These flytings came to be extraordinarily popular, and it is hard to draw a line between the *volkspoesie* and the *volksthümliche;* learned allegory, which was early on the ground, has the mark of Cain upon it, and cannot be missed. Probably Böckel[4] is right in looking on the winter and summer songs as originally communal, with those dialogues between soul and body, which one finds in nearly every literature of Europe, as a learned and allegorical imitation; a combination of the two kinds is not unusual.[5] So one passes to all man-

[1] *Love's Labour's Lost*, V. 2.

[2] Ritson, *Ancient Songs*, 3d ed., pp. 113 ff. The text is a sort of dramatic description. See also T. Wright, *Songs and Carols;* and Brand, under "Morris Dancers." The refrains are unfortunately seldom recorded, but they are the foundation of the little drama.

[3] Used as refrain in ballads; see Child, I. 19 f., *e.g.:*—

Sing ivy, sing ivy . . .
Sing holly, go whistle, and ivy . . .
Sing green bush, holly, and ivy.

[4] *Deutsche Volkslieder aus Oberhessen*, p. xi. His list of references is valuable.

[5] At a harvest-home at Selborne, 1836, Bell (pp. 46 ff.) heard two countrymen recite a "Dialogue between the Husbandman and the Servingman"; "it was delivered in a sort of chant or recitative," though the rhythm is good for such

ner of debates,[1] — riches and poverty, wine and water, peasant and noble, priest and knight, down to Burns's *Twa Dogs;* but it is the old communal sap that keeps holly and ivy green, and an old communal rite, the driving out of winter or of death, lingers in the verses which German children still sing to the dance:[2] —

> Weir alle, weir alle, weir kumma raus,
> Weir brenge enk'n Tod hinaus;
> Der Summa is wieder kumme,
> Willkummen, lieber Summe![3]

Refrain and chorus of labour among savages have been noted here and there in the foregoing pages; to collect them to any extent would be useless. They are found everywhere, and show that stage of development at which the repetition of a single sentence, often of a single word, affords unmeasured delight or ease. Individual singing is almost unknown in many savage tribes,[4] and the refrain in its function as deputy of the older chorus, is less common than the chorus itself.[5] Where the savage is still mainly a hunter, mainly a warrior, the refrain is insistent whenever a connected bit of descrip-

doggerel; what suggests the older refrain is that the rime (second and fourth lines of each stanza) has to be either with "husbandman" or with "servingman" throughout. The odd lines have interior rime.

[1] See Jeanroy's chapter, "Le Debat," in *Origines de la Poésie Lyrique en France*, pp. 45 ff.

[2] Böhme, *Kinderlied*, pp. 332 ff. See p. 347.

[3] See Firmenich, II. 15, where children in the Palatinate on "Rose-Sunday" go about and sing: —

> Ri, ra, ro
> Der Summertaagk iss do!

See *ibid.*, II. 34.

[4] Letourneau, *L'Évolution Littéraire*, p. 21.

[5] "Choruses are about all the Indians sing. They have probably four or five words, then the chorus. 'They have brought us a fat dog'; then the chorus goes on for half a minute; then a repetition again of the above words 'they have brought us a fat dog.' . . . Tukensha, a rock, or grandfather, is often appealed to in the choruses for aid." Answer to question about Indian poetry by Rev. Mr. Fletcher, who lived several years with the Winnebago Indians. He says, too, "there are no Indian poets in this country." Schoolcraft, IV. 71.

tion breaks away from the choral song, as if artistic poetry could not yet walk by itself; and where he has begun to till the soil, or even merely to gather plants and fruits, there is the chorus and there is the refrain of a rude harvest-home. For the hunter and warrior we may quote Heckewelder's account.[1] "Their songs are by no means inharmonious. They sing in chorus; first the men and then the women. At times the women join in the general song, or repeat the strain which the men have just finished. It seems like two parties singing in questions and answers, and is upon the whole very agreeable and enlivening. . . . The singing always begins by one person only, but others soon fall in successively, until the general chorus begins, the drum beating all the while to mark the time." Their war-dance is described in the familiar terms; but Heckewelder adds a more interesting account of the feast which under agricultural conditions would be a harvest-home. "After returning from a successful expedition," he says, "a dance of thanksgiving is always performed. . . . It is accompanied with singing and choruses, in which the women join. . . . At the end of every song, the scalp-yell is shouted as many times as there have been scalps taken from the enemy." As to the rhythm, Heckewelder makes a statement much clearer than the accounts given in Schoolcraft's question and answer, for he does not undertake to express Indian metres in terms of civilized poetry, but simply says that "their songs . . . are sung in short sentences, not without some kind of measure harmonious to an Indian ear."

These Indians, however, were not in the absolutely primitive stage, and the artist had elaborated dance, speech, song; in short, like European peasants of isolated communities a

[1] "Account of the History, Manners, and Customs of the Indian Nations who once Inhabited Pennsylvania and the Neighbouring States," *Transact. Amer. Philos. Soc.*, 1819, pp. 200 ff.

century ago, the redskin was at that point of poetical development where improvisation is a general gift, and every one is expected to compose his bit of song, leaning, of course, on the chorus, on refrain and repetition, and on those traditional phrases which even more than modern speech realized Schiller's lines about the poet: —

> Weil dir ein Vers gelingt in einer gebildeten Sprache
> Die für dich dichtet und denkt, glaubst du schon
> Dichter zu sein?

"The Indians also meet," says Heckewelder, "for the purpose of recounting their warlike exploits, which is done in a kind of half-singing or recitative . . . the drum beating all the while. . . . After each has made a short recital in his turn, they begin again in the same order, and so continue going the rounds, in a kind of alternate chaunting, until every one has concluded." It is easy to see that while the chorus of war is an eminently communal performance, asking an exactness of consent which makes strongly for rhythm at its best, the conditions of nomadic and belligerent life must breed excellent differences, set apart the great warrior, the great orator, and work in certain ways toward communal disintegration and the triumph of the artist. Agricultural communities, on the other hand, foster the choral and social side of poetry, and discourage individual feats. So even with the Indians; witness that "cereal chorus," as Schoolcraft calls it,[1] at the corn-husking, sung whenever a crooked ear is found by one of the maidens: —

> Crooked ear, crooked ear, walker at night, —

with additions and variations. This crooked ear, *wa-ge-min*, is the symbol of a "thief in the cornfield," and may have some relationship with Mannhardt's corn-demon.[2]

[1] Quoted above, p. 255, from *Indian Tribes*, V. 563 f.

[2] *Die Korndaemonen*, Berlin, 1868. See also his *Roggenwulf und Roggenhund*, Danzig, 1866.

Older views of the American savage show him in the war-like guise, to be sure, but with poetry overwhelmingly choral. Lafitau,[1] who says that commerce with the white man has materially changed the savage's customs, is determined to paint him in his unspoiled state. During an eclipse, for example, all the tribe dance in a peculiar manner, filling the air with lugubrious cries; that rhythm is in them, though it is no song in Lafitau's ear, is proved by the dance, which, of course, compels a rhythm, and by that picture of the girl who shakes pebbles in a calabash, "trying meanwhile to make her rough voice accord with this importunate jingle."[2] Singing and dancing are the chief features of Indian social life, and constitute the main charm of the life to come; improvised songs, even speeches, occur, but general singing and dancing make the background of their poetry and fill their festivals.[3] Everybody improvises, and has his special song,—a trait noted among the Eskimo; the dancers always sing, and apparently the singers always dance; the verse is measured, but has no rime, and individual songs are always supported by an accompanying *he! he!* in cadence from the throng, a sort of burden. Dramatic songs of war are common; and Lafitau gives a case marvellously like that Faroe ballad of the luckless fisherman, with satirist and victim in full view, although here the latter is passive, and is often forced by the laughter and scorn of the tribe to break away and hide his head in shame.[4] Song-duels, too, as among the Eskimo, are frequent, with throwing of ashes, which makes Lafitau call on Athenæus for a parallel among the ancient Greeks. But, after all, what sticks in Lafitau's mind about Indian dances is the fury of them and that wild *he! he!* which gave them cadence, but which often "made the whole village tremble and shake." The war-dance is described in terms familiar to the reader of later accounts.

[1] Work quoted, I. 25.
[2] *Ibid.*, I. 248.
[3] *Ibid.*, I. 517 ff.; II. 189 f.
[4] *Ibid.*, I. 525.

Lery gives an older story, but in the same spirit as that found in Lafitau. Of great interest is the Huguenot's account[1] of a festivity which he and one Jacques Rousseau saw and heard performed by five or six hundred savages in a certain village. The men retired into one house, the women to another; Lery and his friend were shut in with the women, about two hundred in all. From the house of the men came a low murmur, like that of folk at prayers; and the women, pricking their ears, huddled together in great excitement. Then the noise grew in volume, and the men could be heard singing in concert, and often repeating their interjection, *he, he, he, he;* the women now began to reply in kind, crying, *he, he, he, he,* for more than a quarter-hour, leaping, meanwhile, and foaming at the mouth, till it was quite plain to Lery that the devil was entering into them. But this was not all. From another house a mob of children now tuned the hallowed quire; and the Huguenot, despite his year and a half in those parts, is free to say he felt a desire to be "en nostre Fort," doubting the sequel of all this coil. Suddenly the women and children were quiet; and Lery could now hear the men singing and shouting "*d'un accord merveilleux*," so that these "sweet and more gracious sounds" heartened him to go near the house of the men. He made a hole in the soft wall and looked in; then, with two friends, he went inside, saw the dance, and heard the songs, which ran on without stop. All the men stood in a close circle, but without clasping hands or stirring from the place, bent forward, moving only the leg and the right foot, each having his right hand on his buttocks, the arm and left hand hanging, and so danced and sang. It seems to have been a communal dance, like that of the Botocudos, save that certain priests — *caraïbes* — richly arrayed, holding in their hands "little rattles or bells made of a fruit bigger than an ostrich

[1] Jean de Lery, *Histoire*, etc., pp. 268 ff.

egg," had evidently extraordinary powers. There is a remarkable picture by way of illustration,[1] showing the naked dancer, bent over, as described, with a priest behind him, a parrot on a perch just above the dancer's shoulder, and a monkey at his feet, — these doubtless an exuberance of the artist.

The social foundation, the communal dance, the incessant refrain, the festal excitement, are here plain outcome of primitive conditions in survival; the priest, and the ritual functions which are left to one's guessing, show that mingling of ceremonial tradition and art which is bound to spring up with even savage culture. Despite this mingling, however, the overwhelming characteristic of the whole affair is communal, and the songs are in close tether to the refrain. An excellent summary of American savage songs and American savage poetry in general has been already quoted in part from a paper by Dr. Brinton,[2] and may be used here as a conclusion of the whole matter. Repetition is the groundwork of this poetry; it is always sung; it has no rhythm, — no metre, that is, — no alliteration, but depends on two kinds of repetition. Either one verse is repeated indefinitely, or a refrain is used. "The refrain is usually interjectional and wholly meaningless; and the verses are often repeated without alteration four or five times ever." This is the case with Eskimo poetry. Now and then, each line "is followed by an interjectional burden." A little ballad may be quoted from Dr. Brinton's paper [3] to show how events passed into poetry, without forming what could be called in any sense narrative or epic verse. About the year 1820, the Pawnees captured a girl and put her to the torture; but a Pawnee brave, of generous vein, made a daring rescue and flight. After three days he came back; and as the thing was so mad, it was counted inspiration, and no one harmed him. Whereupon this song was sung: —

[1] Opposite p. 274. [2] See above, p. 253. [3] On pp. 25 ff.

Well he foretold this,
Well he foretold this,
Yes, he foretold this,
I, Pitale-Sharu,[1]
Am arrived here.
Well he foretold this,
Yes, he foretold this;
I, Pitale-Sharu,[1]
Am arrived here,—

and in this song, leaning so hard on the event, so bare of statement, so woven in with the life of the actual day that lapse even of a year or so must have brought need to its hearers to be edified by the margent,[2] so dependent on the refrain, so suggestive of an accompanying dance and of gestures to make the little drama real, it is not unfair to say that one has at least some of those factors which went to make the beginnings of poetry.

The refrain has been considered as the main communal element in songs of labour; here are its functions in communal play, primarily a combination of consenting cries and movements in the festal dance. The song that always went with a dance got its name thence, and was called a ballad; and in the ballad, whether strictly taken as a narrative song, or as the purely lyrical outburst for which there is no better term than folksong, this consenting and cadenced series of words found its main refuge and record. The subject is complicated enough, and asks a volume to put it into any semblance of order; all that can be done here is to group the main facts in their relation to primitive poetry. Unless one holds fast to the idea that refrains represent the original choral song of the mass, one begins to explain them by their modern features, and thus, while accurate as to a certain

[1] The name of the brave.

[2] One can readily understand that Stevenson heard his islanders sing, in chorus of perhaps a hundred persons, legendary songs about which not two of these singers could agree in their translation. *Letters of R. L. Stevenson*, II. 152.

stage of poetry, falls into error on the historic and genetic side. Ferdinand Wolf[1] gives an admirable account of the refrain, an admirable definition, but with a wrong inference of origins, when he assigns it to the participation of the people or of the congregation in songs which were sung to them by one or more persons on festal occasions, where the throng repeated in chorus single words, verses, whole strophes, or else in pauses of the main song answered the singer with a repeated shout to express their agreement, applause, horror, joy, or grief, — a shout which often lost its real meaning and became a mere conventional choral cry. Hence, says Wolf, it is clear that the refrain is as old as songs of the people.[2] It has been said that this statement is misleading in any genetic sense; it fails to note the growth of the exarch or foresinger into the poet, and to follow the backward curve of evolution to a point where the voice of the foresinger is lost in the voices of the choral throng itself, that raw material from which all poetry has been made. On the other hand, this definition undoubtedly states the facts of the refrain in its mediæval stage of survival from the chorus. In ballads, for example, it is the part taken by the throng in distinction from the part of the minstrel; but there is great difficulty in deciding how

[1] *Lais*, p. 18. Professor Schipper, in his valuable treatise on *Englische Metrik*, I. 326 ff., follows Wolf in this definition; but in both cases the analytic purpose excuses this neglect of the communal origin, and the material presented allows the student to make his own comparisons and supply the neglected considerations.

[2] A. W. Grube, *Deutsche Volkslieder*, Iserlohn, 1866, in his sections "Der Kehrreim des Volksliedes," pp. 1–103, and "Der Kehrreim bei Goethe, Uhland und Rückert," pp. 187–306, follows Wolf in part, deriving refrains from the church hymns (p. 112), but adds a plea for the antiquity of folksong, which is "von Haus aus Chorgesang" (p. 183). So, too, on p. 125, he seems to view the origin of poetry of the people as a statement of contemporaneous events in one sentence — hence not "invented" — which is sung by the throng. He notes the increased power of the refrain with the preponderance of lyric over epic elements: though he neglects the dance and communal conditions generally. The close connection of Goethe (as in the *Ach neige, Du Schmerzensreiche*) and of Rückert (as in the beautiful repetitions of *Aus der Jugendzeit*) with popular poetry, is admirably treated. See pp. 189 ff., 284 ff.

the throng actually sang the refrain. Names are no guide; and the terms, chorus, refrain, and burden are used in no exclusive fashion.[1] Probably one will not stray far from facts if one assumes that whenever a ballad came to be sung artistically, as a part-song in the rough, the refrain — *hey-no-nonny, the wind and the rain*, or what not — was really a burden, "the base, foot, or under-song";[2] as is proved by the scene in *Much Ado*,[3] where no man is in the group to sing this base or foot, and Margaret, wishing a song to which they can dance, cries, — "Clap us into *Light o' Love;* that goes without a burden: do you sing it, and I'll dance it." A passage quoted by many writers from the old play, *The Longer thou Livest the more Foole thou art*, tells how Moros enters, "synging the foote of many songes"; and bits of them follow, an interesting list; a little later, three of the characters are to "beare the foote," and there is much testing of the key. On the other hand, in Jonson's *Bartholomew Fair*,[4] there is the same play of getting key and tune, and Cokes "sings the burden" with Nightingale; but this is simply a couplet recurring at the end of each stanza. So Guest[5] defines the burden as "the return of the same words at the close of each stave." Is this right? For what one most wishes to know, so far as the singing of ballads is concerned, is whether the refrain, constant or intermittent, was sung as the "foot," that is, contemporaneously with the regular lines, or after them, either as couplet or in alternation, — as in —[6]

It was a knight in Scotland borne,
  Follow, my love, come over the strand,
Was taken prisoner and left forlorne
  Even by the good Earle of Northumberland.

[1] See a note in the author's *Old English Ballads*, p. lxxxiv.

[2] See Chappell, *Popular Music*, I. 222 ff., 34, 264; II. 426, 457.

[3] III. 4. See also the Oxford *Dictionary*, s.v. "burden," with the reference to Shakspere's *Lucrece*, v. 1133.

[4] III. 1.

[5] *English Rhythms*, II. 290.

[6] Child, I. 113.

Here the fitness of things indicates intermittent singing of the refrain which thus makes a four-line stanza out of a two-line stanza; this is Rosenberg's theory of the evolution of a ballad strophe.[1] Certainly the refrain came to be used in artistic and late communal poetry to mark off the stanza as the rime marked off the verse. What we now call a chorus, a recurrent stanza, sung after each new stanza, is often a clear case in ballads; for example, in *The Twa Magicians*,[2] that provocative and tuneful cadence of —

> O bide, lady, bide,
> And aye he bade her bide;
> The rusty smith your leman shall be
> For a' your muckle pride.

But there is doubt in regard to the refrain when it is said to be sung as burden, or what Grundtvig calls burden-stem; although there is no doubt that refrains were taken from folksong and chorus and were used as burdens in the ballad.[3] Even the song of labour is used for the refrain:[4]—

> Hey with a gay and a grinding, O!

distorted into —

> Hey with the gay and the grandeur, O!

The question, as Professor Child acknowledged, is extraordinarily difficult even when narrowed down to ballads. It is discussed at length in an unpublished dissertation by the late Dr. J. H. Boynton, who decides for the simultaneous singing of the ballad strophe and the refrain,[5] and incident-

[1] *Nordboernes Aandsliv*, II. 434 ff.; but this evolution is stoutly denied by Steenstrup, *Vore Folkeviser*, pp. 120 ff., in a study of the refrain to be considered below.

[2] Child, I. 403: printed after the sixth stanza, and so till the eleventh, when the chorus is slightly changed to suit the story, and kept so to the end. For the strophic refrain or chorus and its popularity in Old French, see Schipper, I. 328.

[3] Child, I. 209, 214.

[4] *Ibid.*, I. 126 ff., in F., O. See H.

[5] *Studies in the English Ballad Refrain, with a Collection of Ballad and Early Song Refrains.* Thesis presented by John Henry Boynton in candidacy for the

ally for the growth of a four-line strophe out of the early strophe of two lines. Icelandic and Faroe ballads show the most archaic elements in the Germanic group, and "a large proportion of their refrains deal directly with the dance." The "stem" is sung first by the leader of the dance, and is a "lyric in itself," fit to go "with any ballad." Now it is clear that whether the ballad and the burden were sung simultaneously, as Boynton believes to have been the case, or alternately, as certain English ballads seem to require, and as Guest assumed in his definition, this question of musical technique cannot affect the inference that the burden, a "lyric in itself" which serves as refrain, is older than the ballad or narrative song, and has most intimate relations with the steps of the dance. In other words, here is the refrain in its passage from a dominant place as choral repetition of the throng, timed to their steps and deriving its existence from these steps and from the expression of festal delight that prompted them, to an ancillary and subordinate place as choral support to the artistic progress of a narrative in song. This agrees with the records of communal song not only under savage conditions but among the homogeneous and unlettered communities of Europe. Neocorus,[1] a priest who writes about the beginning of the seventeenth century, defending that unschooled song which he still heard at the dances and festivities of his countryfolk of the Cimbrian peninsula, and which still flowed so easily, although much of it was lost that ought to have been recorded and sung, describes their communal dance; it is in a fairly advanced stage, of course, and is led by an expert. First, this leader

degree of Doctor of Philosophy in English, May 1, 1897. In 3 vols., Ms., Harvard University Library. The material is excellently put together; but the genetic and historical elements are not sufficiently brought out. The comparative work is good, and as a study of actual refrains this dissertation is of distinct value. The burden-stem is discussed in section V., pp. 184 ff.

[1] *Chronik*, ed. Dahlmann, I. 176 f. See also II. 559 ff.

comes forward singing alone, or with a colleague, and begins a ballad. "And when he has sung a verse, he sings no further, but the whole throng, who either know the ballad or else have paid close attention to him, repeat and echo the same verse. And when they have brought it to the point where the leader stopped, he begins again and sings another verse." This is again repeated. Presently, with the singing thus under way, a leader of the dance comes forward, hat in hand, dances about the room, and invites the whole assembly to join. Facts which have been given already, and facts still to be considered, show clearly that these leaders of song and of dance are deputies of the throng which once danced as a mass to its own choral singing. On the other hand, as Boynton noted, repetition and refrain may take the form of a genuine burden. In Icelandic ballads, the "burden-stem" was often in a different metre from the ballad stanza; it was sung "to support the voice by harmonious notes under the melody," and "was heard separately only when the voices singing the air stopped."[1] But in the Faroe isles "the whole stem is sung first, and then repeated as a burden at the end of every verse." This is certainly more natural than the process, known in Iceland, where a leader sings the incremental stanzas and the throng keeps singing the burden or accompaniment; although a very familiar ballad might so be sung, and the fact would of course indicate either a shifting of interest toward purely musical ends, as in Elizabethan England, or else a devotion on the part of the crowd to the dance proper and the refrain, while the narrative is left to the leader of the song.[2]

Apart from the manner of singing it under later conditions,

[1] Chappell quoted by Child, *Ballads*, I. 7. "I must avow myself," says Professor Child, "to be very much in the dark as to the exact relation of stem and burden." See also *Ballads*, II. 204, first note.

[2] This technical side of the case is discussed by Valentin, *Studien über die schwedischen Volksmelodien*, pp. 9 f.

the refrain in itself, so far as ballads are concerned, is clearly the recurrent verse or verses sung by the festal crowd; and the nearer one comes to the source of a ballad, that is, to the dancing throng, the more insistent and pervasive and dominant this refrain becomes. That is the fact which nobody has ever denied. Jeanroy,[1] in a careful discussion of origins, concludes that refrains are really fragments of song for the dance, now and then, as he hints, of songs of labour; he regards them solely in their function as lines sung at the end of a stanza, and like other scholars thinks they were "originally repeated by the chorus in answer to the soloist."[2] Elsewhere, however, he grants that this need not have been the universal fashion, and that now and then all the dancers may have sung all the song,[3] a theory fortified by his conjecture that the refrain was once made up of imitative sounds. However, the modern refrain of the dance, best preserved among French and Italians, is a lively lilting couplet, or the like, to which the other riming verses are prefixed in the growth of the actual song, as in the stanzas quoted from Bujeaud:—

Là haut, dessus ces rochettes,
J'entend le haut-bois jouer,
Et vous autr', jeunes fillettes,
Qui allez au bal danser,
Allez, allez, tenez vous dreites,
Prenez gard' de n' pas tomber.

[1] *Les Origines de la Poésie Lyrique en France au Moyen Age*, Paris, 1889, pp. 102 ff. (see note 2, p. 111), and 387 ff. On the etymology of *refrain*, see pp. 103 f.

[2] *Ibid.*, p. 113. Jeanroy will not accept the view of Wackernagel and Bartsch that the refrains preserved in old French lyric poetry are actual "popular" songs, or fragments of them; but he willingly accepts the theory that all refrains were once of a communal kind. These, he thinks, are hopelessly lost. See pp. 115 ff. A few older refrains can be found in foreign lyric which imitated the French; pp. 177 ff.

[3] *Ibid.*, p. 396, note 1. Or, as in old Portuguese song, copied from the popular manner, one part of the dancers sang one verse, and another part, like strophe and antistrophe, repeated the verse with a slight change, usually in the final word

The transition is very evident. In another case[1] the leader calls on the dancers to make some cry imitative of animals, which now serves as refrain; but, wherever found, the test of a really popular refrain, as Jeanroy insists, is that it was made for the dance. Read "in the dance," and communal conditions are even better satisfied.

For the ballad is a song made in the dance, and so by the dance; a mass of those older dance-songs which have come down to us as popular, are later development, are of either aristocratic or learned origin, and simply point back to the communal dance which is the real source of the song. Originally a chorus of all the dancers, it gave vent to the feelings of joy, — in the old *vocero* dance, of grief, — to the common emotion of the throng. An impulse which makes for this song of the dance is simple delight that the season of dancing is begun: —

A l'entrada del tems clar, *eya*;[2]

and so one may trace these invocations of nature to their later form at the beginning of a narrative song like *Robin Hood and the Monk*. This dancing of the round as an expression of feeling on the part of a throng — dancing in pairs, we know, did not reach Neocorus's country, for example, until the middle of the sixteenth century — meets one everywhere in mediæval records, and it has died a reluctant death;

which rimes with the other final word. The connection of this with the *contrasto* of lover and sweetheart, imitated in the dance, of debate, flyting, *tenso*, and the like, would lead too far afield. See p. 207, and below, p. 325.

[1] *Ibid.*, p. 405. This chapter, where Jeanroy traces the growth of artificial forms, like the rondel and so on, out of purely popular refrain and verse, is of distinct value to the student of communal poetry. It completely refutes the claim of superficial criticism, common enough of late, that ballad and folksong are merely dregs of an older art, and that some pretty comparison, say a tramp in an old dress-coat, solves the communal problem. As jaunty and insufferable a piece of comment as can be found anywhere in print is Mr. Gregory Smith's chapter on "The Problem of the Ballads and Popular Songs" in his *Transition Period*, pp. 180 ff.

[2] See above, p. 174. The refrain is very clearly an actual cry at the dance.

unless observation be at fault, even children are ceasing to play the old round games common not many years ago, a city of refuge that seemed at one time so secure. But in those mediæval days one danced in throngs on almost any occasion; and impossible as the story may be if taken literally, there is truth enough for our purpose in that account[1] of Leicester's army in 1173 pausing on a heath, where they "fell to daunce and singe —

> "Hoppe, Wylikin, hoppe Wyllikin,
> Ingland is thine and mine."

Many of the folksongs go little beyond this stage of an exhortation to dance, along with a brief comment on the posture of affairs or on the scene. Such an exhortation as refrain for the dance occurs in the old play of the *Four Elements*, with an interesting context. Says Ignorance —

> I can you thank ; that is done well ;
> It is pity ye had not a minstrel
> For to augment your solace.

and Sensual Desire replies: —

> As for minstrel, it maketh no force,[2]
> Ye shall see me dance a course
> Without a minstrel.

Then he singeth this song and danceth withal, and evermore maketh countenance according to the matter; and all the others answer likewise: —

> Dance we, dance we, prance we, prance we.

Ignorance says it "is the best dance without a pipe he has seen this seven year." But Humanity inclines to think "a kit or taboret" would improve the dance; and the dancers retire to a tavern where they are sure "of one or twain of minstrels that can well play." Humanity now proposes "to sing some lusty ballad"; but Ignorance is against all such

[1] Quoted by Ritson, *Anc. Songs*[3], p. xxxv.

[2] Difference.

"peevish prick-ear'd song," and when he is told that prick-song in church pleases God, makes the often-quoted reply that there is no good reason why it is "not as good to say plainly *Give me a spade*, as *Give me a spa, ve, va, ve, va, vade.*" No; if a song is wanted, one of the good old sort will do; and there follows a list not unlike that of Moros in the play or that of Laneham in the letter, with the trifling exception that this runs into a helpless sort of burlesque. "Robin Hood in Barnsdale stood" is probably a genuine first line, and so are some of the other titles. The main thing is that ballad singing is opposed to prick-song and the new fashions generally, and that a refrain from all lusty throats is better for the dance than pipe or minstrel. The refrain in this case is just the old exhortation to dance. This exhortation is common enough in folksong, alone or as a refrain: [1] —

> Springe wir den reigen . . .
> Saute, blonde, ma joli' blonde . . .

but a pure and simple description of the matter in hand, as communal, spontaneous, and immediate an expression in song as may be, and tied to steps of the dance by the shortest of tethers, is doubtless to be found in the game where a circle of children dance round one of their companions in the ring to this refrain: [2] —

[1] It is useless to pile up references; any collection has such refrains in plenty. This "springewir den reigen" (*Carmina Burana*, ed. Schmeller, p. 178), however, like Neidhart's dance-songs, although it goes with the welcome to May, is conventional already and artistic.

[2] Chambers, *Popular Rhymes of Scotland*, pp. 132 ff. "Another form of this game is *only a kind of dance*," says the editor, without italics, "in which the girls first join hands in a circle and sing while moving round to the tune of Nancy Dawson: —

> Here we go round the mulberry-bush,

and so on. Then: —

> This is the way the ladies walk . . .
> This is the way they wash the clothes . . .

with refrain, or chorus, as before, and imitative actions."

Here we go the jingo-ring,
The jingo-ring, the jingo-ring,
Here we go the jingo-ring
About the merry-ma-tanzie.

Let this be a survival of a wedding ceremony, or whatever the learned will, the refrain, sung with each stanza, and suited of course to the action, is typical of the earliest choral stage.[1] Now so soon as narrative takes the place of this description of contemporary and common action, this exhortation of all to all to do something which they are all doing, then memory, deliberation, arrangement, are needed, and an artist comes to the fore. When a ballad records some doing of the folk, when the epic element takes upper hand, it is clear that a process of separation is inevitable. A ballad of this sort may long remain as favourite song for the communal dance. Thus a lively little thing, found in Flanders and in Germany,[2] is of particular interest, first for the narrative which is the old satire on monk and nun, so popular in mediæval times; secondly for the refrain, which is nothing less than a dance about the maypole, keeping the song itself in some places for this festivity; and thirdly for the wandering of the ballad as a whole, from the fifteenth century down to its modern refuge in a children's game:—

A monk went walking along the strand,—
Hey! 'twas in the May!
He took his sweetheart[3] by the hand,—
Hey! 'twas in the May!
So gay!
Hey! 'twas in the May!

[1] Lucian, in his treatise on the dance, is no authority for primitive dancing and refrain; but it is noteworthy that he gives such an exhortation as a kind of refrain. "The song that they sing as they dance," he says of the Lacedæmonians, § 11, "is an invitation to Venus and the loves. . . . One of these songs is a lesson in dancing (!): 'On,' they sing, 'young people, stretch your legs and dance your best.'"

[2] Coussemaker, I. 328; Firmenich, I. 380, IV. 679.

[3] In the other version "nonnetje," "nönneke," little nun.

Here the dance has held its own with the story; but in most cases, as the foresinger or exarch takes command, the new verses, beginning as incremental repetition in the dance, grow bolder and learn to walk alone; singing is still a condition, but the dance is only an occasion, not a cause; and finally the crowd passes over the bridge of chorus and refrain into a quite passive state of audience, with intermittent echo and applause, utterly disappearing at last behind the sheets of a broadside.

This, of course, is a conclusion at very long range; and there is an extensive period, a large field, where elements of art mingled freely with the old communal motive. For a single example, take the *Bouquet de Marjolaine.*[1] This is a case of incremental repetition, with the same rimes throughout, and an unvaried refrain or chorus which is knitted to each stanza by this pervading rime. The third line of each stanza forms the opening line of the next stanza, so that the story proceeds slowly but surely to the end. The whole can be gathered from one stanza and its refrain, with addition of the following incremental lines: —

Me promenant dans la plaine,
(Tir' ton joli bas de laine)
J'ai trouvé un Capitaine.
(Tir' ton, tir' ton, tir' ton bas,
Tir' ton joli bas de laine,
Car on le verra.)

Then, "il m'a appelé' vilaine"; "je ne suis point si vilaine;" "le plus jeun' fils du roi m'aime;" "il m'a donné pour étrenne" — "une bourse d'écus pleine," "un bouquet de marjolaine;" "je l'ai planté dans la plaine;" — and, for good last, and with that touch of pathos common in these things,

[1] Bujeaud, *Chants et Chansons . . . de l'ouest,* I. 88, from Poitou; reprinted by Crane, *Chansons Populaires,* pp. 87 ff. See a similar song, Crane, pp. 162 ff.; many more could be instanced, and some have been already named.

despite the gay tone, "s'il fleurit, je serai reine"; and so, with the refrain, an end. Full of communal elements, this song is nevertheless of an artistic type and of an aristocratic origin, an offshot of the *pastourelle* and its kin; popular enough, of a certain simplicity and beauty, it is not directly communal in its tone; it has gone among the people, and yet, though it was imitated from purely communal refrains, like other and older songs treated so successfully by Jeanroy, it has not come directly from the people. In fact, the communal refrain of the dance is seldom in such independent case as this infectious lilt; when it is not a survival, as in children's games, its best chance for life is as parasite to a narrative ballad or even to a "lyric of sentiment and reflection," as anthologies call them. Thus Ten Brink is undoubtedly right when he takes the refrain as old, traditional, communal, and the stanzas as new and artistic, in that pretty English lyric, *Ichot a burde in boure bryht*, which has the refrain at the beginning, as in many Provençal ballads:—

Blow, northern wind,
Send thou me my sweeting!
Blow, northern wind, blow, blow, blow!

Compare this with the artistic refrain of *Alisoun*, from which it differs so widely, and with the refrain of the Cuckoo Song, in its recorded form part of an elaborate composition, but doubtless taken from the "nature" refrain of a dance. The ballads and folksongs of Europe are of course in the transitional stage. They ought to be sung, but many of them may have been recited; they echo the cadence of a dancing throng, and have often timed the dance, though they are separable from such company. It must be borne in mind, however, that many ballads in which one would not now suspect such uses, were employed to regulate the slow steps of a dance. Narrative ballads were in great favour for the purpose; Faroe islanders danced to the stories of Sigurd, and the Russians, whose folksongs are always choral and without instrumental music, dance the *khorovod* to a narrative song, — in fact, the word means a blended song and dance; while even the Robin Hood ballads, if we may believe the *Complaynt of Scotland*, as well as some ballad of Johnny Armstrong, were sung at the dance of the shepherds. Savages sing narrative poems to the dance, and so do Melanesians.[1] One can therefore understand the statement made by Steenstrup,[2] that every genuine ballad has a refrain, though this may not be recorded; for the refrain is the tie which binds a ballad to its parent dance. As one retraces the path of the ballad, the refrain grows in importance, slowly pushing the leader or soloist nearer and nearer to the throng, until he is lost in it; and a repetition of cadenced choral cries becomes the main factor of poetry. As every one knows, those cadenced cries were regulated by the dance; and to this important factor in early poetry, already considered under the head of rhythm, we must now turn.

Dancing, most momentary of all the arts, as A. W. Schlegel called it, in Wagner's words "the most real," seeing that the

[1] Waitz, *Anthropologie*, VI. 606.

[2] *Vore Folkeviser*, pp. 75–112, "Omkvaedet." Geijer denied that the refrain is necessary to a ballad, but Steenstrup's argument is convincing; out of 502 Scandinavian ballads which he examined, not more than 20 lacked a refrain. The ballads in Child's collection point the same way, at least for the older and shorter ballads; the *Gest*, of course, and others of that sort, as well as broadside copies, have passed from the lyrical stage. But even these must go back to an earlier song with a refrain. Of the two-line ballads, the older form, there are 31, and of these only 7 lack the refrain in their present form. Of the 305 ballads in the collection, 106 in at least one version show evidence of refrain or chorus, — more than a third; while of some 1250 versions in all, about 300 have the refrain. This count was made very carefully by Mr. C. H. Carter, of Haverford College. Of course, Wolf had long since proved that the refrain is characteristic of all early poetry in the vernacular, and played a leading part in popular verse everywhere, from its first collection in the fifteenth century down to the present time. See his *Lais*, pp. 27, 191.

whole man is concerned in it, "from head to foot," with motions and gestures that give it tone, and rhythm that gives it speech,[1] was also the primitive and universal art, the sign of social consent; consenting steps, with mimicry of whatever sort, timed a series of rude cries which expressed the emotion of the moment, and so grew into articulate language. But the song detached itself from dancing long before dancing could shake off the choral cries and the refrain. Among Tasmanians and Australians songs already existed apart from the dance; but there was no dance without a song, and the dances were prevailingly of the whole horde or clan. Survivals of this primitive stage, and the early history of dancing in all quarters of the world, afford good warrant for the conclusion of Böhme;[2] "no dance without singing, and no song without a dance," is his axiom for earliest times. Moreover, this proof of the connection of song and dance in the primitive horde, a bond which one or two writers have lately tried to sever, but without success, disposes of Mr. Herbert Spencer's attempt[3] to explain the dance as a modification of the old movement of obeisance.

Dancing is universal among savages; and if a few cases occur which make against this doctrine, one may safely assume, as Ribot does, and even Wallaschek,[4] that they are

[1] "Das Kunstwerk der Zukunft," *Schriften*, III., pp. 87, 89. See also Ribot, *Psychology of the Emotions*, p. 334, who calls dancing the "primordial art," and shows that here is the transition from mere movement to æsthetic activity.

[2] *Geschichte des Tanzes*, p. 4. This is the best treatise on the subject, though mainly confined to Germany. *A History of Dancing from the Earliest Ages . . . from the French of Gaston Vuillier, with a Sketch of Dancing in England*, by Joseph Grego, London, 1898, is of scant use for the student of origins and development. Dancing "was probably unknown to the earliest ages of humanity," a bold assertion, is followed by another, that "it is certain that dancing was born with man." Information of value can be found, however, on special topics; *e.g.* on the *branle*, p. 100, and its connection with children's games.

[3] *Sociology*, II. 123.

[4] See also Yrjö Hirn, *Förstudier*, pp. 89 f. Dismissing exceptions, he declares that "dancing in its widest sense is as universal as laughing and weeping."

due to insufficient observation,[1] or else, at the worst, that they belong to tribes with hardly any claims of humanity, degenerates, retrogrades, who have no social order and consequently no dance. Again, the primitive form of the dance is to be found in the choral throng; but it must be borne in mind that even rudest tribes can develop an art of complicated, traditional, and ritual character,[2] which in its turn breeds the solo and the professional artist in dancing. However, the choral dies hard even under civilized conditions; among savages it is prominent everywhere and in full vigour. Waitz,[3] speaking of tribes in the South Seas, says that song there is mainly choral, and dancing, affair of the community as a whole, is as universal as song, often passing into mimicry and a rude drama. Everywhere, too, song is accompanied by dancing, and when women thus dance and sing they clap hands or slap the hip in time with their steps and words, after the manner of their sisters in mediæval Europe. Musical instruments are few. Chamisso noted now and then what he took to be degeneration of song into mere howling; but we know there is a more excellent way to explain these festal and cadenced cries. Dancing is in order at each important moment for the community, — when strangers arrive, when war is imminent, at feasts of every sort. As with these natives of the South Sea, so with other and more savage tribes. It is useless to insist in detail upon the African love of dancing, which goes on every evening and in every village for hours at a time. "The natives of Obbo began their dance by all singing together a wild but pleasant-sounding melody in chorus,[4]" is only one of many descrip-

[1] No dancing in Iceland, says Kerguelen, who visited there in 1767. See Pinkerton, *Voyages and Travels*, I. 751. Volumes of proof could be furnished for refuting this light-hearted assertion.

[2] See Bastian, "Masken und Maskereien," *Zeitschr. f. Völkerpsych.*, XIV. 347.

[3] *Anthropologie der Naturvölker*, VI. 78 ff.

[4] Wallaschek, p. 189.

tions of this favourite communal diversion; but the legends and the complicated artistic dances which exist side by side with the choral song and the communal dance warn one that while primitive ways survive on the Dark Continent, there is a lower stage of song and dance to be found elsewhere. Like the Botocudos in South America, the Australians are on a quite elementary level with regard to dance and song; they attach more importance to the gesture than to the articulate word, so far as the telling of stories or the describing of events is concerned, and they know scarcely any individual performance.[1] Dance and song are of the horde, the clan, as a whole. Choral shouts, refrains which repeat a word or a short phrase indefinitely, and so time the steps of the throng, make the original social art; with the aid of gesture, mimicry of labour, of feats of hunting, this passes into kangaroo-dances, erotic pantomimes, sham fights, and all the rest. Perhaps, as Hirn[2] suggests, the dance of the Weddas, or Veddahs, in Ceylon is as primitive as anything of the kind; although Ehrenreich's account of the Botocudos[3] shows little if any advance. A spear is stuck into the ground to serve as centre for the ring of dancers, who move with swaying of legs and arms to the cadence of their own singing, — call it rather shouting, — while they keep exact time by slapping the naked stomach.[4] From this communal dance and song, emerges after a while, as in the case of the Botocudos, an individual performer; and it is clear that elaborate dances, such as those

[1] Letourneau, p. 28.

[2] Work quoted, pp. 95 ff. He refers to Hartshorne, "The Weddas," *Indian Antiquary*, VIII. 316 f.; E. Tennent, *Ceylon*, II. 437 ff.; and E. Schmidt, *Globus*, LXV. 15 f.

[3] See above, p. 95. It is interesting, however, particularly in connection with the idea of rhythm as the chief factor in the social process, that these Veddahs live mainly in pairs; "except on some extraordinary occasion they never assemble together," and this dance is evidently their chief means to express a social union. See Bastian, *Der Völkergedanke . . .*, p. 72.

[4] See also the Brazilian dances noted by Lery, above, p. 312.

given for the benefit of Captain Cook and other foreign visitors, are an outgrowth of this primitive huddling in mass with concert of cries and movements. It is significant that instinct of the clan calls for some concerted dance and song as necessary preface for war or any similar doing of the community as a whole; in long range of development this is the war-dance of our own Indians, often described, where a general chorus serves as background and stimulus alike to the volunteers who step forward singly and promise, in chanted and improvised song that times their steps, deeds of individual valour in the impending fight. So, perhaps, the *gab* of romance, the *gilp* or *gilpcwide*[1] of Germanic warriors, was originally made not only, as we know it, in the mead hall, but to the chorus of the tribes and with the steps of a dance. At close range, however, and with the foe in sight, it was a communal and general gab, a choral performance; witness the interesting account of Captain Cook.[2] In the first voyage, some four hundred islanders, about to attack the captain and his friends, but hesitating, at length "sung the song of defiance and began to dance." Such was a particular case; and in his general statement, Cook says that New Zealanders, before they begin the onset, "join in a war-song, to which they all keep the exactest time"; and while he does not mention the dance here, it is evidently implied, for his scattered accounts of skirmish and fight are full of it. A curious case is what would seem to be a war-dance in a boat which was attacking Cook's ship; as it approached, the savages in the boat varied menaces with peaceful talk, "till, imagining the sailors were afraid of them, they began the war-song and dance, and threw stones on board the ship." Then Cook goes on: "In the war-dance their motions are numerous, their limbs are distorted . . . they shake their darts, brandish

[1] *Béowulf,* 631 ff., 2631 ff. The *béot* is the same thing; *Battle of Maldon,* 213.
[2] Pinkerton, *Voyages and Travels,* London, 1808 ff., XI. 535, 543, 648.

their spears . . . they accompany this dance with a song, which is sung in concert; every strain ending with a loud and deep sigh. There is an activity and vigour in their dancing which is truly admirable; and their idea of keeping time is such that sixty or eighty paddles will strike at once against the sides of their boats, and make only one report." Concerted singing, this communal initiative, goes not only before war, but before embassies, messages of peace, greetings, and the like; and the dance is clearly an original prop of this song, now and then retained, but often omitted. In Cook's last voyage,[1] "a double canoe, in which were twelve men, came towards us. As they drew near the ship, they recited some words in concert, by way of chorus, one of the number first standing up and giving the word before each repetition," — a "solemn chant," Cook calls it. Readers of these and other voyages in the South Seas, know how singing rather than speaking takes the foreground of private as well as of tribal life; a chief coming on board the ship hails it with a song to explain his visit, and there is the case of the islander who told in song his story of life aboard an English ship, and, asking the native who had met him what news there was from home, put his excited questions in rhythm and got the equally excited answers in rapid chant. Behind this individual song is the chorus; with the chorus is nearly always the dance; wherever the dance, there is song. Musical instruments the islanders knew, of course, — drums, perhaps, best; but as Cook says[2] of a great dance which was given for him, it did not seem "that the dancers were much assisted by these sounds, *but by a chorus of vocal music, in which all the performers joined at the same time.*"

[1] Pinkerton, *Voyages and Travels*, pp. 652, 723.

[2] *Ibid.*, p. 667; no italics in the original. So, p. 654, twenty young women dance to their own singing, and in many other cases; the fact is beyond dispute. For a dance of more complicated character, but with chorus and refrain, see pp. 678 f.

Indians of the Western continent have the same tale to tell, and it has been told in part already by Lery, Lafitau, and the older travellers. A century and more ago, Carver[1] noted that the savages of North America "usually dance either before or after every meal";[2] and "they never meet on any public occasion, but this makes a part of the entertainment. . . . The youth of both sexes amuse themselves in this manner every evening." At the feasts and other dances, "every man rises in his turn, and moves about with great freedom and boldness, singing, as he does so, the exploits of his ancestors. During this the company, who are seated on the ground in a circle, join with him in making the cadence, by an odd tone, which they utter all together, and which sounds '*Heh, heh, heh.*'" This they repeat "with the same violence during the whole of the entertainment." "The women dance without taking any steps . . . but with their feet conjoined, moving by turns their toes and heels. . . . Let those who join in the dance be ever so numerous, they keep time so exactly with each other that no interruption ensues."

In recent times the intricate dances, ritual and ceremony which, of course, reach back in far tradition, have been studied and recorded; but this is not a primitive phase of the art,[3] and even among the Moqui and Navajo tribes of

[1] *Three Years' Travel*, etc., Phila., 1796; the travels were in 1766–1768. See pp. 171 ff., 220.

[2] See Lescarbot, *Histoire de la Nouvelle France*, Paris, 1609, pp. 317 ff., an account of the tribal dances of the Algonquins in honour of a victory, with interesting particulars. So, too, pp. 691 ff., another account, with a dance where they "do nothing but sing *Hé* or *Het!* like a man cutting wood, with a movement of the arm; and they dance a 'round' without holding one another or stirring from one place, beating their feet upon the earth." So, says Lescarbot, they make fires and jump through them, like our French peasants on the eve of St. John, who shout and dance the whole night. His fifteenth chapter, pp. 765 ff., is on *Danses et Chansons*, and accents the dance after a feast. Here, too, he says, "après la panse vient la danse." Savages, he says, always sing to their dancing.

[3] It is unfortunately not superfluous to suggest that the dances described by Homer are anything but primitive, though they retain some primitive traits. The

New Mexico, where instrumental music is common, now and then the dancers furnish their own music, each one rolling out "an *aw*, *aw*, *aw*, *aw*, in a deep bass tone."[1] So in ancient Mexico, where civilization of a sort had long held sway, the dances "were almost always accompanied by singing"; this, however, was "adjusted by the beating of instruments."[2] But this public dance is no longer communal in the old way; ritual of the clan becomes a state religion, while dance and song are not only lifted but expanded. There is a sense of ritual, to be sure, about the dance of a small community, as when among the Bechuanas, to ask a man "what he dances," is the same as asking to what clan or tribe he belongs, a phrase curiously akin to Gosson's remark[3] that "to daunce the same round" means to be of the same flock. But all this belongs only to the primitive horde or the late homogeneous community; the dance of such a little clan about their growing crops yielded to traditional and solemn rites, and the spontaneous singing and dancing which Vergil recommends to his farmers[4] is really a more primitive stage of the art than the seemingly older ceremony of the Arval brothers, which had already hardened into ritual and belonged to a close corporation under control of the state. Tribal dances become expia-

dance pictured on the shield of Achilles (*Il.* XVIII.), youths dancing and fair maids, hand in hand, is a *ronde*, to be sure, in form, but a society affair as well, with full dress, complicated figures, and a "divine minstrel" for the music. However, the vintage dance to the Linos song, described in the preceding verses, holds, like our harvest refrains, an older fashion.

[1] Ten Broeck, in Schoolcraft, IV. 84.

[2] Clavigero, *History of Mexico*, trans. Cullen, London, 1787, I. 399 f., a description of the great public dances.

[3] *Schoole of Abuse*, p. 34.

[4] When M. Gaston Paris, *Les Origines de la Poésie Lyrique en France au Moyen Age*, p. 42, says he has found no dance among the old Romans except the professional dance, he overlooks the fact that this rustic dance in procession about the fields is proof of similar dances for pleasure. It is no professional affair which Vergil has in mind: *det motus incompositos et carmina dicat.* Surely the dances were not danced by slaves.

tory and religious acts at a very early stage of culture; it is easy to see that the records would preserve such a dance only when it had lost some of its spontaneous character, and taken on a ritual form. Germanic, Slavic, and Romance peoples have the communal dance surviving as a religious act; and it was one of the hardest tasks for councils and bishops to stop this dancing of the congregation within the church itself. Often they allowed it in a modified form. As a part of ritual, choristers still dance before the altar of the cathedral at Seville; sixteen boys in blue and white form "in two eights," facing each other, and the priests kneel in a semicircle round them. Then "an unseen orchestra" begins to play, the boys put on their hats and sing the *coplas* in honour of the Virgin: —

O mi, O mi amada
Immaculada! —

"to a dance measure." After this they begin to dance, "still singing," a "kind of solemn minuet."[1] This is done at the feast of the Immaculate Conception. In the sixteenth century boys and girls danced about an image of Christ set upon the altar of German churches, singing Christmas songs, while their parents stood by, also singing and clapping their hands in time with the dance.[2] From these good folk to the German barbarians "running in a circle" round the goat's head and "singing diabolical songs," as seen and heard by Gregory,[3] is no long step backward in development if it is in chronology. When the children were at last driven from the churches, and when the old ring-dance was at last forgotten by their elders, even in the fields and about the fires of St. John's Eve, the little ones made a brave rescue and kept up

[1] Described by Mr. Arthur Symons in *Harper's Monthly Magazine*, March, 1901, p. 503.

[2] Pfannenschmid, *Germ. Erntef.*, p. 400.

[3] See above, p. 301.

the ritual in their games. Now even these are vanishing. Outside of Europe, sacred and even national dances of the throng go this same path of development and decline. The Hebrew communal dance passed into traditional forms;[1] and there are other dances, outside of religious cult, which acquire a fixed form and are passed down as of tribal and even national significance. One thinks of the Pyrrhic dance;[2] indeed, a study of the sword-dance in all its varieties, and from this double point of view, communal and national, would be of great interest. Savages, as Donovan remarked, imitate in their dancing now the movement of animals, now the clash of arms in war, and again, though not to the extent asserted by Scherer, erotic gestures.[3] For the second sort, a gymnastic motive, the sense of preparation and drill for future fighting, and a festal or reminiscential motive, combine to produce such an exercise as the sword-dance, a convenient name for this group, although the sword itself is not always in evidence. Chronology is here of no account; for earliest

[1] See the suggestive treatment of this subject by Posnett, *Comparative Literature*, pp. 117 ff., with his references to Réville and Burnouf.

[2] Silius Italicus, naming the troops which Hannibal led out of winter quarters, comes to the Gallician contingent, and describes their youth —

> barbara nunc patriis ululantem carmina linguis,
> nunc, pedis alterno percussa verbere terra,
> ad numerum resonas gaudentem plaudere caetras.

Lemaire (*Bib. Class. Lat.*, Sil. Ital. *Punic.*, III. 345 ff.), explains this as a heroic ballad which the soldiers sing, as they dance and strike their shields, when going into battle. He refers to the classical passages for this as well as for the Pyrrhic dance; but see note at the end of this chapter. The perhaps similar custom of the Germans, noted by Tacitus, is treated in a masterly way by Müllenhoff. See the next note but one.

[3] Pantomime, as early form of dance leading to poetry and drama, was noted by Adam Smith, *Essays*, p. 151. For older literature, see Blankenburg, *Zusätze*, I. 153 ff. Erotic dances were exaggerated by Scherer into the protoplasm of all poetry, *Poetik*, pp. 83, 114; and are more moderately treated by Hirn, *Förstudier*, pp. 88 ff., and Grosse, *Anf. d. Kunst*, pp. 21 ff. It is a developed art, of course, that Lucian has in mind in his treatise on the dance. See, however, Lucian, §§ 36, 63, 65.

records may show a well-defined and almost national exercise such as Tacitus noted among the Germans, and very late examples can be found of the purely communal sword-dance, with flyting, songs, refrain, and rustic acting, as in the Revesby Sword Play;[1] while Xenophon tells of a little drama, enacted by soldiers of the ten thousand, combining the weapon dance, the imitated fight, and other elements, in terms which could be matched by many an account given by traveller or missionary of a similar affair among quite savage tribes.[2] It is easy to see how one of the many paths from this dance of mimicry, exercise, and rhythmic shouting, would lead to the narrative song or ballad, and how such a ballad would long cleave to a particular traditional dance. The Phæacians have a narrative song sung to them as they are dancing, and when two dance alone, tossing the ball,[3] "the other youths . . . beat time"; but an older and more communal habit is found in the dances of the Faroe islanders, where the gestures and expression of face show how keenly the folk feel what they sing;[4] in the Icelandic *rimur*, narrative songs which went with the dance; on the Cimbrian peninsula, where ballads about the battle of Hemmingstede were used for the same purpose; in scattered rural communities[5] of Europe; and among savage tribes the world over. It has

[1] Manley, *Specimens of the Pre-Shaksperian Drama*, I. 296 ff., from the Folk-Lore Journal, VII. 338 ff. The date of the play is 1779. For the Germanic sword-dance, see Müllenhoff, *Festgabe für G. Homeyer*, "Ueber den Schwerttanz," p. 117. A bibliography of this subject is printed in the *Zeitschr. f. Völkerpsychol.*, etc., XIX. 204, 416; especially see p. 223; and other references may be added from Paul's *Grundriss*, II. i. 835, for the German. For the sword-dance in Shetland noted by Scott, see Lockhart's *Life*, ed. 1837, III. 162. For other gymnastic plays, see the two books of Groos, *Spiele der Thiere* and *Spiele der Menschen*.

[2] See Bruchmann, *Poetik*, p. 212.

[3] Skill, of course, and rivalry are early provocatives of art in the dance. As to ball-playing as a part of it, references could be given for all times and climes.

[4] See *Old English Ballads*, p. lxxvi.

[5] Such as the author of the *Complaynt of Scotland* watched at their dancing, and noted the songs.

been made clear to probation how the narrative ballad grew out of a tribal or communal dance; and it is equally clear that there was an even shorter path from dance to drama.[1]

From this point of view, it is easy to understand why the dance plays such a part in the beginning of nearly every national literature, not only in the Dionysian origins of Greek drama, but in less obvious ways. The same ecstasy, indeed, appears again and again in a kind of panic dance; in the summer of 1374 along the Rhine and in the Netherlands, and again in 1418 at Strassburg, communal excitement went quite mad in the St. John's or the St. Vitus's dance, vast crowds of men and women leaping and shouting, garlanded, singing, as they reeled, a refrain which might belong to the usual dances of St. John's Eve:—

> Here Sent Johan, so, so,
> Vrisch ind vro,
> Here Sent Johan!

until they fell exhausted, but still raving.[2] These panic dances reproduce in some features the mad dance of mænads and all that "wild religious excitement," that "Bacchic ecstasy," which lay behind the Hellenic drama, and anticipate as mad a dance of as wild an ecstasy, though not religious, when the mob of Paris dances the *carmagnole* to its own singing; but all this belongs to the pathological side of the case, and one turns to the harvest-field, and to the village oak, where merry dances often set a rhythm heard in later and nobler verse. Not long ago, poetry of every kind was thought to start in some religious rite, and a god or goddess lay hid under the most harmless rime of the yokel; of late, however, a wholesome tendency has prevailed to stop the

[1] See below, Chap. VII.

[2] See Uhland, *Kl. Schr.*, III. 399 ff., and 484 ff., who gives other well-known instances of this panic dance, as well as the *tarantella* of Italy. The shaman, of course, even among a tribe as low as the Veddahs, dances himself into a fit.

search of sky and storm-cloud and other far-away haunts for an explanation of the rustic dance and of the rustic refrain. On one hand, the chase, war, whatever concerned the routine of nomadic life, and on the other hand, among agricultural folk, the round of seedtime and harvest, days of plenty or of want, and in both cases, the common joys and sorrows of mankind, are now thought to be a better reason for communal dance and song. Primitive man did not go about with his eyes fixed upon the heavens; and it is not the goddess of spring and sunshine transferred to those harvested crops as signs of her presence which explains a Nerthus or a Ceres, but rather a slow inference from local delight in harvest up to a great feast of gathered and related tribes, involving wider ideas of divinity and arriving by easy stages at the abstraction of one beneficent deity sending out her largess of sun and quickening showers. The dance, then, with nomadic tribes was a triumph, an outburst of communal elation, dealing in its mimicry with scenes of the war or hunt, and cadenced by shout and song that echoed a clash of arms; with the agricultural community it was a harvest-home, with recapitulation of the rural year, imitated acts of sowing, planting, watching, reaping, storing, which survive in some sort to this day. In both kinds of life, nomadic and agricultural, the dance was an essential part of such rites as the wedding and the funeral, and is still considered in this way by peasants in remoter Europe. Thus in Dalmatia and Montenegro,[1] the *kollo*, that is, circle, "the figure of all their dances, though the steps differ," is danced at weddings. "Twelve or thirteen women . . . danced in a circle, singing a slow and rather plaintive song . . . while waiting for the bride. . . . In the meantime, the men . . . walked in procession to the court before the church door, and danced in a circle." Evidence of this sort is everywhere; it has been studied under the refrain;

[1] See book of this title by Sir J. G. Wilkinson, London, 1848, I. 399.

but the festal idea may be repeated here in comment on the meaning of our old English word and suffix *lâc*, and the related Gothic *laiks*,[1] German *leich*, originally the combination of word, song, and dance — or march — in one communal act,[2] with an easy transition into the idea of battle, the "play of spears," where, indeed, this communal act always served as prelude, as well as into the idea of feast, ceremony, merriment. A festal song and dance after the fight, easily turned into ritual and thanksgiving to the gods, but once mere fighting the battle over again, was called in Norse the *sigrleikr*.[3] Further philology would not be in place; enough that the earliest songs and poetry of Europe appear everywhere hand in hand with the dance,[4] and that this dance is partly the triumph of victorious war, partly a triumph of peace and plenty, always, however, a festal and communal affair.

In considering this communal dance of Europe, one finds that it is practically inseparable from song, and the song is mainly sung by those who dance. In modern Greece, even, Fauriel[5] found that "every new dance was the result of a new song, of which it formed the mimicry; it was never danced without this song, and fell with it into oblivion." A study of the refrain showed how close this bond between song and dance must have been; and one sees how slowly and reluctantly the separation takes place, most reluctantly, of course, in the games of children. It must also be borne in mind that dancing by pairs is of comparatively recent date; Neocorus, one will remember, says it was unknown among

[1] It translates "dance" in Luke xv. 25.

[2] See Kögel, *Gesch. d. deutsch. Lit.*, pp. 7 ff.

[3] *Sigelēoð* in Anglo-Saxon, sung after a victory, was doubtless the same thing. Kögel notes that *leikr*, *leik*, in Norwegian dialects down to this day, means both "war" and "dance"; and he conjectures that *winelâc*, in Anglo-Saxon, goes back to an originally erotic dance, as it may go forward to a children's "kissing-game."

[4] Wolf, *Lais*, pp. 18, 183 f., puts too much stress on the singing of church music, though he concedes popular origins; p. 22.

[5] Work quoted, p. cxvii.

his peasant neighbours between the German ocean and the Baltic until the middle of the sixteenth century, while Bladé makes this way of dancing a stranger to the Gascon country-folk as late as seventy years ago. What they knew and practised was the old round, danced once to the songs of the dancers, but now dominated more and more by instruments;[1] the song, when used, is led by a soloist who improvises a line or so which is repeated by the dancers in chorus, with a refrain for all stanzas. This round, of course, is the *carole*[2] of Romance literature, known later as the *branle*, a dance or march of many, hand in hand, with chorus or refrain to time the steps;[3] it was the main amusement of aristocratic folk, but derived directly from popular usage. Such an aristocratic dance is described in the *Romaunt of the Rose*.[4] Dante refers[5]

[1] Bladé, *Poésies Populaires de la Gascogne* (Vol. III. is devoted entirely to songs for the dance), III. i. ff. "En général on ne danse aux chansons que faute de mieux," although even now, at times, "they bid the music cease, and dance to the sound of their own voices." The dancing is literally a round, a circle.

[2] See Wolf's note, *Lais*, pp. 185 f. On this *carole* or *ronde*, danced mainly by women, but now and then by men and women, see Jeanroy's chapter, already quoted, and the additional suggestions of M. Gaston Paris, *Origines d. l. Poés. Lyr.*, pp. 44 ff., really a review of Jeanroy's book. "Ce qui caractérisait surtout les caroles, c'était le chant qui les accompagnait," says M. Paris. The only use of instruments, and these very simple, was to mark the rhythm. Dancers turned to the left.

[3] An early reference, from "Ruodlieb," may be added to show the connection of dance and song; the passage occurs in a description of the dancing bears (III. 84 ff., ed. Grimm-Schmeller, *Lat. Ged. des X. u. XI. Jhrh.*, p. 144) :—

> cum plebs altisonam fecit gyrando choream,
> accurrunt et se mulieribus applicuere,
> quae gracili voce cecinẻrunt deliciose,
> insertisque suis harum manibus speciosis
> erecti calcant . . .

The bears dance, then, along with the singing and dancing women; Grimm calls them *spielweiber*, and quotes an ecclesiastical prohibition (*ibid.*, p. xv); but part of the description, witness the *plebs*, will pass for a communal dance.

[4] In the translation ascribed to Chaucer, vv. 759 ff., "Tha myghtist thou karoles sene," etc.

[5] *De vulg. Eloq.*, II. iii. See note in Howell's translation, London, 1890. Crescimbeni, *L'Istoria della volgar Poesia*, Venez., 1731 (written in 1697), quotes,

to the practise of singing with the dance; and if we had his chapter on the *ballata*, we should have riches. On the dance-song of these Romance nations, and its absolutely communal origin, enough has been quoted already from such authors as Wolf and Jeanroy; and it would be waste of time to heap up evidence of the English ballad[1] as it was danced in Elizabethan fields, and when the youth went out to "mix their songs and dances in the wood." Dances of this sort we have already noted not only among shepherds, but in the Elizabethan theatre; besides the refrains of labour and merriment to which the actors danced, ballads were in demand. A good instance is in the old play of *Like Wil to Like*,[2] where Nichol Newfangle, the Devil, and Tom Collier are on the stage. Says Nichol, —

> Godfather, wilt thou daunce a little before ye go home to hell ? . . .
> Then, godfather, name what the daunce shall be.
>
> "Tom Coliar of Croydon hath solde his cole."
>
> Why, then, haue at it by my father's soule.

[Nichol Newfangle must have a gittorn or some other instrument (if it may bee), but if hee haue not, they must daunce about the place all three, and sing this song that followeth, which must bee doon also althoug they haue an instrumenth.]

And the song follows. Jigs were songs, largely improvised, and sung by actors as they danced; they came after the play.[3] It was the fiddle, says Mr. Baring-Gould,[4] "which

though in disapproval, Minturno for the primacy of *ballate* (p. 148): "ballads," says M., because "si cantavano ballando," which is the root of the matter.

[1] It has been repeatedly noticed that older English dances are known by the ballads sung to them. Even some of the tragic ballads were used for the dance; but one must think of gay little songs and refrains as staple for the merry rounds; nothing else will fit the seasons when "maydes daunce in a ring."

[2] 3^b^, Bodley copy of 1568. See also the refrain for a dance in the *Four Elements*, above, p. 322.

[3] See *Kind-Harts Dreame*, ed. Rimbault, Percy Soc., 1841, p. 38, and note, p. 79.

[4] *English Minstrelsie*, I., p. ix.

banished the ballad as a song-accompaniment to a dance. Nevertheless, as a very aged fiddler told me. . . in his early days the lads and maids always sang whilst dancing to his music." On the stage this substitution was more immediate and thorough; so that in the days of George II, when Nancy Dawson "produced the novelty of singing as she danced," she took the town by storm; though one may conjecture that it was the survival, not the "novelty,"[1] in the case which thus aided her charm as a woman and her grace as a dancer. For rural England, like rural Europe, showed reluctance enough in giving up the good old way; a Scottish parson, moreover, writing in 1793, tells of a large stone, set up in one of the islands, about which he saw "fifty of the inhabitants" gathered on the first day of the year, and "dancing in the moonlight" with no other music than their own singing.[2] About such stones, but by preference about the village linden,[3] folk danced to their own singing in Germany down to modern times; and as the dance was an even movement in a ring, the dancers hand in hand, it was quite possible for them to sing the ballads which seem to us grotesquely unfit for the lively springing of single performers as well as for the rapidly gliding couples. Leaping, and livelier motions generally, followed the dance in a ring; but it was to the latter that ballads were sung and in the first instance composed.[4] The dances which go mainly to a refrain represent of course an older stage than those

[1] In 1767 a "young lady from Scotland" sang as she danced, at the royal theatre in Copenhagen; but there, too, in 1726, a Stockholm dancing-girl had done the same thing. "Novelty" is not the word. See Steenstrup, *Vore Folkev.*, pp. 8 f.

[2] Brand, "New Year's Day."

[3] Mannhardt, *Baumkultus*, in many places; Pfannenschmid, *Germ. Erntej.*, pp. 271 ff., 580 ff. For love-songs and the dance, Uhland, III. 391 ff., and notes, 471, with valuable account of the manner of dancing, and of the leader, the *voresingen* and the *voretanzen*.

[4] See Böhme, *Altd. Liederb.*, p. xxxv.

which are danced to a ballad, to a narrative song; the early dance knows only present action, and exhorts or describes, as in the Flemish dances[1] now mainly relegated to children.

As Mr. Thomas Hardy is so fond of reminding his readers, this is a merry, dancing world no more; even youth can hardly make shift "to revel in the general situation" as all men used to do. *Weltschmerz* is to blame, no doubt, and there is Mr. Baring-Gould's fiddle, which has done a deal of mischief. Rivals to the human voice, successful rivals, were early at the dance, — harp, lyre, pipe, what not. South Sea islanders were fain, not of these, but of the drum. With the dominant note of alien music came a desire to break up the ring, to dance in pairs, or even to listen and look on. Meddlesome bishops and officials of every sort were bound to destroy this communal dance as a place of scandal; and we have seen how the chimney and the clean, warm fireside and the lamp drew sober folk from the village dances and left these to the baser element. One can take quite seriously that petition[2] of the would-be peasant to restore legal sanction to the village dance; and one is interested to hear the petitioner complain that it is the violin now where once was the bagpipe, — and once, too, he might have added, the echoing refrain. No, the dance as well as the dancing song, the ballad proper, is going out of date;[3] and not only the dance in this communal and social meaning, but the very fact of rhythm, which is the soul of the dance. Children play these games less and less, although the kindergarten makes some stand in the matter;

[1] *'T Boertje*, Coussemaker, pp. 329 f., and *'t Patertje*, already quoted.

[2] *Pétition pour des Villageois que l'on empêche de danser.* Par Paul-Louis Courier, Vigneron, . . . Paris, 1822, addressed to the Chamber of Deputies, asking that the folk of Azai may dance on Sundays "sur le place de leur commune." Despite the mystification, there is some serious intent behind this fooling.

[3] In Germany itself: cf. Meyer, *Volkskunde*, pp. 158, 160, 163.

and even in music, as Bücher[1] points out in those pages to which we have so often referred, teachers and artists are fain to give rhythm an ancillary place and put melody, harmony, in the foreground. One feels little displeasure, says Bücher, at the sight of unrhythmic movements; and what would be said of an orator who, like his Athenian brother, should address a political assembly as his "fellow dancers"? But the decline set in early; even in Sir Thomas Elyot's day,[2] dancing is "that exercise whiche of the more parte of sadde men" — serious folk, that is — "is so litle estimed." So, too, in imperial Rome. When the Romans hired mimes to dance for them, some lover of the old ways might have said of the communal dance, expression of social union and social equality and the strong, compact state, what the stern old orator said of his profession when he first heard hired applause in the courts of law: *centumviri, hoc artificium periit*, — "judges, oratory is doomed!" In both cases one is dealing with the decline of communal force and the growth of individual power.

Our business, however, is with the past. It is clear that movements of labour, particularly in a reminiscent festal act, and movements of the communal dance, furnished the raw material of poetry. In all cases the primitive dance, or what seems to come nearest to that state of the art, is a dance of masses of men for one purpose and to one exact rhythm.[3] Equal sets of movements gave the verse, and sets of these sets gave in time the strophe. Communal interest,

[1] *Arbeit u. Rhythmus*, pp. 103 f.

[2] See note, end of chapter.

[3] Grosse, *Anf. d. Kunst*, p. 218; Donovan, *Lyre to Muse*, pp. 91, 127 ff.; Jacobowski, *Anfänge d. Poesie*, p. 127. This author's discussion of circle and straight line, as of women and of men in the dance, and of other formations, is a bit fanciful although interesting and suggestive. See, too, Donovan on the ring of folk (choral) about a centre of interest, — altar or the like. Work quoted, p. 204.

resulting in the communal expression, added contents to form; and shout, movement, cadence, are all born of this absolutely social and communal impulse. To use the good old word, here is the poetry of nature; facing this communal material, what are we to say of the changes wrought upon it by individual art? [1]

[1] The development of the dance into different kinds of poetry is foreshadowed by many of the older writers, although the first really comparative treatment of the subject must be assigned to A. W. Schlegel in the lectures at Berlin a century ago. Herder has some valuable remarks on the subject in his early essay *Vom Geist der ebräischen Poesie*, following, of course, many hints of Lowth. Two hundred years ago, Burette, a really learned writer, drew up his "Mémoire pour servir à l'Histoire de la Danse des Anciens," published in the *Mém.*, Acad. of Inscript., etc., I. 93 ff., Paris, 1717. Movement and imitation caused the dance, which is "nearly as old as man," and sprang from joy. Cadence is the mainspring; avoid, he says, Lucian's prattle about the stars. Wedding, festival, vintage, harvest, — look to these, says Burette, in quite modern spirit, for the origins of the dance. He traces metres to the rhythm of songs sung by the dancers. Another article of this writer investigates ball-playing, often combined with dance and song. Another writer on the dance was John Spencer, D.D., master of Corpus Christi College (1630–1693), the founder of the science of comparative religions; his "Dissertatio de Saltandi Ritu," is printed in the *Thesaurus Antiquitat. Sacrar. complectens selectissima clarissimorum Virorum Opuscula in quibus Veterum Hebraeorum Mores, Leges, etc., illustrantur*, Vol. XXXII., Venet., 1767. Spencer studies the dance of the Hebrews, and his references are valuable; he is comparative, and uses dances of modern Turks to illustrate his subject. Hebrews got some of their festal dances from heathen, — the *saltationes promiscuas;* for erotic dances he thinks to have been early and everywhere. For a man of his date, he concludes very boldly "probabilius est, sacras choreas agendi morem, ex antiquissimo gentium usu primitus oriundum," and so came to the Hebrews. The festal dances, where Jews bore about branches and sang a choral full of repetitions and with a constant refrain, he compares with pagan affairs of the sort; the *pæan* is compared with refrains like *Hallel* and *Hosannah.* In fine, this is sharp, clear, comparative work, and good reading still. From Joannis Meursi *Orchestra sive de Saltationibus Veterum* . . . Lugd. Batav., 1618, not much is to be learned except a list (alphabetical) of the old dances, with references to the classic passages. Most of the articles are short, but the Pyrrhic Dance has twelve pages. An early essay on dancing, with considerable scope for its time, is inserted in Elyot's *Governour*, edited by Croft, London, 1880, from the edition of 1531, I. 202 ff. Elyot seems to be the first Englishman who wrote about the art.

CHAPTER VI

SCIENCE AND COMMUNAL POETRY

We have Dr. Johnson's word for it that one does well "to see great works in their seminal state, pregnant with latent possibilities of excellence; nor could there be any more delightful entertainment than to trace their gradual growth and expansion." So science came to think; and all the works of nature and of man have been treated in this spirit to the convincing of sane minds everywhere, except in the domain of poetry. There one still clings to a paradise and a perfect poet at the start, — perfect, that is, because he had all the functions and privileges and opportunities of the latter-day bard, and stood to his public as a poet stands to the public of this age. A study of facts, records as well as survivals, leads us to no such perfect primitive bard; at the end of the path we see no dignified old gentleman in flowing robe, with a long white beard, upturned eyes, and a harp clasped to his bosom, but rather a ring of savages dancing uncouthly to the sound of their own voices in a rhythmic but inharmonious chant. This, however, is only saying that poetry, like all human institutions, like the earth itself, goes back to rude and barren beginnings; and the lowest stratum of poetry to which one can come either by sight or by inference is only what one ought to expect from the doctrine of evolution, applicable in this case as in any other case. With a sense not intended by Browning, "rock's the song-soil rather," and even fossil signs of life are few. But it is precisely here that Johnson's unconscious praise of these studies should be borne in mind. Not the bard come down from Olympus, with majesty in his mien and the light of divine song shed about him, singing to his rapt hearers of the deep things of life, is the nobler view: nobler by far is the sight of those little groups gathered on the marches that lay between the old beast and the new man, facing inexorable powers which had crushed out life upon life before, and whole systems of life; dimly conscious of a force that treads down the individual and dooms the solitary to defeat; dimly conscious, too, of the resisting power that lies in coherence, union, common front in a common cause; marshalled by the instinct of kind into a tentative confederation of single resources; and so beginning the long battle which humanity is still waging against foes unseen as well as seen. The first cry of emotional consent along with the consenting step, the cry that remembered a triumph found in instinctive common action, and felt itself to be prophetic of a triumph yet to come; this concerted step and shout which seemed the expression of concerted purpose, of communal will, force, effectiveness, has more in it even for the man of sentiment than can be found in any flight of poetry in later time. But we are not seeking sentiment in the case; and having come in this rude dance and song, so it would seem, to the beginnings of poetry, we ask what was the beginning of this beginning. If one must have a formula for the process, it need not be in those intolerant terms of personal initiative and gregarious imitation upon which M. Tarde insists so strenuously, but rather in the mild and quite as scientific terms of consent, the consent of instinctive individual gestures and sounds due to the perception by a group of human beings that common action makes unity out of diversity. Art is of social origin; that is the thesis of Guyau in his well-known book; and the social sense precedes any relation of master and pupil, leader and followers. It is overwhelmingly probable that rhythm, the simplest form of social consent, was the earliest form of a discovery which made social progress possible. Still, this probability must not be taken for granted.

The question, like the democratic thought of a century and more ago, has an outer and an inner circle.[1] For the latter, let us ask whether poetry, queen of the arts, is an art in the sense of something invented by the artist, not only in details, but in essence. The arts of life belong to the artist; but is the artist anterior in every way to his art? Is there no spontaneous, instinctive background? In the first place, one must guard against a fallacy of terms. The invention of a tool, for example, even though it be "organic projection," is different in kind from the invention of a poem, which, by the principles of æsthetic, has no one practical end in view, — for theory, at least; in reality, the inventor of a poem nowadays has a practical end in view, the sale of his verse, and Scherer carried this commercial idea back to the very origins, setting up a primitive literary market, with supply and demand, poet and public, bargains, sales, entertainer and audience, on the very tree-platform of our hairy ancestors. But Scherer fell into absurdities. Gigadibs the literary man does not thrive in those regions; and one cannot reduce the primitive choral to terms of artist, invention, public, sale. If anything has been made clear in preceding pages of this book, if anything can be made clear in the study of improvisation about to follow, if there is any certain curve of evolution in the course of poetry, it is that the passive element, the audience, the receptive public, disappears inevitably as one recedes from conditions of the present time, and that the throng as a productive active body assumes more and more the functions now regarded as belonging almost exclusively to the individual. Invention itself has been reduced to a convenient absurdity, for this very article of rhythm, by M. Kawczynski, in his

[1] See above, p. 128.

essay on rhythmic origins.[1] Nobody denies that an Alcæus may invent an Alcaic strophe,[2] that another master may hit upon the elegiac couplet; but this vivacious essay declares that rhythm itself was invented by some thoughtful benefactor of the race, some genius of prehistoric times. A book published in the same year, the *Æsthetics of Movement*, by M. Souriau,[3] had made temperate protest against Mr. Herbert Spencer's doctrine[4] of the universality of rhythm in the realm of nature, and had asserted that rhythm, exceptional in nature, is nevertheless "the constant law of muscular movements," and not the result of will. But this spontaneity of rhythm in the motion and muscular exertion of man, this tendency in each of our motor organs "to adopt a fixed rhythm which becomes its normal movement," is precisely what M. Kawczynski will not allow; he is bent upon banishing "the false system of spontaneity" from its last place of refuge and will hound it off the face of the earth. Not only was this or that dance invented, this or that march and walk; dancing, marching, leaping, yes, walking, are inventions all. This is very clear language of M. Kawczynski, but it is a trifle too clear; one asks for a bill of particulars, — first for an explanation of the inventive process, and secondly for an account of the imitation; and here one meets difficulties. The individual mind plays about general instincts, modifies them, develops them into a thousand forms, precisely as it does with the raw material of nature. It invents a dance as modification of the general instinct to dance; it invents the steam-engine, but is not yet credited with inventing steam and iron. So one easily

[1] *Essai Comparatif sur l'Origine et l'Histoire des Rythmes*, Paris, 1889.

[2] Even this may be questioned in a literal sense. "Formen," says Usener, *Altgriechischer Versbau*, p. 111, "werden nicht geschaffen, sondern sie entstehen und wachsen. Der schöpferische Künstler erzeugt sie nicht, sondern bildet das Ueberkommene veredelnd um." He is speaking of the popular four-accent verse found in so many languages.

[3] *L'Esthétique du Mouvement*, Paris, 1889, Cap. iv. See pp. 54, 65.

[4] In the *First Principles*.

understands the invention of a distinct song; but what of singing? Or say of breathing? The Dogberry who says that these things come by nature, and asks how they could come by art, is pained to find the advocate of invention wrapping himself in a cloak of biological mystery not unlike the theological garment donned, under similar questions, by Jacob Grimm himself. We shall see that in the outer circle this question is answered by M. Tarde with a reference to the cell; ultimate individual invention is an affair of the individual cell; while the process itself is a mystery, described only in the most modest and euphemistic hints, and to stare at it would be the part of peeping Tom. M. Kawczynski makes no effort to explain invention, but simply asserts it; and although imitation is a clearer case, yet even here he says things which are not good for the interests of his theory. He is safe so long as he keeps to general terms and describes all literature as a gigantic system of borrowings, — German from Roman, Roman from Greek, Greek from Egyptian mayhap, and Egyptian from creditors unknown, all imitation, with here and there a bit of invention going on decently behind closed doors. But M. Kawczynski dares too much, and blunders in the particular case. A witness should be taken from the box when he tries to help his cause by making German Siegfried an imitated compound of Jason, Achilles, and Perseus; by naming Otfried as the founder of really Germanic literature; by making alliteration in Norse an imitation of German, which got it from Anglo-Saxons, who got it from the Irish, who got it from the Latin; and by calling Germanic verse itself an imitation of the classic hexameter.[1] "Historic influences," one is told, "are stronger than the natural and proper gifts of any people"; but are not natural and proper gifts themselves the strongest of historic influences? This question is worth a glance by the way.

[1] *Essai*, pp. 102, 104.

No one denies the great part played in poetry by imitation; but it is not the only element in the case. True, it is the most obvious element. Comparative literature, as a science, is young. The task put before its followers was plain enough; they had first of all to sift the material, to note where deep has called unto deep in the influence of one poet upon another, as well as to follow the fortunes of a primitive bagman's jest carried on the old trading routes from land to land and starting up at last as *conte* or *schwank* in a hundred scattered communities, in cloister, school, and court. But this is not all, and the task is not done even when one has struck the balance between the borrowings of a poet and what one suffers to pass as his individual and original genius. Abused as the terms have been, the genius of time, place, community, is still a factor in the growth of any literature; and M. Gaston Paris, who has done so much for the study of sources, is emphatic on this point. In several passages, notably in a discussion of the method to be followed in studying poetry of the people,[1] he sets a bound to the theory of borrowings, and insists upon the common fund or "patrimony" of national tradition. Steinthal, too, is not altogether negligible with his query; why assume, he asks,[2] that because Europe imported so much, she must have been herself sterile? That old Aryan patrimony, to be sure, as source of myth, legend, poem, rite, is out of favour, perhaps definitely abandoned; but Comparetti,[3] who approves this abandonment, is full of zeal for the development of all poetry, provided it has the spontaneous and native note, within the limits of its own nation and its own tongue. Borrowing is, after all, incidental, however conspicuous in fact; and it would be a wild system of economics which should explain the industrial life of the

[1] *Mélusine*, I. 1 ff. See, too, *Poésie du Moyen Age*, pp. 77, 89.
[2] *Zeitschr. f. Völkerpsychol.*, XVII. 113 ff.
[3] *Kalewala*, p. 38.

world as purely a matter of exchange, of debtor and creditor, without any hint of agriculture and manufactures. One sees all the faring of ship and car, the tumult of docks, drays, storehouses, the stir in counting-rooms, banks, exchange; what of plough and mill and mine? It is just these, so to speak, that one fails to see in such clever literary balancing of accounts as certain scholars have made in the study of Scandinavian ballads. Take a holiday throng of the unlettered mediæval community, intent upon song and dance, all dancing and all singing; will no one tell us what they sing? A score of scholars. They produce the ballad, — no easy feat, — and for this alone deserve lasting gratitude. As they find it, it is not likely to be merely a local affair, for such things seldom come upon record, although it is quite clear that perhaps the majority of ballads in this class were of purely local interest. Very likely, however, it is borrowed, and the scholar — again, no easy feat — traces the loan to its source. The form of the stanza may be imported, too, with its simple air; and even now and then the peculiar rhythm of the lines may be an echo of alien song. Here, then, is imitation; it need not have been imitation, and in some other place was doubtless a home product throughout; but here imitation must be conceded. Our ingenious literary accountant, however, is emboldened to take another step; the impulse which drives that throng to express its feelings by rhythm, movement, cry, he takes away from instinct and sets down to the credit of some other community; the very dancing and singing, that is, he regards as an imitated, borrowed thing. Rosenberg, in his book on the *Intellectual Life of Scandinavia*,[1] tries to prove that "dancing and singing to the dance" came to Norsemen from the Celts; and to make this probable, he has recourse to that perilous figure, the universal negative. There were no dancing-songs, he says, in oldest

[1] *Nordboernes Aandsliv*, II. 437 ff.

English; dancing-song and refrain, he argues from records notoriously imperfect, were also unknown to the early German, and came to him as a Celtic export, although the German was the first to use these forms in narrative.[1] That is, the Germans had at first no song for the dance, but got it from the Celts, who in their turn had not used the narrative song for dancing, and by way of barter imported it, as among the Bretons, from a German source. The refrain and the dance, novelties both, came with viking spoils into Scandinavian life, made things "lighter and more gay," and "for the first time gave ladies the chance of active participation in social enjoyment." In Iceland, Rosenberg goes on to say, there was no dancing until about the year 1200;[2] though folk there took hugely to the thing when they once had it. Moreover, "all agree that this dance and song was at first an exclusive prerogative of noble families." A thousand years, then, one is to conceive the case, foot and voice went never paired in Norland, dance and refrain were unknown, until example came from the South! *Tantae molis erat;* to set folk dancing to their own songs needed such ponderous machinery and such a stretch of time! Had Rosenberg's comparative literature only made itself comparative beyond the shreds and patches of written records, beyond the narrow range of Europe and the mediæval limits; had he only taken Adam Smith's or Lord Monboddo's interest in African natives like that one who danced a war dance before the genial Adam and his friends, compelling all hands to leap upon chairs and tables for safety! Rosenberg and scholars of his class are

[1] The refrain of two lines, he thinks, was added to the two-line stanza of narrative ballads; and so resulted the common ballad stanza. This is denied by Steenstrup.

[2] "Proved" by that old primitive-Aryan process now something discredited: *danz* is an imported word (meaning both song and dance). See Vigfusson's *Icelandic Dictionary, s.v.* More formidable, but far from final, is the silence of the sagas.

not comparative enough; they forget wider and more important reaches.[1] The habit of turning an event or a situation straightway into improvised verse with gestures and dancing, is so well attested in the accounts of savage life, so well attested in cases where isolated and unlettered communities in modern Europe have been left to their own "literary" devices,[2] that in the face of such evidence the assertion that Norse folk waited a thousand years for a hint from the Celts before they began to dance to rough chorus and refrain of their own singing, falls like a house of cards. Borrowing money is not a sign of bankruptcy; and the valuable affirmative evidence of literary loans which these scholars give us is half spoiled by the absurdity of their universal negative in regard to native production. For example, we know that Finns, in very recent times, borrowed a store of Swedish ballads, and that the name *veisa*,[3] used in Finnish for a ballad, is taken from that source; but, as every one knows, the Finns had their own native songs. Suppose, now, that these native songs had long since disappeared, as they doubtless would have disappeared under the circumstances of primitive Scandinavian ballads; and how cheerfully the literary accountant could have assured his reader that there were no Finnish songs whatever until those Swedish loans were made!

Let us go back now to the main question, and take its outer circle. Here one is told to blot from one's dictionary such words as *instinct*, *spontaneity*, *homogeneous;* but, with these well erased, how is one to speak of that group

[1] A similar denial, not only of the original character of recorded ballads, but of the ballad habit itself, is made for Denmark by Professor G. Storm in his otherwise valuable book, *Sagnkredsene om Karl den Store og Didrik af Bern hos de nordiske Folk*, Kristiania, 1874, pp. 174 f.

[2] See below on the *schnaderhüpfl* and *stev.*

[3] Comparetti, *Kalewala*, 1892. pp. 3, 264 ff. The very name of the Finnish song is probably borrowed; but its original and native character is successfully defended by Comparetti, pp. 37, 272, against the attempt of Ahlqvist to prove alliteration in Finnish verse a loan from the Scandinavians.

of primitive men huddled on the frontier of civilization? They have no instincts, no spontaneous gestures and cries; they are not homogeneous, and no homogeneous expression can come out of them. They cannot borrow; for they are opening the first concern of its kind. What are they doing, then? Getting ready, one is told, for a game of follow-the-leader, the game of all civilized and uncivilized beings, and the law of all animate things. Here is a formula not merely valid in the explanation of literary progress, but the last word of philosophy itself. It is labour lost to set up the spontaneous, communal impulse as a factor in solving these problems of primitive poetry, if the spontaneous and the communal are impossible ideas, mere superstitions, props on which rationalism once leaned in passing from the grosser explanations of ghosts, gods, what not, but now broken and cast as rubbish to the void. By the theory of M. Tarde, for example, there is no spontaneity possible; rhythm in its widest sense, dancing, even tears and laughter, breathing, all cease to be outcome of emotion common and instinctive; they are imitation by one individual of another individual, or, to take refuge in biology, of one cell of another cell. The microcosm is here no figure of speech; in this little world of man is a commonwealth of individual cells, with crossing and varied interests; an inventive, masterful cell takes the lead, sweeps along most of the other cells, which imitate and obey, opposes and destroys others, adapts itself by compromise to a few more, — and this is man, just as it is society: invention, imitation, but no spontaneity. Invention is the rare and difficult factor; imitation is the constant factor.[1] That

[1] Set forth in Tarde's *Les Lois de l'Imitation*, Paris, 1890; but the best recent summary of his views is *Les Lois Sociales*, Paris, 1898. Special problems of the crowd as imitative, dangerous, weak, are treated in his *Essais et Mélanges Sociologiques*, Lyon-Paris, 1895. See also "Les deux Éléments de la Sociologie," in *Études de Psychologie Sociale*, Paris, 1898, an address delivered in 1894 before the first international Congress of Sociology.

is, to put the case more concisely, Tarde attacks two theses, the assertion of spontaneity in a throng and the assertion that development is from the homogeneous to the heterogeneous.

All this is not so new as it seems to be. It is early eighteenth-century philosophy translated into late nineteenth-century science. It is a reaction from a reaction; for Wilhelm von Humboldt, Hamann, Herder, and the rest, "tired of kings," tired of the "great man," turned to man himself, to humanity, nature, to great forces revealed in human institutions everywhere. Speech, said Humboldt, is no invention; it is an energy, a power. At the beginning, says M. Tarde,[1] "a savage genius" in a single family, invented the earliest form of language; and families everywhere came to borrow this anthropoid's linguistic fire. M. Tarde is suavely bent on exterminating the idea of nature. Even Darwin had said speech was half art, half instinct; and an early Darwinian, Lord Monboddo,[2] believing that "everything of art must be founded on nature," derived language from "natural cries." Nature, says M. Tarde, is a superstition; and with it he tosses away instinct and spontaneity. The solution for every possible problem of man's destiny he seeks in one of those *cerveaux de génie*, savage or civilized, heterogeneous factors of life, like the masterful cell from which all has come and to which all shall yet return. All social adaptation is reduced to the work "of two men, of whom one answers, by word or by deed, to the question, verbal or silent, of the other." Men are alike, think alike, do alike, not by any law or by any instinct of species, but by this fact of imitation; any group, large or small, will consist of two parts, one learning and one teaching, one producing and one con-

[1] *Les Lois de l'Imitation*, p. 279. So p. 48, — "A l'origine un anthropoïde a imaginé . . . les rudiments d'un langage."

[2] *Of the Origin and Progress of Language*, I. 318 ff.

suming, "one actor, poet, artist, and the other looker-on, reader, amateur."[1] The group of two individuals, the harmony of it, Tarde now pushes back to an earlier harmony between two ideas in the brain of the individual inventor; and this is to stretch into the infinitesimal. How, he cries in an eloquent passage,[2] how can a Spencer, as well as the man in the street, go on treating this infinitesimal as of no moment, as a homogeneous, neutral thing, with naught in it spiritual and distinct? Why make the vast range of space your theatre of existence? Within this despised infinitesimal, mayhap, lie the chances of death or immortality, the secret of being itself. And we call this ovule, this part of the ovule, this part of the part, — undifferentiated![3] Darwin is right in his general theory of descent, but he is wrong in his explanation, thinks M. Tarde; for the true cause of the species is "the secret of the cells, *the invention of some early ovule endowed with peculiar and rich originality.*" What, once more, what of our little group of primitive men, their instinct of kind, their spontaneous gestures and steps and cries, their homogeneous character and therefore homogeneous expression? Seek out the masterful cell in the masterful brain of the masterful leader of that sorry set of imitators, and it will tell all secrets of civilization and human progress, poetry and the arts included. There is no "society" for M. Tarde, and, for the sake of dignified and decent thought, no *milieu*, no "they,"[4] — that figment of nonsense in the phrase "they say," — no "social forces." Instead of explaining the small by the great, the detail by the

[1] He concedes that a different relation exists when two are working together at the same thing (*Lois Soc.*, p. 129); although here are "model and copy," suggestion at least.

[2] *Ibid.*, p. 159.

[3] He sees light ahead for a world now hung in Schopenhauer-black; the infinitesimal shall cheer us. *Ibid.*, pp. 87, 105, 110.

[4] *Lois Sociales*, pp. 40 f. This passage will repay close attention.

mass, he explains a group of similar things by the accumulation of minor elementary processes, the great by the small, the mass by the detail. There is for M. Tarde no genius of a race, of a language, of a religion; at the best, this genius of the people is a label for the individuals, or a sort of composite photograph. Hennequin[1] argued in the same way against an English type in literature, against a Norman or a Gascon type in French; it is worth noting that his arguments and Tarde's philosophy were anticipated at one of the Magny dinners in January, 1866. "Taine asserted," so the *Goncourt Journal* reports, "that all men of talent are the product of their environment. We took the other side. 'Where are you going to find,' we said, 'the exotic root of Chateaubriand, — a pineapple growing in the barracks!' Gautier came to our support, and maintained that the brain of an artist was the same thing under the Pharaohs that it is now."

M. Tarde, however, with his followers, is by no means in undisputed possession of the field, whether in sociology or in literature. Gumplowicz[2] declares that "the behaviour of collective entities is determined by natural and sociological laws, and not by the motives and natural qualities of individuals." Moreover, as he says, the horde and the social group make a unit, and this is unlike its parts; it cannot be inferred from its parts. Social thought came before individual thought. Some of the best scholars in sociology have come out frankly for dualism; and in the opinion of

[1] *Critique Scientifique*, pp. 191 ff. Carstanjen made a fierce attack on the *milieu* in art, and, by implication, in literature: *Vierteljahrsschrift f. wissenschaftl. Philosophie*, XX. (1896), 1 ff., 143 ff. He explains the art of the renaissance by the artists of that time, and not by their environment. For a fine defence of the *milieu*, however, see the late M. Texte's book on *Jean-Jacques Rousseau et les Origines du Cosmopolitisme Littéraire*, pp. xvii. ff.

[2] *Outlines of Sociology*, trans. F. W. Moore for the Amer. Acad. Pol. and Soc. Sci., June, 1899, pp. 45, 88. See the translator's abstract, p. 7.

Dr. Barth,[1] dualism has now been proved for the past and recognized for present and future. Professor Giddings[2] takes this view and offers proof; he puts the consciousness of kind before invention and initiation, for society, as he says, is an organization and not an organism. Perhaps a majority of French scholars hold against M. Tarde; and while Germany has been rampant for individualism, a distinct reaction has set in with the work of Bernheim, of Lamprecht, and of Barth himself. As Ranke grew older, says Lamprecht, he grew less willing to lay stress on great personalities in history, which, he thought, must more and more find its account in the movement and condition of masses. Comte is not discredited in the spirit of his theory, whatever has become of the details; and, turning to psychology, one finds Wundt[3] actually defending the social mind, so vehemently attacked by Paul in his *Principles.* Wundt says there is such a thing as the *volksseele,* the sum of experiences in a multitude; and the products of such communal experiences, due to the coexistence and mutual working of many minds, cannot be explained by conditions of the individual mind. Language, myth, and custom, he says, are the three products of this mind or soul of the people; and it is not hard to find room for poetry in the province lying between speech and myth.[4] The problem thus stated and studied by Wundt has been undertaken by several other writers, notably by M. Le Bon,[5] and even, in a hostile spirit,

[1] *Die Philosophie der Geschichte als Sociologie,* Leipzig, 1897, I. 183, 213 f.

[2] *Principles of Sociology,* New York, 1896.

[3] "Ueber Ziele und Wege der Völkerpsychologie," in *Philosophische Studien,* 1888, IV. 1 ff., particularly pp. 11 ff. and 17.

[4] In his *Völkerpsychologie* (Vol. I., Leipzig, 1900, has appeared), he undertakes to study the making of these three products, which he calls a *gemeinsames Erzeugniss.* See pp. 4, 6, 24 f. A sensible plea for the *volksseele,* "which need not have any mystical connotation," was made by Gustav Freytag in the introduction to his *Bilder aus der deutschen Vergangenheit,* I. 13 ff.

[5] *Psychologie des Foules;* and in English translation, *The Crowd.*

by M. Tarde himself. Von Hartmann[1] studied the "collective mind" as long ago as 1869, and fitted it into his philosophy of the unconscious; while the *Journal of Demopsychology and Philology*, of Steinthal and Lazarus, fought a losing fight for demos in the old days from 1860, merging at last into the *Journal of the Ethnological Society*.[2] It is the fashion to laugh at this old journal, and it had its defects; the student of poetry, however, will do well to bear in mind that Ten Brink,[3] in his spirited account of communal song as the basis of English poetry, expressly declares that he "learned the most" about his subject from an article by Steinthal in the same periodical. Again, there is Bastian for ethnology; obscure in expression, hazy in thought, he backs his pet idea of the *völkergedanken* with a range of ethnological facts which no one will neglect or despise. These are positive considerations; and with them must go a negative but valuable result due to the failure of Tarde, Kawczynski, and others, in applying their arguments to facts. Take M. Tarde's signally unfortunate illustration of his idea that invention is the only initial power with which one reckons in literature, — that poetry, for example, always "begins[4] with a book" — a book! — "an *épopée*, some poetical work of great relative perfection, . . . some high initial source." And what are the examples of this law of poetic origins? "The *Iliad*, the Bible, Dante." Here is sheer absurdity. Each of these cases tends to prove the exact opposite of what M. Tarde would have it prove. Did he

[1] "Das Wesen des Gesammtgeistes," *Studien und Aufsätze*, pp. 504 ff.

[2] Significant is the change from *Völkerpsychologie* to *Volkskunde*. The new journal is edited by Professor Weinhold, and began in 1891.

[3] In Paul's *Grundriss der Philologie*, II. i., 512 ff. See also Ten Brink's *Beowulf*, pp. 105 f.

[4] *Débute*. See *Lois de l'Imit.*, p. 233. He is arguing against Spencer's doctrine of the development of the arts, and implies the same "high initial source" for music, architecture, and the rest.

come to this fatal idea, that all great literature starts with a great book, by reading Hugo's preface to *Cromwell?*[1] Worse, even, is his assertion that "modern literature begins with the *Romance of the Rose*."[2]

The theory of M. Tarde, noteworthy as it is, and salutary as some of its appeals must prove in correcting romantic extravagances, cannot be upheld even as a theory, and breaks down lamentably when applied to poetical facts. A saner belief would accept the immense part played by imitation, but would refuse to give it sole possession of the field. It is the clash of communal and individual tendencies,[3] of centripetal and centrifugal, with which M. Tarde forgets to reckon; now the individual invents, rules, awes, masters, and the throng follow like sheep, and now again this throng is — not *are* — tyrannical to such a degree that the philosopher of that epoch cries out that there is no individual initiative, all is law, natural forces, social forces, — and so comes to an extreme as illogical as that of M. Tarde. It is true that a work of art is not a mere registry of popular sentiment, of environment, of the temper of the time; it is also true that the artist cannot take himself out of those influences. Art is social, and without society would not exist. It is simple recognition of facts to assert that art, like religion, law, custom, serves as an index for tendencies which underlie the thought and emotion of an epoch; it works below the surface, this movement, and is often belied by all signs that can be read on the surface,

1 "Enfin ce triple poésie découle de trois grandes sources, la Bible, Homère, Shakspeare."

2 *Lois Sociales*, p. 49.

3 The abstract question is foreign to the present purpose; but it may be urged that one is wise to take neither the extreme position of Buckle, Gumplowicz, and Bourdeau, — who said that if Napoleon had been shot at Toulon, Hoche, or Kleber, or some one, would have done what Napoleon did, — nor yet the equally extreme stand of Tarde and his school. Some sensible remarks on the whole matter may be found in Bernheim's *Lehrbuch d. historischen Methode*, pp. 513 ff. of the second edition, Leipzig, 1894.

until suddenly these change too, and the period has registered its characteristics after the fashion of a clock which moves its hands only at the end of each minute. It is true, moreover, that this movement must belong to the body in which it takes place; yet it is also true that the movements of communal thought, as Wundt pointed out, are different in kind from the movements of individual thought.

But this is too fine-spun stuff for that group of primitive men concerned with their first effort at song. Granted the communal force with which we would endow them, what of the instinctive step, gesture, cry, — can these really be instinctive and not mere imitation of a leader?

As to instinctive utterance, that idea, though somewhat rudely shaken, still stands.[1] There are instinctive sounds, and man is or was no exception to the rule. The social influence, assumed by everybody as real cause of articulate speech, would work not upon a new sound "invented" by some primitive genius, but upon the instinctive sounds uttered by each unit of a throng. That individuals discovered or invented modifications of these sounds, no one will deny; but the conditions of primitive life were those of a horde, with individuals at a minimum of importance, so that the earliest progress in speech and poetry was due to the almost unconscious changes made by a festal throng under the excitement of social consent, — a very different thing from invention and imitation as the terms now hold. Whether one wishes to carry farther this mutual influence of man upon man in a throng equally active in all its parts, or not, is of little moment. The conditions of progress in

[1] See Lloyd Morgan, *Habit and Instinct*, Chap. II. Solitary chicks hatched in an incubator can be heard chirping, all in the same way, before they break the shell, and with no chance of imitation in the case. Weismann, "Gedanken über Musik," *Rundschau*, LXI. (1889), 63, remarks that a young finch brought up alone will sing the song of its kind, "but never so beautifully as when a good singer is put with him as teacher." The concession is enough.

speech and song were immediately communal, in strong contrast to the isolated, individual, mediating conditions of such progress at the present day. All we ask of biology is the concession of instinct; at the basis of human poetry, that vast edifice of art, and, as it seems to the modern man, of nothing but art, lie instinctive utterances, homogeneous, if one may judge by chick and bird,[1] and subject to their first modifications not from individual effort but from social consent and the enormous force of communal emotion.

Psychology, too, joins biology in allowing that instinctive forms of utterance and expression in primitive times may have led to that *gemeinsames dichten* in chorus, refrain, dance, which is claimed for nature and opposed to art. Imitation, in any sense that concerns the argument in hand, is after all a matter of deliberation, reason, choice; but the expression of emotion in children as in savages is rapid, instantaneous, instinctive. "Except fear," says Ribot,[2] "all primary emotions imply tendencies to movement, sometimes blind and violent, like natural forces. This is seen in infants, animals, savages, the barbarians of the first centuries of our era. . . . The passage of emotion into action, good or bad, is instantaneous, rapid, and fatal as a reflex movement." Panic fright, where animals are almost paralyzed, is, indeed, a matter of rapid suggestion and imitation in cases where the cause is not apparent; but panic elation is active, a movement, a sympathy, an instinctive consent of voice and limb. Moreover, the throng is always to be kept in mind,

[1] Morgan, work quoted, p. 90. Even Mr. Witchell, for whom the song of birds is traditional, grants that call-notes, alarm-notes, and all such utterances are instinctive. See Morgan, p. 178, and Romanes, *Mental Evolution in Animals*, pp. 222 f.

[2] *Psychology of the Emotions*, p. 265. The part assigned to imitation in seemingly spontaneous expression of emotion in a child, Baldwin, *Mental Development in Child and Race*, pp. 260 ff., does not affect this study of emotion in throngs.

and the analogy of children in a family, as well as of savages brought among civilized folk, is to be held resolutely back; it is no analogy at all. Who played the suggestive part of parent, of grown or civilized people, to the imitation of a mass of human beings in those earliest days? Horde conditions are too easily forgotten, and psychology needs to take them more into account, just as it is taking instinct again into favour. Beginning about 1850, a movement against instinct is plainly traced through the writings of men like Bain and A. R. Wallace; but the feud was carried too far, and Professor Karl Groos, in one of the best books[1] which have lately appeared on this subject, notes the reaction not only in Wundt, but in Lotze, Spencer, Sully, and Ribot, against this effort to blot the word instinct from our dictionaries. Groos, who has ample respect for imitation as a leading force in development of both body and mind, refuses to give it absolute rule. Play, he says, is not imitation, "but, if the phrase will pass, a foreboding of the serious occupation of the individual";[2] and again, "particularly in the most important and most elementary forms of play, there can be no question either of imitating the animal's own previous activity, *or of imitating the activity of other individuals.*" Mr. Lloyd Morgan allowed that his young moor-hen, with imitation out of the question, executing "a pretty and characteristic dance," showed instinct "even in the narrower acceptation of the term." Now if this solitary activity is "congenital" and "instinctive," imitation must also yield some ground to instinct in gregarious play of animals and in communal play

[1] *Die Spiele der Thiere*, Jena, 1896, p. 8. See, however, *Spiele der Menschen*, pp. 4, 365 ff., 431, 446 ff., 511 f.

[2] So Noiré explained the case in the section on the development of language in his book, *Die Welt als Entwicklung des Geistes*, Leipzig, 1874. Like Donovan, too, he assumed that the first words were uttered under pressure of communal excitement, elation, joy, social sense. He assumes that social conditions quite overwhelmed the individual, who hardly existed as such. See pp. 266 f.

of men. When Wundt[1] says that human life "is permeated through and through with instinctive action, determined in part by intelligence and volition," he states in scientific terms the old dualism of nature and art, of throng and artist, at which the rationalists of criticism have directed so many attacks. That fascinating book, Hudson's *Naturalist on the La Plata,* gives evidence about gregarious play among animals.[2] All mammals and birds, he says, have "more or less regular or set performances with or without sound, or composed of sound exclusively . . . performances which in many animals are only discordant cries and chorus and uncouth irregular motions," yet, "in the more aerial, graceful, and melodious kinds, take immeasurably higher, more complex, and more beautiful forms." Again, "every species, or group of species, has its own inherited form or style of performance; and however rude and irregular this may be . . . *that is the form in which the feeling will always be expressed.*" Plainly, for whatever reason, the individual is here under the control of the species; and imitation cannot be the sole explaining cause either of the impulse or of the performance. In fact, as Groos concludes,[3] in regard to play "the instincts are sole foundation. Foundation, for not all play is pure work of instinct; on the contrary, the higher one proceeds, the richer and more delicate grow those psychological elements which are added to the simple impulse of nature, ennoble it, elevate it, and now and again almost conceal it. But the foundation is instinct."

What Professor Groos has not done in his interesting books is to give adequate importance to the choral and communal fact; he neglects the antithesis between common action and

[1] Quoted, p. 328, by Morgan, from *Lectures on Human and Animal Psychology,* p. 397.

[2] See Wallaschek against this idea, above, p. 100.

[3] Work quoted, p. 21.

imitated action in a social group. This choral impulse may be referred to a pleasure in common, instinctive action, rarely noted by psychologists, which is a quite different affair from the pleasure of imitating as well as from the pleasure of seeing or hearing a thing done. Groos himself notes that the mass-play of birds is like the mass-dance of primitive men which sprang from sexual excitement. Still, in the table[1] printed at the end of his earlier book one sees how completely he leaves the choral and communal case out of account. He recognizes in the first column of this table the representation of self, the personal impulse, but not as a social expression by social consent; these forms of play should differ according to the solitary or social character of the performance, and this again not simply in terms of personal instinct and communal imitation. There is a social or communal personality, at all events where human society is in question, created by any combined action and deriving from the instinctive, not necessarily imitative acts of indi-

[1] Work quoted, p. 340. Play is thus tabulated: —

Selbstdarstellung.	Nachahmung.	Ausschmückung.
Persönliches.	Wahres.	Schönes.
Beim Thier: Bewerbungskünste.	Nachahmungskünste.	Baukünste.
Beim Menschen: Erregungstanz. Musik. Lyrik.	Nachahmungstanz. Mimik. Plastik. Malerei. Epik. Drama.	Kunstgewerbe. (Gartenbaukunst.) Architectur.

Compare with this the table given in Mr. Baldwin Brown's useful book on *The Fine Arts*, p. 36.

viduals as conscious parts of a whole. Society is not the sum of individuals, but the mass of them, differing as a mass in its parts from these parts as individuals, plus the greater or less influence of generations of previous masses, — in traditions, custom, and the like. Dead and living form a combination partly organic and vital, partly immaterial; against this stands the centrifugal, thinking, protesting, innovating individual. But even ignoring tradition, the difference holds. If I vote with a party, and "it" gains, my joy is not mine plus the joy of all who voted with me, but mine because I am a part of the voting body. How much stronger the direct case under almost exclusively communal conditions! Communal elation, quite apart from personal elation, any one can still study in his own mind, but under conditions which make his elation a thing of shame to his intellectual, critical self. This shame, which breeds the "mugwump" and breaks up political parties, barely existed in primitive life, — so sociology concludes with no dissenting voice. Communal elation, instinctive expression in consent, began, by Donovan's reckoning,[1] in the spontaneous "play-excitement" of a festal throng, which may or may not have parallels in the play of beasts and birds; here were human fellowship, homogeneous conditions, "a common cause of excitement," and a common expression of it in the social consent of rhythm. Donovan, too, has a table[2] to illustrate all this; "play-excitement," instinctive, drifts into "habits of movement" and into song; individual song-making is a later affair, and is developed "out of the racial memories." So great a factor was this communal elation, this play-excitement, in the making of poetry. But life has never been all play; poetry echoes, perhaps even clearer than in the case of play, the stress and

[1] *Lyre to Muse*, pp. 127 f. Mr. Baldwin Brown, *The Fine Arts*, p. 23, also regards art in general as an outgrowth of festal celebrations.

[2] At the end of his *Lyre to Muse*, p. 209.

pain of human effort. As was shown in preceding pages, Bücher laid stress upon the instinctive cries and motions of labour, the rhythm of individual and social work. Rhythm, he insisted, "springs from the organic nature of man"; it is automatic, instinctive,[1] and nowhere so much as in labour. Nor were the realms of play and labour very far apart. Treading the grapes of Dionysos, treading the wild dance of Dionysos, — there was little space between the two activities, and no distinction at all so far as rhythm and instinctive motion were concerned. In brief, whether one takes the instinct of play, as preparation for work, with Groos, or the play-excitement, with Donovan, or the instinctive rhythm furnished by work pure and simple, with Bücher, there is ample recognition in each case for the spontaneous, and in two of the cases for the communal, as essential elements in the beginnings of poetry. The conclusions of psychology[2] and sociology are still in tune with the dualism hinted long since by Aristotle, and stated just a century ago by A. W. Schlegel. Aristotle referred the beginning of poetry to two instincts, — imitation and "the instinct for harmony and rhythm"; but the art itself came only with individual effort. "Persons . . . with this natural gift little by little improved upon their early efforts till their rude improvisations gave birth to poetry. Poetry now branched off in two directions *according to the individual character of the writers*."[3] So, too, he speaks of tragedy, which, like comedy, "was at first mere improvisation," festal excitement of the throng;[4] and there is the same hint of communal spontaneity coming under artistic control when Aristotle notes that "Æschylus diminished the importance of the chorus,"

[1] *Arbeit und Rhythmus*, pp. 17, 25, 82.

[2] In Ribot's *Psychology of the Emotions*, e.g., p. 332, ample justice is done to spontaneous emotion and expression.

[3] See Butcher's translation, pp. 15 ff.

[4] So Butcher explains, p. 252: "a wild religious excitement, a bacchic ecstasy."

and when he speaks of a time when "poetry was of the satyric order, *and had greater affinities with dancing*." Would there were more historical work of this sort from that "honest and keen-eyed observer," as Schlegel calls him! Could the dualism be more plainly set forth? Döring[1] points out that Aristotle distinguishes two kinds of dithyramb; one is natural, spontaneous, improvised, and this is nothing, in his eyes, but the raw material of poetry; the other is the dithyramb of art. Schlegel's position has been defined already, but part of a brief[2] for a lecture which was never written out, may be noted as in point; he is more generous to the ruder stage of verse than Aristotle seems to be. "The idea of a natural history of poetry . . . End of this. *Transition to art and to the consciousness of it. All primitive, original songs inspiration of the moment*." Now the evidence of ethnology has set this last remark upon the surest base;[3] no fact is better established for savage poetry. Creatures of impulse, without individual thinking, without individual plan and purpose, with uniform and circumscribed conditions, with homogeneous natures, they are swayed by communal emotion to a degree which seems incredible to the man of culture. Schlegel himself had an eye on this sort of evidence. Speaking[4] of the songs before Homer, he calls them "quite artless outpourings of lyrical impulse"; they were "made up of a few simple words and outcries, constantly repeated, such as we find to-day among savages." Again, returning to the dualism of instinctive and artistic, one may note his happy phrase for

[1] *Kunstlehre des Aristoteles*, Jena, 1876, pp. 83 ff. Gerber, *Die Sprache als Kunst*, I. 32, follows Aristotle in denying that improvisations are ever poetry, which is enthusiasm plus deliberation and selection.

[2] *Vorlesungen*, I. 356 ff. Compare I. 340.

[3] Waitz-Gerland, *Anthropologie*, I. (2d. ed.), 345.

[4] *Vorlesungen*, II. 117, 119. He calls the Homeric epos an artistic improvisation as compared with earlier spontaneous, instinctive improvisation. See also II. 20.

it when he speaks[1] of "the change of nature-purpose into art-purpose."

A deeper study of this change, a study of the beginnings and development of Hellenic poetry, was made in one of the earlier and saner works of Nietzsche,[2] written while he was still in philological harness and before he broke with Wagner. Art, he thinks, depends on the enduring strife and occasional reconciliation of two opposing forces which the Greeks embodied in Dionysos and Apollo. Apollo finds expression in sculpture, in the individual work of art, Dionysos in the impersonal art of music; the genius of Greece united these two in Attic tragedy. Apollo is the personification of that *principium individuationis*, the deification of man as artist, as the solitary boatman whom Schopenhauer imagined[3] driven and tossed in this frail bark of individuality upon a sea of troubles. Now "individual" is as much as to say bounded, definite, restricted; hence the Hellenic dislike of exaggeration, its love of artistic reticence and restraint, and that "Know Thyself" as final word of the god who is simply a deification of the individual. But there is the other side. From time to time, say in intoxication, which has its god in all popular mythologies, or in those great upheavals of communal emotion due to victory, to love, to the coming of spring, rises the Dionysian impulse and shatters all sense of the individual. Such a movement made the chorus of the Greeks as well as the St. John and the St. Vitus dances of mediæval Europe. Man the individual, so Nietzsche puts it in his own dithyrambic style, sinks back, a prodigal son, into the bosom of that nature which he has deserted. "By song and dance man shows

[1] *Ibid.*, III. 141, — a mere note for his lecture.

[2] *Die Geburt der Tragödie*, oder *Griechenthum und Pessimismus*, 3d. ed. 1894; the immediate title, however, is *Die Geburt der Tragödie aus dem Geiste der Musik*.

[3] *Welt als Wille*, etc., I. 416. Nietzsche, pp. 22, 35 f.

himself a member of the higher unity; he forgets how to walk, to talk; he is on the way, dancing and leaping as he goes, fairly to fly aloft. His gestures tell of the magic which holds him. . . . *He is no longer artist, he is art,*" — and all this in the communal, Dionysian frenzy, the folk as a whole, and the individual lost in the throng. *Turba fit mens.* Here in spontaneous song, dance, gesture, of the crowd is the opposite of that reticent, deliberative Apollinian art; "this demonic folksong" is set over against the "artist of Apollo, chanting psalms to his harp."[1] The Greek dramatic chorus, Nietzsche goes on to say, is simply the old Dionysian throng, once transformed by their spontaneous excitement into satyrs,[2] pure nature and instinct, now conventionalized and brought under artistic control; the separation of chorus and spectators is artificial, for at bottom there is no difference between them, and all make a single body of dancing and singing satyrs, — that is, the greater part of the throng now dance by deputy.[3] We are absurdly narrow, he thinks, in applying modern ideas of authorship to primitive conditions. "Dionysian ecstasy," — and Nietzsche's fantastic style[4] should not hide the soundness of his idea, —

[1] Lyric and folksong, according to Nietzsche, p. 48, are outcome of music. "Diesen Prozess einer Entladung der Musik in Bildern haben wir uns auf eine jugendfrische, sprachlich schöpferische Volksmenge zu übertragen, um zur Ahnung zu kommen, wie das strophische Volkslied entsteht."

[2] The usual references for Bacchic or Dionysian orgies are Livy, IX. 4 ff., where minute particulars are given; Strabo, bk. X.; Athenæus, X.

[3] In Nietzsche's mystic phrase, the chorus "auf seiner primitiven Stufe in der Urtragödie," is "eine Sebstspiegelung des dionysischen Menschen . . . eine Vision der dionysischen Masse."

[4] See pp. 60 f. This artistic power is his definition of the poetic process. Professor Giddings, on hints of Mr. Spencer, has drawn a picture of solitary, primitive man arguing a spirit from the phenomenon of his shadow and of the echo of his voice. It may be pointed out that communal shouts and cries, echoed from the rocks, would be more likely to rouse a belief in that horde of spirits with which the primitive human horde thought itself surrounded. Early religion was social, communal; individual meditation, a process of individual thought, was utterly subordinate to communal thought. Even now superstition is a lingering "they say."

"Dionysian ecstasy can give to a whole throng this artistic power of seeing itself ringed about by a host of spiritual forms with which it feels itself essentially one." This passing into another character on the part of a throng, homogeneous of course and instinctive, is the beginning of the drama, and differs from the work of the rhapsodist. "All other choral lyric of the Greeks," says Nietzsche, "is only the Apollinian solitary singer intensified; but in the dithyramb there stands before us a community of unconscious actors[1] who see one another as transformed." The drama, in short, came from the union of a Dionysian spontaneous, communal song, in itself chaotic outburst of passion, and the ordering, restraining, artistic, deliberative spirit which breathed order into this chaos and is known as the spirit of Apollo. Thinking on the functions of this artistic, Apollinian spirit, one is reminded of De Vigny's definition of art, as "la verité choisie"[2]; while it is clear that in the cadences of his verse, and in the emotion that surges through it, the poet is still a part of that Dionysian throng. In a word, the Apollinian process, which is the only process one now connects with one's idea of art, or of poetry, intellectualizes and therefore individualizes emotion. An instructive essay by Dr. Krejči[3] regards the fundamental dualism of poetry as a contrast between the involuntary or mechanical element, and the element of logical or voluntary creation. As we follow back the course of poetry, he asserts, the voluntary and creative element decreases, while there is a steady gain in the automatic, the mechanical, and the spontaneous, — a gain which is made still more probable by Bücher's theory of rhythm. If one could see the conditions and hear the songs of a primitive time, one would find poetry, so Krejči makes bold to assert, entirely

[1] "Eine Gemeinde von unbewussten Schauspielern," p. 61.

[2] *Journal d'un Poète*, p. 38.

[3] "Das charakteristische Merkmal der Volkspoesie," *Zeitschr. f. Völkerpsychol.*, XIX. (1889), 115 ff.

swayed by the unreflective, mechanical, and spontaneous element.[1] In this sense, Apollo is thought mastering emotion, art in control of that spontaneous, chaotic, and yet rhythmic expression of the Dionysian throng.

Instinctive and spontaneous expression, then, is to be assumed for primitive song; but the communal idea involves something more. It demands a homogeneous body of people. Again tradition points this way, as in the case of rhythm and of the dualism between nature and art; again, as before, voices are raised in protest; again M. Tarde is in the field with a formula directly opposed to the formula of tradition; and again we must turn to modern science for some definite answer, only to find it fairly in favour of tradition and backed in this respect by ample evidence from ethnology and literature. Modern psychology, it seems, leaves one free to conceive a throng of primitive men so homogeneous that a common emotion would call out a common and simultaneous expression. Thoughts diverge, and thought, or purpose, controls modern art as it controls modern emotion; but primitive folk did little thinking, if one may here trust ethnology and the savage, backed by the controlling evolutionary facts of literature.[2] Savage thinking is limited to the few objects of the savage world, and any effort beyond this is painful; the wild man complains of headache the moment he is forced to "think." Deliberation implies memory, and purpose regards future complications; but we saw that the Botocudos have no legends, and we know how accurately care for future needs marks progress in culture; barring those ancestral shadows, as with Eskimos, it is true of all savages that they have no history at all. So utterly disappears our sharp individual thinking as one touches savage life. Herodotus was surprised to find a tribe "that had no name"; but,

[1] *Zeitschr. f. Völkerpsychol.*, XIX., p. 120.

[2] See Schultze, *Der Fetischismus*, pp. 30 ff., with his authorities.

as Schultze notes, Bushmen now do not know one another by any individual appellation. The language of all savage tribes reflects this lack of individual thinking in our sense; and it is to tribal emotion, instincts of tribal life and their social expression, that one always looks for what must pass as the intellectual life of the savage. The individual savages do not think, but they feel; and feelings, unlike thoughts, tend to converge. Nor, again, a most important point, is the communal elation of the primitive throng to be confused with the imitation of a modern crowd, yielding, after individual mental suicide, to the suggestions of a leader who does the thinking while the crowd acts out his thought. Ethnology records the fact, but few if any scholars have noted its significance, that savages are formidable and command civilized respect in proportion as they act in mass and as a unit, while modern man is contemptible in the mass; modern man is formidable as an individual, while the individual savage is little better than an idiot. Detached from the throng in which and by which he thinks, feels, acts, he is a silent, stolid fellow, into whose silence romantic folk like Châteaubriand and Cooper have read vast philosophies, and from whose forced conversation, uncentred and mobile as a child's, missionaries have drawn most of their conflicting and suspicious statements about savage myths, customs, beliefs, and ways of thought. Evidence about savages in the mass, about their communal life, on the other hand, is nearly all straightforward and consistent. Hence a conclusion of vast reach and meaning for the beginnings of poetry: just as individuals are superior now, just as the mob, the masses, the *profanum volgus*, what not, are objects of contempt in these latter days,[1] so

[1] Two famous utterances voice this feeling. Swift loved his Peter, Paul, John, and the rest; he hated the human race at large. This for the outer circle. As for crowds, Schiller put the antithesis in a distich: —

> Jeder, sieht man ihn einzeln, ist leidlich klug und beständig;
> Sind sie *in corpore*, gleich wird euch ein Dummkopf daraus.

this mob, these masses, were far and away superior to individuals in conditions of primitive life and at the start of social progress. By the very terms of the case, and in the struggle for existence, social man was forced to win the early fight by social consent, and this was the overwhelming fact to which all individual considerations had to yield. This superiority attached, of course, to what the mass did and said and sang as compared with individual utterance. Human nature remains unchanged, but human conditions are always changing. One must not treat primitive man, with regard to the conditions and outcome of his life, in terms of modern man. The mob, the masses, exist for us mainly as the raw material of social and political factions. Lack of bread, of work, or the infringement of fancied rights, leads to a common and intense emotion, the first requisite of mass movement; a leader of some sort, with a plan which comes of more or less thinking, sways the mob to a definite act. But the behaviour of a mob, the doing and expression of a mob, are now in sharp antithesis to that doing and expression of individual men at the bidding of individual thought, of deliberation, plan, and definite purpose. Conditions of primitive life, so all evidence goes to prove, reversed this order; and it is a totally evil process when one transfers the value of a modern mass of men to the communal throng, the horde, if one will, which began our social progress. Hence the error in Tarde's ingenious argument.[1] Attacking the idea that a mass of men ever created language, he conceives the mass in terms of a mob, language in terms of our highly intellectualized and individualized speech; and he applies the same impossible test to religion and to poetry. Who, he cries, "ever saw a masterpiece of art . . . planned and wrought out by the collective inspiration of ten or a hundred poets or artists?" None of us, certainly, save in some form of survival hard to

[1] "Foules et Sectes," in *Essais et Mélanges Sociol.*, p. 4.

recognize, has seen such a thing. Primitive man, on the other hand, knew nothing of a poetical masterpiece in M. Tarde's sense. When communal "inspiration" was dominant, when the throng absorbed the individual, when thought hardly dared to show its solitary visage before a solid communal emotion, the masterpiece of art, that is, of individual planning, hardly had a place; under modern conditions of individual thinking, communal emotion is just as unproductive in the æsthetic realm. The masterpiece waited for the master; and one remembers M. Tarde's delusion about the origins of all poetry in some "great book." In stating his case for the artist, which is perfectly true for modern conditions, he is really stating the case, by implication, for primitive communal song.

But was this throng really homogeneous? Are the facts in accord with this theory of communal conditions and the outcome of them? Mr. Spencer, as every one knows, laid down the law that all social progress is from the homogeneous to the heterogeneous;[1] and M. Brunetière has adopted this principle as a guide to the study of literary development,[2] regarding it as the one doctrine of evolution, held by Spencer as by Haeckel, which stands the test of criticism and is beyond the reach of doubt. The history of culture, so M. le Bon thinks,[3] points the same way; "counter to our dreams of equality, the result of modern civilization is not to make men more and more equal, but to make them

[1] *Principles of Sociology*, I. 459, 704 f. Tribe to nation, I. 584. Rise of professions due to "specialization of a relatively homogeneous mass," III. 181. See II. 307 ff. In the *First Principles*, §§ 125, 127, he had defined the process as "change from an incoherent homogeneity to a coherent heterogeneity," and had applied the idea not only to the primitive union of poetry, music, and dancing, but within poetic limits to that undifferentiated song which held in germ the epic, the lyric, the drama.

[2] *Revue des deux Mondes*, 15 Feb., 1898, p. 880; "le passage de l'homogène à l'heterogène," that "idée mère, l'idée substantielle de l'évolution"; or in Haeckel's words, "gradual differentiation of matter originally simple."

[3] *L'Évolution des Peuples*, pp. 37 f. See also pp. 43, 167.

more and more different." Comte assumed that the common trait of biology and sociology is this passing from the whole to the parts; and although Mr. Spencer, with his doctrine of cells, has largely set Comte aside, that part of the old system is intact. Popular books, supposed to sum up the best results of science, are to the same effect. In primitive times, says Reclus,[1] "all felt, thought, and acted in concert. Everything leads us to believe that at the outset collectivism was at its maximum and individualism at its minimum. The individual," he declares, "was not the father of society; society was the mother of the individual." Studies of prehistoric man, as in the stone age, point to a sameness of individuals now quite impossible to imagine.[2] Hennequin is not with Tarde on this point; the primitive community was homogeneous, and its members "were all nearly exactly alike in body and in mind."[3] Gumplowicz is explicit for the beginning of society in homogeneous hordes.[4] A recent writer who has made a study of the horde and the family in primitive development,[5] and who is by no means of the extreme school, — he rejects promiscuity, for example, — declares the horde to have been the starting-point of social progress. Grosse, casting about for a state of savage life which shall give the best idea of the life of primitive man, finds it in a "homogeneous, undifferentiated mass," thus backing Spencer at least in his sociological assertion;[6] and

[1] *Primitive Folk*, p. 57.

[2] So the reviews summarize the doctrine of A. H. Keane, *Man Past and Present*, 1899.

[3] *Critique Scientifique*, pp. 112, 115.

[4] In the *Rassenkampf*, and especially in *Outlines of Sociology*, trans. Moore, pp. 39, 124, 139 note; on p. 142 he names the factors which made a horde homogeneous.

[5] Dr. Richard Mucke, *Horde und Familie in ihrer urgeschichtlichen Entwicklung*, Stuttgart, 1895.

[6] Grosse, *Formen der Familie*, pp. 30 ff. See p. 39. He takes as "representatives of the oldest form of social life" those scattered tribes which subsist

the best authorities bear out this view. The hordes which serve, in lack of better ethnological material, as the type of primitive man, are small and scattered; they have no arts, no division of labour; individual property is almost unknown, and the one piece of property, their hunting-ground, belongs to all the adult males in common. As little difference of rank exists as of property; seldom are there any leaders, and where, in a few cases, these are found, their authority is pitifully small. The only individuals who break this "homogeneous and undifferentiated" monotony are the supposed possessors of a magical power.[1] So runs the certainly unprejudiced account of Grosse. Even by Sir Henry Maine's extreme patriarchal views, the family itself, the first social group, was a homogeneous and undifferentiated mass in those characteristics with which the student of poetry must deal. Mr. Tylor's group of Caribs,[2] with uniformity of physical and mental structure, amply bears out the communal and homogeneous argument for earliest song; but perhaps the shortest way with dissenters is a passage by Waitz,[3] where he sums up the evidence for this uniformity of the individuals in a horde and in social groups of a low order. All their relations of life, he says, are simple, and are bent in one direction, the procuring of food; there is a maximum of instinct and common appetite, and almost no

entirely by hunting; we know nothing so primitive, and while checked in culture, these tribes are probably not degraded (32 f.). The statements in the text are based on careful arrangement of the statistics, a very important point. See Mucke, *Horde und Familie*, pp. 181 ff. Spencer describes the "small, simple aggregates," coöperating "with or without a regulating centre, for certain public ends," of which the "headless" kind must be regarded as the primitive type; and gives a list of these not very different from the list of Grosse. *Prin. Soc.*, I. § 257.

[1] Grosse refuses to extend this lack of individual power to promiscuity in sexual relations. That precious theory was doubtless carried to an absurd point; but the reaction may likewise go too far, and the case of those Andamanese (p. 43) with their "absolute conjugal fidelity even unto death," uncannily suggests Sir Charles Grandison and even Isaac Walton's mullet.

[2] *Anthropology*, p. 79.

[3] *Anthropologie*, I. 74 ff., 349 ff.

stir of mind such as follows the division of labour; and this uniform mental habit works upon the outward person, so that, physically as well as intellectually, the single man fails to stand out from the mass. Waitz, who quotes Humboldt to the same purpose, thus explains why the Romans, with their complicated civilization, found the Germans all looking alike, all of one type.[1] Wherever the horde is visible, even in a comparatively civilized case, as with the Scottish clans, there the resemblance of individuals, the emphasis of a type, is unmistakable; and it is precisely under these conditions that we find the survivals of communal song. Primitive man, moreover, dependent on the nature about him, and acting in his horde like other creatures in the face of a power which they fear, surrounded himself with a like horde of spirits,[2] themselves as little differentiated or distinguished in any way as the human horde which conceived them. Even under the highest civilization such conditions of the horde survive in communal worship. True, the informing power of Christianity is its individualism, its "flight of the one to the One"; but the litany, the general confession, the spirit of congregational worship, are suggestive not so much of the "O God, I" as of the "O Spirits, We," — homage once paid by all the living souls to all the souls of the dead, and still lingering as a shadowy survival in two great festivals of the church. Religious emotion is still the strongest communal element in modern times, particularly when it takes the form of a great revival.

Against all this in general and Mr. Spencer's theory in particular, M. Tarde, as was noted, set up his theory of the infinitesimal and the cell; against the narrower idea of differentiation in poetry, — epic, lyric, and dramatic regarded as developments from an earlier compact form in which the

[1] Waitz, I. 446, answers objections to this view, and disposes of the idea that civilization levels mankind.

[2] See above, p. 372, note 4.

three were still united, — Professor Grosse,[1] who was so bold in his assertion of homogeneous life, asserts heterogeneous poetry from the beginning. Yet he presently lays down[2] the larger truth, which carries with it a confusion of his own particular denial on poetic grounds. "In the lowest stage of culture," he says, "art appears, at least for us, simply and only as a social phenomenon. . . . In the higher stages, however, along with the influence which art exerts upon social life, there comes more and more into view the value of art for the development of individual life. . . . *Between the individual and the social function of art is a deep antithesis.*" In other words, he proves by his admirably selected facts, throughout the whole book, that the art of primitive times was mainly social, whereas the art of modern times is mainly individual. Moreover, he is very sure that primitive society was homogeneous. The inference is inevitable. Dr. Wallaschek, we saw, set down the "collectiveness of amusement" as main characteristic of primitive life. These things cannot be said in one breath, only to be followed in another by such amazing contradictions as the implication of Grosse[3] that the egoist in man is the first of poets, or the jaunty talk of Scherer about primitive poets and their public, their royalties, their authorship, when only a few pages away he tells us that "mass poetry," poetry of the throng, is the differencing element in primitive æsthetic life. Posnett, to whom all students of poetry are under deep obligations for his vigorous sketch of comparative literature, does justice to the communal element in early song and reduces the individual, heterogeneous element to a minimum; his formula for poetic development is "the progressive deepening and widening of personality."[4]

[1] *Anfänge der Kunst*, p. 224. [2] *Ibid.*, pp. 300 f. [3] *Ibid.*, p. 236.

[4] *Comparative Literature*, p. 72. See pp. 89 ff., 155 ff., 347 f., and the whole chapter on "The Principle of Literary Growth." He glorifies sympathy as the

It is to be conceded that a superficial view reverses this order of progress. What does one meet oftener in history and song, —

> O nimis optato saeclorum tempore nati,
> Heroes, salvete, deum genus ![1] —

than talk of a "heroic" age in the remote past, and of the commonplace, average-ridden present, the epoch, as Le Bon calls it, of crowds? Against the mediocrity, the hustings, the juries, the lynching-bees, the "suffrage of the plough," the dead level of uninteresting masses, there floats up a vision of the knight on his quest, of the solitary hero at odds, like Hercules, with divinity itself, of the good old king who sits to judge his people in the gates. Have not we moderns the homogeneous mass, and was not the individual a child of the early world? Wilhelm von Humboldt[2] finds the secret of Homer in his "sense of individuality" and "individualizing impulse." Haym, a careful writer, talks of the individualism of the Middle Ages as opposed to modern times. Blémont[3] admits that democracy is individualism, but contends that it makes for anything rather than for individuality, and simply levels human life; the mind ceases to be free, and men act in masses, simplify everything, make life monotonous. Against this, however, one needs only to recall that quotation just made from Le Bon; the process seems to be toward sameness, but is really toward diversity. Men may dress alike, may show concerted action, may discourage the unusual and set up a god of averages; but the individual is stronger than ever before, and he does more thinking for himself. Men move in masses, true; but it is less and less the herd instinct and more and more the voluntary coherence of thinking

poetic mainspring; but he fails to study the dualism in terms of actual throng and actual artist. The spirit and plan of the book, however, are worthy of the highest praise, whatever its shortcomings in detail.

[1] Catullus, lxiv. [2] *Werke*, VI. 26. [3] *Esthétique de la Tradition*, pp. 69 ff.

minds. Instinct has yielded to thought. The history of civilization is the making and unmaking of communities; society means more than it ever meant; but this is not denying the fundamental law of progress from homogeneous to heterogeneous, from communal to individual and artistic. One must not juggle with these terms. It is true that an army, a group of men for any purpose, which marches as one man, is the end and not the beginning of communal effort. It is true that the savage is notoriously fitful; there is anything but splendid purpose in his eyes; combined action, under certain conditions — that is, conditions of civilization — is difficult even for members of one tribe; their prevailing force seems to be individual and centrifugal; the bond that binds them to the community often seems slight beyond belief; as to their feelings, just now assumed to be almost a unit, "emotional variability" is the report of many a traveller.[1] This has been extended to primitive life, and to the moral side of the case; early man, says Pulszky,[2] was ruled by "unqualified selfishness," and asserted "his individuality in every respect." The same author speaks of "a gradation, the first word of which is selfishness, and the last, public sentiment." Where in all this coil of caprice and incoherence is the homogeneous community expressing a common emotion by a common utterance? The answer is clear enough. Escape from this caprice, this incoherence, this centrifugal force, is found primarily in social consent, in the communal utterance which began the long struggle against purely selfish ends; and communal utterance begins, as has been shown, in the consent of rhythm. Strong as the selfish impulses were, so strong the need for at least an incipient

[1] Spencer, *Sociology*, I. 56 ff., 70 f., II. 271, note; Grosse, *Formen der Familie*, p. 57, with quotation from Petroff's book on Alaska; Schultze, *Fetischismus*, pp. 51 f.

[2] *The Theory of Law and Civil Society*, London, 1888, pp. 106 f. See above, p. 26.

check upon them in social action; and from social action and utterance sprang all those altruistic virtues which Pulszky lauds — patriotism, piety, duty to kin and to the race. The end of society is to take brute man and make him a civilized man, to let "the ape and tiger" in him die; man when nearest ape and tiger, at the beginning of social union, was individually brutish, stolid, selfish, idiotic, fitful, in a word, individually bad; and just so far as he submitted to social consent, lived for the horde, the clan, kin, country, so far he was socially good. Hence it is easy to see that in this homogeneous society all the beginnings of civilization, art, poetry, religion, would be overwhelmingly homogeneous, social, communal; the condition of their existence was the abnegation of the individual man in favour of the social man. In a word, society itself began in this social consent, and since it had such tremendous forces of selfishness arrayed against it in the primitive individual instincts,[1] the only way in which it could make its way was by utter suppression of the individual in so far as he was a party to the social bond itself. Hence a contradiction that is only apparent. The savage as a creature of animal instinct is as capricious and centrifugal as one will; as a creature of social act, emotion, thought, he has no individuality, and puts none into his expression; for it was precisely this tuition of social consent which little by little gave him the impulse to deed, feeling, deliberation, as member of society. Here is the solution of the problem. Arab boatmen who can not pull ropes in unison,[2] sing and dance together with a consent that astonishes the traveller. They

[1] Professor Baldwin, *Social and Ethical Interpretations*, p. 214, puts the beginning of the social period just after man's release from the animal. See too his appendix. Ribot, work quoted, p. 281, says the gregarious life — of animals in hordes, that is — "is founded on the attraction of like for like, irrespective of sex." See this whole chapter on "The Social and Moral Feelings."

[2] See, however, the case of New Zealanders who work in large numbers and in perfect accord by singing their song *totowaka*. Wallaschek, *Prim. Mus.*, p. 43.

are capricious, fitful individuals in regard to the new kind of work, but compact, communal society in regard to the festal consent which united their wandering hordes thousands of years ago. Descriptions of the savage state easily bear out this contradiction and this solution, if one will analyze the facts; and this is why one finds Spencer and Grosse asserting on one page the homogeneity and collectiveness of savage communitics, and on another page the heterogeneous, capricious, individual, selfish traits of the savage himself. In literature we do not so clearly see both sides. Throng-poetry is rarely recorded; one merely describes a village or tribal chorus, — and takes down the individual song. Luckily, however, the "collective character" of primitive amusement is made as certain as such things can be, by the ethnological evidence considered in the chapter on rhythm, by the evidence of popular survivals collected in the chapter on communal song and dance, and by the evolutionary curves of poetry itself. Considering all this evidence, one escapes the snare laid in one's path by the idea of individualism in the savage. That "emotional variability"[1] is individual indeed, and disappears precisely as the communal expression of emotion comes into play. It has been proved, too, that, like speech, rhythmic utterance and rhythm itself in the sense which Bücher gives to it, are not so much the outcome as the occasion of social union. The sense of this union, "the consciousness of kind" as Professor Giddings calls it, is at bottom a sense of order, and the "instinct for order" is best

[1] Even Mr. Spencer points out that this is no bar to communal consent, *Sociology*, I. 59; for the variability implies "smaller departure from primitive reflex action, . . . lack of the re-representative emotions which hold the simpler ones in check." Bastian, too, has shown that in the formation of society out of individuals, the social element as such, the social whole, must precede the element of social individuality or of the individuality within the mass. This is what one gathers from Bastian's books in general; in one case, *Die Welt in ihren Spiegelungen unter dem Wandel des Völkergedankens*, p. 413, he applies this idea to the priority of social property as compared with individual property.

expressed in rhythm; rhythm, it was seen, is not invention and imitation, but discovery and consent. Anterior to any process of invention and imitation, which is a social act, must be the condition which makes this act possible, — a consciousness of kind and a social consent. Instinctive emotions of a homogeneous horde felt in common on a great occasion gave birth to a common expression in which the separate individuals discovered this social consent. Invention and imitation, begun as early as one will after this social consent, gave them the conditions of their activity; but they must not be put before it, nor, for considerable stretches of social development, could they be said to have an important place, since they grew with the growing importance of the individual in society. If one may dogmatize on the matter, one may think of three gradations in social progress. First, there is the consent due mainly to external suggestion working on instinctive movements: in the dance it is due to that festive joy of victory and that "rhythmic beating" outward, that rhythmic impulse inward, which Donovan describes; and in labour, as Bücher thinks of it, it is either the consent of a solitary labourer with the labour itself, or, more often, the consent of several labourers with those instinctive and necessary movements. Vocal and significant cries went with the movements in each case. Secondly, but contemporary with the other, one may figure a less festal occasion and a more active personal agency; five or six men marching abreast fall into step and find the labour of marching is lightened, — not a very different matter from the dance, but less communal and more unrestrained. Imitation comes slightly into play, but it is wholly subordinate to consent. Thirdly, imitation and invention get their rights where the individual discovers or invents an isolated act, in various degrees of artistic and social significance, from the jump over an obstacle by the leader in a row of men marching in Indian file, the sheep-over-a-fence process, as Mr. Lloyd Morgan calls it, up to the clever throwing of a spear, the tying together of two vine branches, the fashioning of a spear-head, which are invention outright, triumph of individual thinking, plan and deliberation detached from communal emotion. The leader is on hand; the "headless" hordes have heads. Spontaneity, instinct, the automatic, still dominant in communal dance and song, in reminiscential rites of every sort, have yielded in active life to thought and purpose of the individual, to division of labour, to that power to plan a protracted piece of work and carry it out in detail which makes for progress. But before this formula of invention and imitation can apply, before one talks of the leader and the led, there must be a coherent body which can resolve itself into these relations of parts; and precisely here is the beginning of society in social consent, and here, too, the beginning of poetry in communal and rhythmic utterance.

One thus faces a seeming paradox in the conception of poetry as at once the highest expression of the differentiated, deliberate, artistic individual, and, at the same time, the fullest expression of a homogeneous, spontaneous, automatic mass; the paradox vanishes at once if one will only see in rhythm consent and emotional cadence of a dancing, singing multitude, and in artistic phrase and thought the deliberate control and plan of the individual, — Apollo in the foreground, and the background filled with a festal Dionysian throng. Why refuse to see this social background, or, in another figure, this communal foundation of poetry? Guyau puts beyond doubt the essentially social character of the art, even under modern conditions; but one makes a phrase, and returns to the old way. A long succession of deliverances on solitary genius has befogged the critical vision and blotted this lodestar of social conditions from the sky. In other fields such a mistake is unknown. The student of political science would never deny that a representative in Congress, as his name implies, is the deputy of a throng that once, say in the forests of Germany, would have come together as a compact legislative body and settled questions of state. But in poetry the poet ends and the poet began, a creature of solitude, now in commerce with the immensities and infinities, and now holding out his hat to the public for a *honorarium*,— the public's only part in the poetic process. If the public is brought in, it is to explain the poet, as with Sainte-Beuve and Taine, or to explain the gentle reader, as with Hennequin. Poetry is a whisper, a confidence, to this gentle reader. When the throng, not to speak of the silence about its active functions in poetry, catches up a poem that it likes, and roars it, as it roared Mr. Kipling's *Absent-minded Beggar*, over all England, this is very salt in the wounds of the critic, who declares, with some justice, that here is no "poetry" at all; while the same author's *Recessional*, with its individual appeal, its recoil from popular sentiment, its assertion of thought over emotion, is set down, and rightly, as "poetry of a high order." Judging poetry by the standard of modern conditions, which are wholly individual, artistic, intellectual, the critic is right. The war-song of to-day, all lyrics of the throng, have a hollow and unreal ring in them; even Tennyson's *Light Brigade* somehow gives the effect of armour which is laced with bonnet-strings. The real song of war in an age of communal poetry was heard at that moment which Müllenhoff calls the supreme moment of all Germanic life, when the images of the gods were brought out, when the wedge was formed,— leaders of battle at the thin forward end and women and children in the rear,— the whole community at hand; with the hurling of Woden's spear, all swept into the fight, chanting the great chorus of war. Here is the folk communal in organization to great extent, but not quite homogeneous; not a leaderless horde, but still holding to elements of that primitive life; here is still poetry of the people.

Communal elation still furnishes the main cause of poetic utterance; the utterance is immediate; and development of the individual has not yet sundered the making and the hearing of a song.[1]

[1] Perhaps there is some connection between the fervour and merit of French war-songs like the Marseillaise, the *Ça ira*, and the fact that French literature as a whole is averse from undue stress upon the individual and does not suffer, whatever its other defects, from "too much ego in its cosmos." Texte points out that Jean-Jacques, Germanic by nature, noticed this trait in the French. "Le *je* . . . est presque aussi scrupuleusement bannit de la scène française que des écrits de Port-Royal, *et les passions humaines . . . n'y parlent jamais que par on.*" How contemptuously M. Brunetière, who has no superior in the appreciation of French literature as a whole, speaks of that new personal note, set in fashion by Rousseau, "most eloquent of lackeys!" See "La Littérature Personelle," in B.'s *Questions de Critique*, pp. 211 ff., and his review of Hennequin's book in the same collection, pp. 305 ff.

CHAPTER VII

THE EARLIEST DIFFERENTIATIONS OF POETRY

THAT primitive horde with its uncouth but rhythmic dance, its well timed but seemingly futile song, has now, let us hope, found its justification as the source of poetry. Not like the dance and song among Botocudos and Veddahs, a thing of degeneration or at least of sterile and unpromising kind, was this beginning of the beginnings; rather a feat of vast moment for the coming race of men, an achievement not to be measured by ordinary phrase. In the long reaches of growth and differentiation which stretch from this beginning to the present time, we are now to take our steps forward; the backward mutters of dissevering power which sought to resolve poetry unto its communal elements must now yield to a record of its progress; and our first task is to catch sight of the poet, the master of his art, as he detaches himself from the throng and sets out upon that path which leads him to his present state of grace. Another and an interesting question concerns the waning communal element, how it loses its hold upon poetical production, and how far it still modifies the poet's work.

Where and how, then, does the poet appear? Coöperation, however unlike what one now understands by coöperation, was the beginning of social progress, and the discovery or perception of rhythm had to play the main part in this first communal act whether of work or of play. Rhythm is the expression of a sense of coherence; and the first coherence was of a kind to suppress the individual: all evidence goes to show this fact. The Veddahs live mainly in isolated pairs, a brutish existence, except when some great tribal interest brings them together; at such a time that monotonous, leaderless dance about the arrow, man clasped close to man in an almost solid ring, — the Botocudos, too, and many other tribes, are pictured as thus forming a fairly compact mass, with only a part of the individual body free to move in unison with the same part of every other body, — is the way by which the clan or horde finds itself in this unwonted relation. Then the individual detaches himself from his singing with the throng, and for a verse or so sings to the throng; but how tentative, how momentary his effort, and how short his range away from the repeated communal chorus! For this individual is not acting as individual, acting freely in isolated life, but as member of a body which is just beginning to be a body and to understand its power of social and therefore of mutual influence. Moreover, as Spencer points out, primitive imagination is purely reminiscent, not constructive; the earliest working of what may pass as poetical imagination, then, is an individual utterance reminiscent of communal utterance and prolonging it with shy and tentative variations. This is precisely what one finds in the song of Veddahs and Botocudos. In the Eskimo singing-house the soloist has come to greater importance; he sings always a song of his own making, while the women join in the chorus "*amna aya*, the never failing end of each verse." In this singing-house "almost every great success in hunting is celebrated . . . and especially the capture of a whale." When the soloist is not singing these adventures, or satiric songs, also great favorites, the flyting or song-duel is in order.[1] Great, however, as the independence of the singer seems compared with a bard of the Botocudos, the chorus is still imperious, and no one singer is eminent. Everybody sings, — not only in chorus, but in

[1] Boas, *Report Bur. Ethnol.*, 1884–1885, pp. 564, 600 ff.

his turn as soloist; and everybody makes his own song. How utterly alien to this conception of early social life is the monarchical idea, the great man idea, human history begun by the tyrant of a submissive band! Take a half civilized state of society, as among the Germans described by Tacitus; here it is evident that democracy prevailed in peace, while in war, with concessions to men of "royal" blood, the strongest and boldest men acted as chieftains gathered in the thin end of the wedge, going into battle as exemplars and leaders, but not as generals, not as commanding, overseeing genius of a deliberate plan. As with government and war, so with property. Grosse[1] notes in those tribes that approach primitive ways few marks of individual ownership, but a mass of marks which denote claims of the horde or clan. So, too, with language, a problem which nobody in these days is fain to undertake;[2] but surely the mystic style of Donovan's article must not hide the soundness of his views,[3] already noted, on the festal origin of human speech. Religion, however, may have offered an earlier chance for centrifugal forces. It is probable that the medicine man, the shaman, with his visions, his abnormal states and doings, closely connected with that perilous stuff which every man of the horde had upon his individual heart in ordinary dreams, furnished the earliest example of a commanding personality acting in such an eccentric way as to make sharpest contrast with the coherence of communal action. Here, said the community, here is a man with a "gift," a man apart; and his use of wild dance and song in exorcism may have begun at a very

[1] *Anf. d. Kunst*, p. 132.

[2] On this baffling theme there is good reasoning in a neglected book by Noiré, *Die Welt als Entwicklung des Geistes*, pp. 240 f. He notes the mnemonic force of earliest words, which were few and used under strong emotional excitement; language was a kind of "thinking aloud."

[3] Stated in different terms by W. von Humboldt, *Werke*, VI. 198.

early date. Later, too, something of the sacred and the mysterious inherent in a shaman's vocation may have been transferred to the poet; priest and singer alike came to refer their ecstasy to a divine source. Yet magical ceremonies, whatever the advocates of prose-poetry may say, offer no good opportunity to observe the actual beginnings of the poet. We can see him detaching himself, not as magician or in special rites, but as a simple singer and dancer, from the singing and dancing throng; and this is the proper point of departure in our study, for the good reason that here is a fissiparous birth. Offspring of the communal chant by the simplest process, his own chant merely continues that of the community, which for an instant or so turns silent and passive for his profit. Again, this first of singers is no artist in verse, favourite of the muses, no man apart, son of the golden clime and solitary wanderer over Parnassus; he is every member of the throng in turn. To prove this vital point, we must not only take ethnological evidence, here conclusive as well as abundant, but must also follow that method which has led to some good results in foregoing pages of this book; we must try to connect the evidence of savage life with those survivals in an advanced stage of culture which by their mere survival indicate the persistence of a habit rooted deep in human history and human nature. We must study by this double light a few facts in regard to that improvisation in which Aristotle found the beginning of poetic art.

The fissiparous birth of individual from communal poetry is confirmed by the process observed everywhere among savage tribes. Solitary performance has come there to a considerable pitch of skill, but it yields always in importance to the chorus, and along with profit and reputation of a sort it often involves a kind of shame. Prostitutes do the individual singing and dancing in many parts of the Orient;[1] singing-

[1] Wallaschek, *Prim. Mus.*, pp. 70 f.

women and dance-girls, even in advanced stages of culture, pay dearly for their eminence; and something of this decline in caste clings to the most respectable solitary performances, now and here, of the skilled "entertainer." The mimes of the Middle Ages were often held to be without the pale, not only of the law, but of the church itself;[1] and while other causes worked to this end, something must be conceded to that attitude of every public to its entertainer or even teacher, — extravagant praise and delight, extravagant rewards, but with it all a sense of aloofness, an inclination to wave away this centrifugal element which has set itself over against the communal body, now an indulgent contempt, where mere pastime is concerned, and now dislike and distrust at an exhibition of independent thought.

It has been repeatedly shown that short improvisations are the earliest form of individual poetic art, and are sung in the intervals of a chorus, or to relieve the monotony of labour, where again they detach themselves from the parent refrain, modify it, add to it, and so build up a song. There is no need to dwell on the evidence for savage improvisation. The African is amazing in his power to turn an event into verse; it is a communal affair for the most part, with a chorus in the background. At public dances the Indians of America improvise, man for man, indefinitely, leaning also on the monotonous refrain. Throughout the South-Sea Islands[2] improvisation of songs is as common as speech; even the children improvise. The lower the level of culture, the more general this gift of improvising; "among the Anda-

[1] I. von Döllinger, *Beiträge zur Sektengeschichte des Mittelalters*, Munich, 1890, II. 623 f., from an old Ms., "de hystrionibus et officiis inutilibus." Priests are instructed what professions bar the granting of absolution, — an interesting passage. "Cum igitur meretrices ad confessionem venerint, vel hystriones, non est eis danda poenitentia, nisi ex toto talia relinquant officia," etc.

[2] See Dana's account of an improvising islander working in California, *Two Years before the Mast*, Chap. XIX.

mans every one composes songs."[1] The same holds of Australia, of far Siberia, and throughout the savage world; moreover in all these cases the habit is not solitary but festal. The oldest poetry known to tradition among the Afghans was improvised in reply to an insulting verse;[2] but the professional singer is on hand, and improvisation has become an art. The history of poetry among civilized races always shows a surplus of improvisation in the initial stage known to the records; so it is with the Greek *skolion*, as well as with dramatic beginnings; and so, to take a different case, with the Arabs, where improvisation long held almost absolute sway,[3] although drama had no place and a subjective spirit reaches back to the earliest tradition. Again, where a literature is undeveloped, although under civilized conditions, improvisation is the main force; in this case are the Basques.[4] In fine, it is not a vain tradition which puts a general gift of improvising verse before the development of any national literature; and Plutarch, in his treatises on Music and on the Pythian Oracle, speaking of a time when all formal utterance was in poetry, and when even men without poetic fire were wont to make verses on any subject, is telling not a fable but something very close to truth. The proof is not far to seek, and comes from ethnological as well as literary sources.

[1] Wallaschek, quoting Portman, p. 278.

[2] J. Darmesteter, *Chants Populaires des Afghans*, Paris, 1888–1890, p. clxxxvi. The Afghans have got to a Browning level in poetry, if we may believe Captain Rafferty, *Selections from the Poetry of the Afghans*, London, 1862. "Shaida's poetry . . . " he says, "is deep and difficult."

[3] Ahlwardt, *über Poesie und Poetik der Araber*, Gotha, 1856, p. 7.

[4] F. Michel, *Le Pays Basque*, Paris, 1857, pp. 214 f. The same is true of the Poles. See Talvj (here spelled Talvi) *Historical View of the Languages and Literatures of the Slavic Nations*, New York, 1850, Part IV., pp. 315 ff. Speaking of the Polish ballads, Mrs. Robinson says, "Their dances were formerly always accompanied by singing. *But these songs are always extemporized.* Among the country gentry . . . the custom of extemporizing songs . . . continued even down to the beginning of our own century."

Improvisation in this early and general sense, however, must be distinguished from the later sort which was purely professional, an art which Schlegel[1] calls "poetic rope-dancing" and sunders from the older and nobler gift, from "natural and partly amœbean, extemporaneous poetry, which was and still is a source of social entertainment." The drama, he notes, began in this way.[2] As a social gift, indeed, improvisation lingers long with civilized folk; a hundred years ago the poet was ready with his "impromptu on seeing Miss —— asleep in the moonlight;" and games were common enough where every one had to make verse. Lady Luxborough[3] wrote to Shenstone: "It is the fashion for everybody to write a couplet to the same tune — an old country dance — upon whatever subject occurs to them." The couplets, it would seem, were satiric; and here, of course, is a late stage of the flyting. Then there was the clever man of society, like Theodore Hook,[4] who would improvise you verses on anything; but this phase of the art is best studied in Italy. It is to be noted that such verses were generally sung;[5] and, indeed, they come close to the professional improvisation which is to be considered below. For the present we are to look at the older and more communal stage, where art is just putting on a show of independence and learning to walk alone.

The question is not of the fact of improvisation in primitive stages of culture, familiar to every student in this field, but of the manner in which improvisation begins, grows, hardens into a profession, and dies out in vain rivalry with

[1] "Etwas über William Shakspeare," *Werke*, VII. 57 f.

[2] He refers to the Homeric hymn to Hermes, vv. 54–56: "The god sang to the playing what came into his mind, quickly, readily, just as at festal banquets youths tease one another with verses sung in turn."

[3] Quoted by Chappell, II. 623.

[4] See the *Greville Memoirs*, III. 122, 202.

[5] Spence, *Anecdotes* (for Italy), pp. 116 ff., 120 note.

song of a more deliberate art. A mass of improvised verse could be quoted which differs from the refrain and chorus of the throng only in respect of a trifling variation in language and a trifling addition to the matter. Leaving this fissiparous offspring, we turn to that form of improvisation which shows an organic structure of its own, and keeps the refrain at greater distance, discarding, too, the more persistent forms of repetition. Mungo Park [1] tells one story of his African wanderings which may be assumed as a faithful report of the facts; for it is to be believed, or hoped, that Park's pen, unlike the pen of many travellers in general, and the pen of Mr. Brooke of Middlemarch in particular, was not "a thinking organ" apt to run into adventures of its own. The wanderer, wet and tired, was taken into the hut of a native woman, who gave him food and a mat for bed, going on with the other women to "spin cotton" most of the night. "They lightened their labour [2] by songs, one of which was composed *extempore*," says Park, "for I was myself the subject of it. It was sung by one of the young women, the rest joining in a sort of chorus. . . . The words, literally translated, were these: 'The winds roared and the rains fell; the poor white man, faint and weary, came and sat under our tree,—he has no mother to bring him milk; no wife to grind his corn. *Chorus:* Let us pity the white man; no mother has he,' etc." Here the young woman seems to lead the chorus and suggest its words, while in the more primitive type of improvisation it is the chorus which supplies the main theme, and the tentative, momentary singer only adds his flourish. Here, too, is the element of the *honorarium;* for Park was so affected that he gave his landlady "two of the four brass buttons which remained" on

[1] *Travels in Africa*, reprinted in Pinkerton, XVI. 844.

[2] Improvisation of labour songs by women, solitary or in bands, is very common. See Bücher, *Arbeit u. Rhythmus*, passim, especially, p. 78, and above, p. 269.

his waistcoat, and surely the poetess could claim one of them for her poetry. We have all read far worse at far higher rates. True, the chorus or refrain is still very potent; the little contemporary event is the sole suggestion of verse which looks neither before nor after; but the incremental factor is less hampered and less timid, and a touch of reflection and sentiment — provided this was not the product of Park's reminiscent mood — is at hand in the sympathy for a motherless man.[1] Australians, too, though lower in the scale than Africans, make songs on the spur of the moment which "refer to something that has struck the attention at the time," and add a bit of reflection. Actually subjective and reflective poetry among such people, now and then reported by missionaries,[2] may be rejected with confidence as either mistaken in the hearing or else as echoed from hymns or pious stories told to an excessively imitative folk. It is still the tribe, clan, horde, for the party of the first part, and an event, an emotion, affecting this body as a whole, for the party of the second part, which gets into the communal verse even when sung by a single deputy. Individual emotion as a thing for itself is nowhere in the case. Indeed, if there were time for it, a raid upon philological ground would show a tendency to avoid the first and second person singular in all primitive speech; surely that observation of Schleicher[3] is not antiquated, along with his other theories, when he says that the varying stems of the personal pronoun point at a deliberate process aimed to avoid expression, "as indeed often in language one finds a shyness to use the *I* and the *thou*." Romanes,[4] too, notes that "in the

[1] Improvisations at dance, funeral, wedding, and the like, among these Africans, are summed up by Spencer in his unfinished *Descriptive Sociology*, pp. 24 f.

[2] See above, p. 20.

[3] *Compendium*, 4th ed., p. 641. Cf. Spencer, *Princ. Sociol.*, II. 151, American ed.

[4] *Mental Evolution in Man*, p. 358, American ed.

earliest stages of articulate utterance pronominal elements, and even predicative words, were used in the impersonal manner which belongs to a hitherto undeveloped form of self-consciousness." Perhaps this belated individual expression came into poetry in the guise of robust satire, which at first clannish and collective, like the songs of the maids about Bannockburn, like the mutual satire of rival villages even now, like the mocking songs sung by African girls at a dance, passed into the particular mood as a kind of flyting. An excellent survival of this clan-satire turned upon an individual member occurs some hundred years ago. Pastor Lyngbye,[1] long a resident among the Faroe islanders, tells, without the faintest desire to advance a critical theory, precisely how a ballad was made in a throng and under circumstances which were primitive in every respect save the accident of date. The whole community meets on even terms to spend a few hours in sport. The expression of communal feeling is first and foremost the dance; and to this dance, as was once the universal custom, they sing their own songs. Now the song may be one about Sigurd or other hero of yore; and in this case one can determine, so far as possible, whether the "common fund or patrimony" of race tradition furnishes the theme or whether the story is borrowed from abroad. But the song is not always about Sigurd; and Lyngbye's simple story of one which is local, spontaneous, communal, should be taken to heart by comparative literary accountants. Some fisherman has had a misadventure, whether by his fault or his fate, and comes to the public dance. Stalwart comrades seize him, push him to the front, and before the whole community dancing

[1] *Færφiske Quæder om Sigurd*, etc., Randers, 1822. P. E. Müller wrote the preface and made the extracts from Lyngbye's journal; so that the evidence is at first hand and by an exact observer. The remoteness of the place is equivalent to centuries in point of time. See, too, V. U. Hammershaimb, *Færφsk Anthologi*, Copenhagen, I. xli ff.

and swaying to a traditional rhythm, stanza after stanza is improvised and sung, first by a few, then in hilarious repetition by the throng; and so, verse by verse, the story of the accident "sings itself," with the hero dancing willy-nilly to the tale of his own doings. Now, adds Lyngbye, if this ballad takes the fancy of the people, it becomes a permanent thing, repeated from year to year. Here, indeed, is what may well pass as "objective" poetry;[1] an absolute antithesis to the subjective and reflective poetry with which modern conditions of authorship have made us so familiar that we ignore the fact of any other kind.

Similar makings and traditions of the improvised song of satire come from the Highlands; witness the words of J. F. Campbell.[2] "It was quite a custom in the Highlands, and that not long ago, to meet for the purpose of composing verses. These were often satirical, and any one who happened not to be popular was fixed upon for a subject. Each was to contribute his stanza, and whoever failed to do his part was fined. Whenever a verse happened to be composed that was pretty smooth and smart, it took well . . . and spread far and wide." Campbell notes the corresponding habit of Icelanders, as told in the *Njalssaga*. All this is still fissiparous offspring of the festal dance and song; but just as all mankind now loves a lover, so in more robust days it may be assumed that all mankind most loved a fight; and the fight in alternate stanzas of a song-duel concentrated attention on the fighting pair, spurred them to independent effort, and brought about an organic, individual song. This flyting is a venerable affair; and every one knows the dual combats in verse so common among the Eskimo, a pretty makeweight to amœbean verse under the Sicilian skies. In Iceland not only were sarcastic verses

[1] See the author's *Old English Ballads*, p. xxxiv.

[2] *Popular Tales of the West Highlands*, 2d ed., IV. 164 f.

made upon one another by professed poets like Gunnlaug Snake-Tongue, but at the dance *mansöngvar*, that is, satiric stanzas exchanged by men and women, were in vogue for every one, and in their Fescennine license often called out futile protest from the church.[1] Civilized Europe itself is covered from end to end by traces of a custom once, it would seem, universal among folk of low and high degree; and it is beyond doubt, save with theorists who decline to look at the evidence of comparative literature, that amœbean verse of the classic kind, rude dramatic beginnings, survivals like the *strambotto* and *stornello* of Italy, the *coplas*[2] of Spain, the *stev* of Norway, the *gaytas* of Galicia, the *schnaderhüpfl* of Germany, all go along with these rough flytings of half-civilized and of wholly barbarous races as offshoots of communal song where the individual singer detaches himself from the chorus and sings stanzas which mainly incline to rivalry with another singer. Moreover, this was once a universal gift. Wherever communal conditions survive, there survive also traces of a time when one could talk of a "folk in verse" as well as of a folk in arms. Improvisation is a fairly easy process with Esthonians, Lithuanians, Finns, where classic tradition is out of the question, just as it is an easy process with the peasant of Italy. The substitution of love for hate or satire, of frank erotic stanzas of the times when the way of a man with a maid was matter of communal interest, is easy to understand, if hard to date and place; even now, rustic love-making at picnics is conspicuous for epithets that might easily be understood as belonging to a quarrel. The publicity of these

[1] Described at length by Möbius in the "Ergänzungsband" for Zacher's *Zeitschrift f. d. deutsche Philologie*, 1874, p. 54. For the *débat*, *tenso*, *sirventes*, *jeu-parti*, *conflictos*, and all the rest on romance ground, see Jeanroy, pp. 48 f., and Greif, *Zst. f. vgl. Lit.*, N. F., I. 289.

[2] For Portugal, see Dr. C. F. Bellermann, *Portug. Volkslieder u. Romanzen*, Leipzig, 1874, p. viii.

amatorious stanzas still survives in games and country revel. A game now played among the young people of Swedish Finland, "Simon i Sälle," was described by a native to the present writer; in a dancing ring of both sexes, with chorus and refrain, a youth steps up to a girl and says he has something to give her. What has he, is the more or less defiant question; and he must improvise his stanza descriptive of the gift, while all the other young men continue dancing forward and backward as he sings, the girls standing. When a girl has to improvise, the other girls dance and the young men stand still.[1] This universal improvising power must be put in the clearest possible light, in order to show that the formula of exceptional bucolic wit, rustic bard, simple but noted singer of the countryside, as offset to the polished singer of a better time and place, is utterly inadequate to explain the beginnings, growth, and decline of what is called popular poetry. Communal labour, of course, echoes in these improvisations as well as communal satire and love. Until recent days, people in the Scottish Highlands gathered at a farmer's door on the first night of the year, singing a few lines in Gaelic, while one of their number dragged a cowhide and the rest beat time with sticks; in this fashion they marched three times round the house. Then all "halt at the door, *and each person utters an extempore rhyme*, extolling the hospitality of the landlord."[2] Workmen in Dunkirk[3] still improvise verses to a favourite tune, singing the chorus with great energy: —

> Ali, alo, pour Maschero !
> Ali, ali, alo, —

and in solo, improvised then and there, a line such as, —

> Il boit le vin et nous donn' de l'eau, —

[1] On ease of improvisation among the Finns proper, see Comparetti, *Kalewala*, p. 17.

[2] Chambers, *Popular Rhymes of Scotland*, pp. 166 f. [3] Coussemaker, p. 271.

with another choral "ali, ali, alo." In fact, when one comes to a certain class of peasant life, improvisation is as universal a "gift" as it is among the savages, and as it was by general consent of ethnologists[1] among all primitive folk. For a glimpse at the past, Cædmon is evidently a case of improvisation — it was expected of the merest hind, one sees — lifted to literary performance. When Anglo-Saxon laws[2] say a priest must not get drunk and "turn gleeman or ale-bard," they mean that he is not to improvise convivial songs, and they have no reference to the professional minstrel; he is to resist a common temptation and refuse a traditional duty of every reveller, much like the duty of the Greek to make and sing his *skolion* at the banquet. So, again, it is inversion and perversion of the plain facts when one thinks of Welsh *pennillion* as scattered brands from the old Eistedfodd fire; it is the growth of a professional class of bards out of the general turn for improvising which is to explain the Eistedfodd, and it is the survival of old and universal habit when Welshmen even now sing one *pennill* after another in rapid alternation. Professor Schuchardt[3] heard such a friendly contest not long ago, and was struck by the close resemblance of these quatrains to the German *schnaderhüpfl* and the

[1] Wallace is thinking of music and song in the nobler sense when he denies them to primitive races; and Wallaschek's answer is conclusive, for it is based on evidence that all goes one way, *Primitive Music*, pp. 277 f. Another absurd reaction against romantic ideas is to deny lyric propensity to primitive folk and substitute an acute sense of "business." So Norden, work quoted, I. 156, says the prayer of early man was anything but a "lyrical outpouring"; it was "a contract with deity, give and take." But emotional fear and emotional thanks precede any such shrewd rationalism as this, if psychology is to be regarded, let alone ethnological evidence.

[2] Schmid, 2d ed., p. 366.

[3] *Romanisches und Keltisches*, pp. 363 f. The four-line stanza, he says, is easy to compose, and one *pennill* suggests another; so that each is half tradition, half improvisation, belonging "to everybody and nobody." This description approaches very closely the hypothetical description given by Ten Brink in his sketch of Old English poetry for Paul's *Grundriss*, of the making of ballads in a more primitive day.

improvised stanzas of Italy. Improvisation is the first step and not the last step in art; theories that the ballad is a belated bit of art taken up by countryfolk after the lords of letters have flung it aside,[1] that songs of the people echo old opera tunes and concert ditties, and all easy little *dicta* of the sort, are confuted by a study of comparative literature both in the genetic and in the sociological phases of it. Peasants who make verse-combats their source of entertainment might be regarded as imitating a troubadour *débat*, if one did not consider how universal and primitive a custom this is known to be. Eskimo song-duels are not borrowed from the troubadours. Italian peasants might be said to derive their *strambotti* from amœbean verse like that of Vergil, were it not for the fact that Roman peasants loved and practised this sort of thing from the beginning. As Horace says, speaking of the old breed of Roman,[2] —

> Fescennina per hunc inventa licentia morem
> versibus alternis opprobria rustica fudit,
> libertasque recurrentes accepta per annos
> lusit amabiliter . . .

a festal and communal affair. This rustic communal interchange of satire in improvised verses works up to the level of art not at first by aid of the poets, but by singers of note, men who began to take a pride in their special gift of improvisation, as will be shown in the following pages. Meanwhile a specimen of the verse-contest under partly communal conditions can be found in an Irish *carmen amoebaeum*, as Mr. Hyde calls it, improvised alternately by a guest and his hostess. The latter has the hard end to carry, as she must finish the quatrain which the man begins; and no wonder she

[1] Mr. Gregory Smith's facile explanation, *The Transition Period*, pp. 182 f.

[2] Ep. II. i. 145 f. See Zell, *Ferienschriften*, II. 122 ff. Soldiers sang in pairs, or in two sections, these alternate mocking verses.

yields, especially as the Blarney Stone has evidently lent aid to her gallant visitor.[1] It is clear, then, that idyll and eclogue in degeneration are not to explain the verse-combats whether of savages or even of peasants; the Roman and Oscan farmers improvised such songs in their *satura* and in their rough comedies, innocent of all literary influences; and the Italian peasant of to-day keeps up this custom wherever schoolmasters and other plagues of civilization bide afar off and leave him to his own communal devices. What Theocritus [2] and Vergil did was to use these rude improvisations as suggestion or even foundation for their art.[3] For rustic survivals these *strambotti* and the *coplas* of Spain, with other quatrains of the sort, made in and for the dance throughout the length and breadth of southern Europe,[4] are less useful for purposes of study in primitive song than the *schnaderhüpfl* and the *stev*, one German, the other Scandinavian, of northern lands. As to the former, J. A. Schmeller's brief account,[5] made sixty years ago, is still authoritative, though much has been written about these quatrains since; most readable as well as most learned is the essay of Gustav Meyer.[6] Collections and

[1] Douglas Hyde, *Love Songs of Connacht*, 1895, pp. 88 ff. The prose translation has less artificial suggestion than the translation in verses.

[2] Athenæus and Diodorus are quoted as authorities for the Sicilian origin of such combats in verse; but Jeanroy disposes of this theory by an effective use of the argument from comparative literature. See his *Origines*, pp. 260 ff.

[3] On the meaning and relations of *strambotto*, *stornello*, *rispetto*, *ritornello*, and the other terms, see Count Nigra's *Canti Popolari del Riemonte*, Torino, 1888, pp. xi ff. He corrects Schuchardt's use of *ritornell* for *stornello*. This latter is really an amœbean form of verse, has but one stanza, and this of three lines; the *strambotto* is one stanza, too, but has four, six, ten, or even more lines. Still, the four-line stanza, as comparison shows, is clearly the primitive form. Southern Italy is, of course, far richer in these songs than Piedmont, the home of lyrical narrative or ballad.

[4] Found, too, in India; but here not in the really communal stage. See Gustav Meyer, *Essays und Studien*, pp. 293 f.

[5] *Bayerisches Wörterbuch*, III. 499, explaining them as *Schnitterhüpflein*, songs of the reapers.

[6] With references to the literature of these songs, work quoted, pp. 332 ff.

discussions[1] are plentiful; and it is to be noted that the name of this sort of verse is not constant, being now disguised as "songlet," "dancer," and the like, and now as *rundâ*.[2] Schmeller defines the *schnaderhüpfl* as "a short song consisting of one or two riming couplets, *but in any case of four lines*, which is sung to certain local and traditional dance-tunes, and is often improvised on the spot by the singer or dancer." Singer *and* dancer, of course, is the primitive form, and this as hendiadys: "the singing dancer." A typical quatrain of the sort, so far as this consideration goes, comes from Vogtland:—

I and my Hans,
We go to the dance ;
And if no one will dance,
Dance I and my Hans.

Hinterhuber[3] describes the modern process; the waltz goes on awhile, then in a pause the throng sings a few stanzas, then the dance is resumed and youth after youth improvises, without ceasing, to a traditional tune. "*They never sing the verses of local and popular poets, but all is original.*" What is of particular interest in this process is the communal scene and occasion, mainly a village dance, the traditional tune, the frequent chorus, and, against this background, the individual performance of the singer. We seem to find here the point of departure for artistic poetry; for in the actual quatrain one seldom meets repetition, that inevitable note of the refrain and of the fissiparous single song which

[1] On the form cf. O. Brenner, "Zum Versbau der Schnaderhüpfl," in *Festschrift zur 50 jähr. Doktorjubelfeier Karl Weinholds*, Strassburg, 1896, who gives fresh references for the various subjects of discussion. He emphasizes the fact that these *schnaderhüpfl* are always sung.

[2] Dr. H. Dunger, *Rundâs und Reimsprüche aus dem Vogtlande*, Plauen, 1876. A *rundâ* is originally "a little song sung while drinking," but is made to include the *schnaderhüpfl;* and in the author's opinion all these forms go back to songs of reapers during harvest. That, however, is of no great moment here.

[3] "Ueber Poesie der Alpenländer," in a reprint from a magazine whose title does not appear.

detaches itself, as among savages, from the refrain; and while the reapers' song may be behind all this rude lyric of the hills, it is no festal recapitulation of communal labour, no echo of work or village triumph, that one hears, but rather the personal sentiment, either erotic or defiant, of the individual singer. Moreover it is always from one person and mainly to one person. Nevertheless, it must have dance, throng, communal conditions through and through, or it is not the *schnaderhüpfl*. So interesting a case as this excuses some breadth and detail in the treatment of it.

The home of the *schnaderhüpfl* is centred in the Bavarian Alps, spreading thence in many directions and to some remote districts, which may all be found described in the careful summary of Gustav Meyer; the concern now is not with the vogue but with the thing itself. It is slowly degenerating and even disappearing, in spite of its tenacity, its vigour, and the love for it felt by the peasants of those conservative regions. As with the rural refrain, so here, lewd fellows of the baser sort lay hold upon it as the communal and universal character of it lapses; near Weimar one may still hear peasants singing these quatrains in a kind of emulation, but the frankly erotic has become licentiously rotten. Here and there, however, it lives in its old estate, but by a very feeble tenure; singing societies, friends from the city, concert tunes, what not, are hounding it from its last retreats. The quatrains now gathered are mainly traditional, not freshly improvised like those of earlier days, and it is interesting to note how many variants can be found of one theme. Direct borrowing occurs, of course; but a more frequent process is the use of a popular initial line which is continued in varying fashion into a corresponding variety of verses. Something like this, but not really the same thing, is or was common in cheap theatrical exhibitions, where some catching but meaningless refrain introduces a series of local "hits." The *schnader-*

hüpfl, however, has a far more dignified way, reflecting a nobler mood whether of joy or of grief. Thus a pair of quatrains, perhaps amœbean in origin, from near Salzburg:[1] —

When it's cold in the winter,
  And snow-tempests whirl,
How cozy and warm
  In the room of my girl!

When it's cold in the winter,
  Go warm you a while;
And the love that is old
  Cannot easily spoil.

Close to the amœbean, and with two lines essentially the same, are these,[2] in mild satire: —

No mountain so high[3]
  But the chamois can pass,
And no youngster on earth
  Can be true to his lass.

No mountain so high
  But the chamois climbs over,
And no girl is so fair
  But she'll take to a lover.

This is improvisation on crutches. Often, however, the standing line has variations; for example:[4] —

[1] Firmenich, *Germaniens Völkerstimmen*, II. 716. I have made these translations solely to reproduce, if possible, the spirit of the original, and have tried to keep the false "literary" note at arm's length.

[2] *Ibid.*, II. 715, 777.

[3] G. Meyer, p. 357, prints a number of such variations on the standing first verse: —

It is dark in the woods
  Because of the crows, —
That my girl will be false,
  That every one knows.

It is dark in the woods
  Because of the firs, —

and so on.

[4] Firmenich, II. 779.

No sea without water,
  No wood without tree,
And no night when I sleep
  Without dreaming of thee.

No night without star,
  And no day without sun,
And no heart in the world
  But beats for some one.

But we are nearing the "keepsake" and "annual" tone; it is well to hold the dance in plain sight and hearing, where one gets either the mood of Eros:[1] —

O sweetheart, be wiser,
And dance with no tailor,—
Dance only with me,
And my love is for thee!—

or the mood of Anteros: —

I thought you were pretty;
  It's false, I declare;
You're goitred and crooked,
  A girl with red hair,—

one specimen out of many, but quite sufficient, for that lyrical exchange of compliments at the dance which has satisfied the sense of humour in rustic and even savage communities everywhere; a nearer echo, even, of the dance, in the spirit of the Miller of the Dee, is in this quatrain: —

I've a cow and a calf
  And a donkey, all three;
And what do I care
  Who the leader[2] may be?

So the dancing youth, at Innsbrück, flinging his money to the musicians for a good turn, likes to proclaim to the throng his own self, not forgetting his guild: —

[1] Firmenich, II. 661. [2] Of the dance, — the *vorsinger*.

What needs has a hunter?
A hunter has none,
Save a girl with black eyes,
And a dog, and a gun.[1]

Or a girl proclaims her lover's prowess:[2] —

My lover's a rider,
A rider is he;
His horse is the kaiser's,
The rider's for me.

So, too, the rude compliment: —

You girl with the black eyes
And chestnut-brown hair,
When you look at me so,
I turn fool, I declare.

Easy and silly, one says. Precisely. Easy because made by everybody and still close to the repeated refrain of the throng, and silly in the old meaning of simple and plain. All the great lyric poets know that they must be silly in this sense, or they are mere ink and paper, divorced from life and the lilt of communal song; Goethe, Burns, Heine, will tell that tale plainly enough, and let one compare Matthew Arnold's *Geist's Grave*, not to speak of Wordsworth's and Landor's triumphs, with the genuine pathos but irritating intricacy of T. E. Brown's *Aber Stations*. Perhaps this bit from Salzburg[3] shows the improvisation, still simple to a fault, working up to the note which one demanded for real poetry: —

My heart is a clock,
And it stops now and then;
But a kiss from my lassie
Can start it again!

[1] Variants of this are found in many places.
[2] Firmenich, III. 39. [3] *Ibid.*, II. 716.

Or with a little pressure on the form, with hint of art, this from Steiermark:[1] —

> You are fair, you are dear,
> But you are not my own;
> You'd be fairer yet, dearer yet,
> Were you my own!

Familiar as a source of quatrains is the youth pleading or querulous outside of the fair one's window, and the maid doubtful or scornful within; there are a few English fragments of this sort which are printed in Chappell,[2] and some are still heard in the rural parts. The Salzburg youth pleads thus:[3] —

> Ah, love, lift the latch, —
> Here the wind is so bleak;
> With thee in the house there
> How cozy and sweet!

From this, with hundreds of the sort, runs a lyrical path, if one could but trace it, to the elaborate ode of Horace,[4] imitated, of course, from the Greek, and its type long become the conventional treatment of an unconventional situation, but no doubt at the start expanded from shorter and more vivid songs of "the excluded lover," of which one finds a scrap in the other and more famous ode on the courtesan's old age: —

> Audis minus et minus iam
> "*Me tuo longas pereunte noctes,*
> *Lydia, dormis?*"[5]

One has heard the Salzburg youth; and the Salzburg maid is explicit in her reply:[6] —

[1] *Ibid.*, II. 737.

[2] "Go from my window," pp. 140 ff., with variations (as "Come up to my window") and parodies.

[3] Firmenich, II. 715.

[4] *Od.*, III. X.

[5] It is well to note here that development is one thing and imitation is another. The authorities agree that a *schnaderhüpfl* cannot be imitated. See Gustav Meyer, p. 351.

[6] Firmenich, II. 717.

Go away from my window,
  And leave me alone;
The door I'll not open
  However you moan,

a striking contrast to the complacency of a *schnaderhüpfl*, said to be one of the oldest recorded, taken down by Tobler at Appenzell, in 1754:—

Mine, mine, mine, O my love is fine,
  And to-night he shall come to me;
Till the clock strikes eight, till the clock strikes nine,
  My door shall open be.

But one must stay by the dancing throng, the rivalry of the singers, the question and answer, a succession of stanzas thus tending to group about a theme given by the occasion and kept in mind by a constant suggestion of rime and repeated or slightly varied verses; from all this it is highly probable that one will learn something of the communal origins of lyric poetry. Thus there is nothing immediate or suggestive of the dance in a detached quatrain with question and answer like this:[1]—

Why crying, my pretty,
  By the tree there alone?
Why should I not cry
  When my sweetheart is gone?

But the dance and the throng are not far away from saucy bits of another type:[2]—

Black-eyed and bright one,
Were I not the right one
For you of them all . . .
If I loved you at all?

Or this:—

You lass with the black eye,
  Now leave me alone;
I'm not your Darby,
  And you're not my Joan.

[1] Firmenich, III. 396.
[2] *Ibid.*, II. 280. This is widespread. See Meyer, p. 356.

Similarly there comes from Carinthia a challenge of youth to youth, with audible lilt of the dance, too often prelude to a grim struggle not in Touchstone's version of the code, but based on Touchstone's theory of "mine own": —

> You will not, you will not my lassie be loving,
> You will not, you will not a simpleton be;
> You'll have to, you'll have to go find you another,
> You know well, you know well my lass is for me!

What now is to prevent these quatrains, whether in question and answer, or in a succession of related and varied harpings on one theme, to form a little poem, a lyric? Professor Brandl says it does not so happen, as if solitude and paper and emotion at second hand always had to be in the case; facts, however, say that the process is not only probable in theory but definitely before one on the record. To begin with, a quatrain of undoubted communal origin, a genuine *schnaderhüpfl*, often finds its way into a folksong; so with this from Alsace:[1] —

> 'Tis not so long ago it rained,
> The trees are dripping yet;
> And I had, I had a lover once,
> I would I had him yet.

There is a pretty little English ballad called *The Unquiet Grave*,[2] which begins in the same tone: —

> The wind doth blow to-day, my love,
> And a few small drops of rain;
> I never had but one true-love,
> In cold grave she was lain. . . .

and the ballad goes on with a dialogue between the lover and his dead sweetheart.[3] On the other hand, amœbean

[1] Meyer, p. 341. The rimes are identical in the original. Meyer gives seven versions.

[2] Child, III. 236.

[3] On this opening touch from nature in the ballads, exemplified in English by the beautiful beginning of *Robin Hood and the Monk*, much has been written;

forms of the *schnaderhüpfl* could easily lead to such alternate stanzas as one finds in the pretty ballad, common in France, to which Child supplies "a base-born" English cousin, *The Twa Magicians*,[1] with a catching refrain suggestive of the dance. So plain is the connection between these *schnaderhüpfl*, the *stev* of Norway, all similar isolated quatrains, and the actual songs of situation, question, and answer, that Landstad declared for the quatrains as *débris* of longer poems. But Gustav Meyer[2] is surely right in his energetic rejection of this way of looking at the process; his proof seems convincing to a degree. Nobody will say that the artistic lyric as we have it, or even the later communal ballad, is made by direct union of scattered stanzas; but it seems clear enough that these isolated quatrains furnish the material for such poems, and that part of the process could be achieved in the grouping of quatrains improvised about a common subject and on a communal occasion. Those repeated questions why the forsaken lass is crying, still echo in a lyric like Scott's *Jock of Hazeldean:* —

> Why weep ye by the tide, lady,
> Why weep ye by the tide?

and it is demonstrable that improvised quatrains give a situation, and so group themselves into a little poem; Meyer[3] quotes such a song of two stanzas which has been made in this way, and yet could be easily foisted upon Eichendorff or some poet of the sort: —

> My lover has come,
> And what did he bring?
> For the evening a kiss,
> For my finger a ring.

but this use of the same device in a *schnaderhüpfl* is very significant, and has aroused little comment. See Meyer, pp. 377 ff.

[1] Child, I. 399 ff. [2] *Essays*, pp. 365 ff. [3] On p. 358.

The ring it is broken,
The love is all gone,
And out of the window
The kisses have flown.[1]

A little more circumstance, a touch of nature, a touch or two of art, and out of the question and answer in improvised quatrains comes a ballad, with the help of that neglected but so unjustly neglected refrain, for which notice has been demanded already as for an important communal element in poetry. So one might guess the origins of the pretty ballad of the sickle:[2] given a traditional refrain of the reapers, and a couple of *schnaderhüpfl* improvised in the familiar strain of question and answer, and why not such a poem?

I heard a sickle rustling,
Rustling through the corn;
I heard a maid, had lost her love,
A weeping all forlorn.

"O let the sickle rustle!
I care not how it go;
For I have found a lover
Where clover and violets blow!"

"And hast thou found a lover
Where clover and violets blow,
'Tis I am weeping lonely,
And all my heart is woe!"

[1] When the Greek youth leaves his home, Fauriel says, his family sing songs of farewell, traditional and improvised, to which he often improvises a reply. Improvisation, too, and presumably once in the village throng, lies at the foundation of the German prentice songs of leave-taking, the eternal note of *scheiden, das thut grämen*, with culmination in that exquisite poem, probably not improvised, *Innsprück, ich muss dich lassen*. The ennobling process is interesting, and is of a piece with the process assumed by A. W. Schlegel for the ennobling of Greek epic out of rude improvisation.

[2] Uhland, *Volkslieder*, I. 78. In spite of the two melodies, I have put the refrain at the beginning, and slightly changed, as in Uhland's B., at the end. The actual song is for the dance. See Böhme, *Altd. Liederb.*, p. 268. Only two stanzas are given,—one for the happy girl and one for the lovelorn, one the *vortanz*, the other the *nachtanz*.

O rustle, sickle, rustle,
And sound along the corn!
I heard a maid, had lost her love,
A weeping all forlorn.

No stress, of course, is to be laid on this particular case, which simply serves to show how unquestioned improvisation of quatrains on one of the little tragedies common in rural life could be combined with the traditional refrain of a reapers' dance, and so pass into popular lyric.

Often this making of a lyric calls in the aid of repetition, and an iterated line serves as thread to tie the quatrains together; such poems have been noted already,[1] and were called more or less artificial. But they certainly suggest now and then the improvisation of quatrains at the dance, and belong there originally; a clear case may be given from Steiermark.[2]

To thee I've gone often
So happy and gay;
To thee I'll go never, —
Too long is the way.

Too long is the way,
And the wood is too thick;
God keep you, my sweetheart,
I wish you good luck!

I wish you good luck,
And all blessings at need, —
For the times when you loved me
I thank you indeed![3]

[1] See above, p. 208. [2] Firmenich, II. 742.

[3] The translation fails to bring out the simplicity of these two stanzas; they run thus: —

Der Weg ös mer z'wait,
Und der Wold ös mer z'dick,
Bhüat di Gott, main liabs Schotzel,
I wünsch dir viel Glück.

I wünsch dir viel Glück
Und es sull dir guat gian,
Für die Zeit, ols d'mi g'liabt host,
Bedonk i mi schian.

Gustav Meyer has followed this combination of quatrains into a popular song,[1] perhaps sprung from improvised collaboration, or else rivalry, at the dance, with a pretty but cynical stanza added in the process of oral tradition,— itself a quatrain heard singly in Tyrol, while the others, also sung separately, seem to be of Swabian origin. The song may follow as a farewell to these *schnaderhüpfl*, now rapidly passing into a memory of simpler days.

When the Dingelstädt bells ring,
  The street seems to shake;
And I wish you good luck
  For another fine mate.

And I wish you good luck,
  And all blessings at need;
For the times when you loved me
  I thank you indeed.

The times when you loved me
  Need give you no pain,
No thousand times shall you
  Think on me again.

A little bit loving,
  A little bit true,
And a little bit faithless,—
  What else could you do?

"The most genuine of all folksongs, and almost the only kind which is still made," as E. H. Meyer says of it, this *schnaderhüpfl* is a single strophe of four lines,[2] complete in itself, always improvised—though it often becomes traditional—and always in the native dialect; it is not a fragment

[1] *Essays*, p. 370; and see also Kögel, *Gesch. d. d. Lit.*, I. 7, who thinks that Scandinavian *ljóð* (plural) meant once a series of these strophes composed by dancers and so coming to be a *lied*. E. H. Meyer, *Volkskunde*, p. 317, notes the independent quatrains combined into an *almlied*.

[2] Also G. Meyer, *Essays*, pp. 370, 375.

of some older and longer song, but rather lends itself to combination into a popular lyric of oral tradition.[1] Careful comparison shows that similar quatrains, probably of similar origin in the dance, occur not only in Welsh, in Italian, French, and Spanish, in Lithuanian, in Hungarian, in Roumanian, Greek, Russian, Polish, everywhere in European speech, but even in Syrian, in Malay, and such distant languages. It is known in Chinese. Most closely related to it are the *stev* of Norway, of which Landstad[2] gives a small collection in his book of Norwegian ballads. Granting that the real *stev* must be improvisation, he is too quick to connect them with the old scaldic poetry and with earlier and longer poems, regarding these quatrains — he hesitates, however, in stating the case — as wreckage of ancient ballads and once an effort of the bard. The theory of *débris*, thus tentatively asserted, is successfully answered by Gustav Meyer, as it is by a consideration of the *schnaderhüpfl* quoted in these pages; and it fares no better here than it does when applied to Italian *strambotti* and the artistic work of Theocritus and Vergil. Indeed, Landstad's own account of the *stev* confutes his theory about them. Making these quatrains, he says,[3] was once a universal social custom, and lingers even yet.[4] His picture of the peasants gathered for a winter evening's amusement, guests and especially the older people sitting at tables which run along the walls, men at one end, women at another, while the young people dance in the middle of the room; the "drinking" staves sung as the ale cups go round, where women often answer to rough but jolly quatrains from the other end of the tables, and where every person must sing his stave; the rude compliments and vivac-

[1] *Ibid.*, pp. 377 ff.

[2] *Norske Folkeviser*, Christiania, 1853. See especially pp. 365 ff., 423 ff.

[3] *Ibid.*, p. 366.

[4] Lundell, Paul's *Grundriss*, II. i. 730, says that even now any adult in Iceland can make verses.

ities of the dance: all this points to a survival of primitive custom. Traditional verses often serve to open the contest nowadays, but improvisation begins with the personal combat, and the fun grows fast. These older staves have a standing refrain for the second and fourth lines of the quatrain;[1] but the modern kind are like the *schnaderhüpfl* and are improvised throughout. A touch of "sentiment and reflection" is not unusual; for example:[2]—

> I know where to look for my bridal mirth, —
> In a coffin black deep down in the earth;
> I know where my bride-bed soon shall stand, —
> Deep in the earth in the grit and sand.

Verse of this sort points to the improvisations already treated in part under the *vocero*[3] and to the songs which go with refrains of labour, not so much the swift and jovial verses of flax-beaters and other workers in bands, as the often tender and melancholy songs of women grinding at the mill.[4] But enough has been said and quoted to show that improvisation, as it detaches itself from communal refrains, tends to be individual, sentimental, reflective, and so artistic and lyrical in the modern sense. The quatrain sung by youth to maiden in the dance is still communal in its connotation; detached, it smacks less and less of the public occasion, tries a deeper note of sentiment, has more and more of the reflective and confidential; so one can come to the mingling of passion and art in an ode of Sappho, in a lyric of Burns. Moreover, parallel with this change of quality, runs a process of grouping into songs. The scattered traditional stanzas, once improvised as isolated quatrains, gather at first in pairs, —

[1] Landstad, pp. 370 ff.

[2] *Ibid.*, p. 376.

[3] The *vocero* is far less individual than this quatrain or stave just considered, because the former is an outburst rather of public grief than of private emotion.

[4] See above, p. 269.

the prevailing type is question and answer, — to which a stanza or two is added explanatory of the situation and the season, often with that refrain which is recognized as belonging with the original occasion; and this is the communal lyric, or, as it is called in a stricter use of the term, folksong. Henceforth, the difference between a folksong and a lyric is mainly between oral, traditional origin and the deliberate and artistic composition of recorded literature.

This study of the beginnings of lyric has dealt mainly with sentiment, hostile or erotic, as expression of an individual, slowly detaching itself from expression and interests of the clan. But reflection, another note of what passes now for lyric poetry,[1] the element of thought, comes into poetic expression just as sentiment comes, and seems to be of equal date. As the individual erotic song may go back to the concerted dances, cries, gestures, of a whole horde, at periods of sexual excitement which were probably once of uniform occurrence, so the reflective note of a lyric poem could be traced to early communal thinking. "Communal thinking" is perhaps a vile phrase; comment on doings and interests of the horde, as distinguished from those chanted verses merely descriptive of the event or fact, ought to be less open to objection. As a feat of primitive epic, the statement of what the horde has just accomplished, whether in hunting or in war, has been found to be a constant element in the songs sung by savages to their communal dance; while gesture, shout, recapitulation in cadenced movement, of the same feat, has the dramatic note. Now it is well known that little sen-

[1] Definitions are notoriously unsatisfactory in poetics. Contrast Schleiermacher's formula for lyric as poetry plus music, *Aesthetik*, p. 628, with the laborious definition in R. M. Werner's *Lyrik und Lyriker*, Hamburg and Leipzig, 1890, p. 10, based mainly on the subjective element. Confusion of form and conditions, which makes lyric poetry one with music (see Döring, *Kunstlehre d. Aristoteles*, p. 88), with inner meaning and purpose, has caused most of the trouble. In one sense the old choral was the very foundation of lyric. The congregational psalm of the Hebrews is lyric, and so is the solitary cry of the modern poet.

tences detached from the story or acting of the event, but suggested by it, belonging to it, are often sung by these same savages, now in chorus, and now in individual improvisation. "Good hunting to-day!" sang the Botocudos; which is a very different matter from particular recapitulation of the hunt, as in a buffalo-dance or the like. These sentences, like gnomic poetry at large, are of most ancient date;[1] but it is clear that they soon passed under control of the acute thinker, and shunned the fellowship of choral song: —

Einsam zu denken, — das ist weise ;
Einsam zu singen, — das ist dumm.

It is also clear that this element of thought and meditation would help very materially the change from a sung to a recited verse, and hasten, wherever it could act upon poetry, the disintegration of communal song. Of course, an alliance with sentiment was inevitable; the acute thinker deserted verse for prose and science, and with the lapse of communal singing and the rise of solitary reading, lyric came to mean three things: a subconscious harmony of rhythm, legacy of the consenting throng; sentiment, as the expression of individuality, fostered by this confidence between solitary poet and solitary reader; and reflection, which is now the comment of the individual on the doings of the world as a whole, on the burden and the mystery, that final horror, expressed by Leconte de Lisle, at the idea of unending human woe, —

Le long rugissement de la vie éternelle.[2]

[1] *Uralt*, says Usener, *Altgr. Versbau*, p. 45. See above, p. 95.

[2] As Matthew Arnold reminds us: —

Sophocles, long ago,
Heard it on the Ægean.

For the prevailing tone of lyric is sad, and Euterpe treats her poet as Genevieve treated Coleridge: —

She loves me best whene'er I sing
The songs that make her grieve.

This at one end of the chain, and the Botocudos' choral reflection, "Good hunting to-day!" at the other; a link midway, perhaps, is the half individual, half choral expression of pity which those African women put into their song about Mungo Park, and dwelt upon in their refrain.

So much for the beginnings of modern lyric poetry, as an individual and artistic expression, compared with the lyric of a communal dance, the iterated refrain of a throng. "Modern," of course, is a relative word; and the whole process has been hinted rather than described. Holding fast, however, to the facts of earliest and rudest improvisation among savages, holding fast to the facts of universal improvisation as observed among European peasants, and to the making of single songs out of groups of these improvised stanzas, we are warranted in asserting that the process is one from communal to individual conditions, and begins on a level of general, if not equal, ability to make and sing verse, preferably in the form of a single couplet or quatrain, which is at first subordinate to the chorus of the throng, then meets it on even terms, and at last, losing its general origins and its particular individuality and coming to be part of an artistic poem, drives the discredited chorus from the field.

As regards epic poetry, the relations of the ballad and the choral refrain have been studied in preceding pages. This ballad, or narrative song, holds far more closely than the lyric to conditions of communal making. It abhors sentiment and reflection, for it keeps to the impersonal, public path; it is averse even from the arts of variation save in the form of incremental repetition, and it clings to the communal refrain and to the communal dance. For this reason the ballad is without rival among recent forms of poetry as a field for the study of surviving communal elements; joined with the materials of ethnology, it gives the soundest reasons for constructing that curve of evolution which marks the steady increase of lyric, individual, emotional, and reflective characteristics in poetic progress. With its relations to the epic there is here no space to deal in any satisfactory way.[1] The epic, however, is now conceded by every one to belong to times which by no means can be confused with the beginnings of poetry; M. Tarde and his theory that literature begins with a "great book" like the Bible or the Homeric poems,[2] can hardly expect an answer on any serious and scientific ground. The narrative song or ballad goes back, of course, to that universal gift of people in low levels of culture, the power to turn a contemporary event into song, into the rhythm of the communal dance, as is still done by Samoans and by nearly all savage tribes. All was momentary in this initial act. The rhythm was there in cry and beat of foot; the event was there; and the bridge of articulate words to connect these two elements was of the shortest and simplest kind. The variation, the incremental repetition, are obvious advances; but it is worth while to note that the almost endless repetition of a verse or two, describing some event or situation close at hand, is diminished in corresponding ratio to the growing power of tradition, as if the memory of yesterday's poetry, of last year's poetry, gradually took the place of this contemporary repetition, — the "stretched metre" coming in course of time to be the "antique song." Every-

[1] The claim of Usener may be noted ("Der Stoff des griechischen Epos," *Sitzungsber. d. Kais. Acad. d. Wiss. zu Wien*, Bd. 137, pp. 18 ff.), where he puts the ceremonies at the hearthstone, primitive ancestor-worship, as the real beginning of epic song. The offering to an ancestor must have been made "with music, prayer, and song." Hence the epos. It is true that a lyric of this sort is older than any epic, — the epic which Hegel pushed forward as earliest form of poetry, just as the renaissance had put it above the drama in dignity, — and may well have helped the later epic process. But the evidence of ethnology shows that rude songs at the tribal dance, which refer to tribal doings, must be far older than any ceremonies of the primitive *hausvater* at his family altar.

[2] A. W. Schlegel said that the Homeric poems were improvised; but he distinguished between rude communal improvisation and that of incipient art. *Vorlesungen*, II. 119 f., 243.

where among savages, when the improvised song at feast and dance finds favour, it is passed down as part of the traditional stock. And so one comes to that state of things where, as Ten Brink has put it so well, song oscillates between production and reproduction, that is, between improvisation and memory. This is the period of the early epic. When deliberation and conscious art come in, and yet the old alliance of spontaneous production and living memory is not broken up, then is the golden age of epic verse; then Homer, whoever or whatever he may be, can work out the perfect union of art and nature.

Turning to the drama, one asks whether improvisation can also be found in this form of poetry, taking it, as in the case of epic and lyric, out of communal control into the province of individual art. Aristotle has answered the question in that interesting account of Greek drama quoted above; and he has distinctly affirmed the passage from a communal origin in a wild chorus through rude improvisations up to the triumphs of Hellenic tragedy. Nietzsche, in a book also quoted above at considerable length, has studied this transition as a contrast of the Dionysian and Apollinian elements of poetry. Latin drama, of course, is a copy of the Greek; but the imitations of a foreign and finished model were preceded among the Romans by rude improvisations at the festivals of the countryfolk, where anything like copy and importation must be ruled out of the case.[1] In Italy this rude improvisation of comedy lingered later in survivals that were of course mingled with many literary influences; so too the rough drama of the fairs in France,[2] the popular plays in Germany, and

[1] Livy, VII. 2, gives an account of this change.

[2] See Maurice Drack, *Le Théâtre de la Foire, la Comédie Italienne, et l'Opéra-comique*, Paris, 1889. Vol. I. has a sketch of the movement — from 1678 on — indicated in the title. It began with the *pièce à couplets*, and passed gradually into modern comic opera. The great popular fair of St. Lawrence, at Paris, was the scene of part of this development.

even mysteries and moralities as played by the guilds, retained much of the old communal character and were long at the mercy of improvised speeches, however fixed and intricate the plot and scenes. Many of these survivals — such as the mummers' plays — became also fixed in the words, but that was when the plays had gone to fossil and the custom itself lingered as by a sort of inertia. Italian comedy for some time had a dialogue "mainly extemporaneous";[1] and as these plays grew into urban favour, the improvised dialogue was graced by a higher tone and a more dramatic purpose, lasting almost into the eighteenth century. The *commedia dell' arte*, in other words, is simply the improvised play of peasants passing into artistic and professional control, but still holding to certain communal features.[2] The realistic elements of dialect, satire of certain professions, and the like, point back to the satiric quatrains and songs at the dance; and the dance is always at hand in farce and low comedy down to this day. In Spain the *coplas* took a dramatic turn; improvised question and answer, with the situation to fit, easily became a kind of drama, although the records are by no means full or accurate, and other influences played a conspicuous part.[3] The dance and play, described in *Don Quixote*,[4] at Camacho's wedding, may be a "beautified" country mask with more or less extemporaneous songs and dialogue. The main point about these popular plays is their testimony that the drama passed from communal chorus, — dancing, song, gesture, and refrain, — by the way of impro-

[1] Garnett, *Italian Literature*, p. 306, traces this comedy back through Tuscan and Neapolitan peasants to the "Greek rustics who smeared their faces with wine-lees at the Dionysiac festivals, and from whose improvised songs and gestures Greek comedy was developed."

[2] Burckhardt, *Cultur der Ren.*, II. 40, thinks that such well-known characters as Pantalone, the Doctor, Arlecchino, may be in some fashion connected with masked figures in the old Roman plays.

[3] Ticknor, *Spanish Literature*, I. 232 f.

[4] Second Part, Chap. XX.

visation, into its new estate of art; even under Elizabeth the theatre was no stranger to extemporaneous dialogue, and that pathetic appeal, in which, perhaps, Shakspere more completely drops his "irony," his objective mask, than anywhere else, not only testifies to a nobler conception of the drama, but to the clinging abuse. It was not the clowns alone who spoke more than was set down for them; though their fooling was most hurtful because they made jests offhand with persons in the audience,[1] and sang irrelevant doggerel verse. Some of these verses have perhaps crept into the text of *Lear*. Often, however, the jester had full license to entertain the crowd by a piece long known as a jig. Tarlton, the famous jester,[2] "was most celebrated for his extemporal rhyming and his jigs," which were a combination of improvised song and a dance, accompanied by tabor and pipe. But the jig was also used for songs in dialogue, with a dramatic leaning; "a proper new Jigg, to be sung dialogue wise, of a man and woman that would needs be married," is preserved among the Roxburghe Ballads. Amplified a little, the jig was carried across the water by English comedians, and meeting similar native forms of more or less extemporaneous verse, with dance and farce, became the *singspiel*.[3] But the improvisation of one's lines to fit the "plot" or *scenario* of far nobler performance was common on the English stage,[4] and may have had Shakspere's indulgence if not his sympathy;

[1] Malone's *Shakspere*, 1821, III. 131.

[2] *Tarlton's Jests* . . . ed. J. O. Halliwell, London, 1844, pp. xviii f. (Shakspere Society). "As Antipater Sidonius," says the comparative Meres, "was famous for extemporall verse in Greeke . . . so was our Tarleton."

[3] See Bolte, *Die Singspiele der englischen Komödianten und ihrer Nachfolger*, Hamburg u. Leipzig, 1893, pp. 50 ff. He prints parallel copies of "Singing Simpkin" and the German "Pickelhering in der Kiste."

[4] "Passages were often left for the extempore declamation of the actors. Sometimes the whole conduct of the piece depended on their powers of improvisation." Symonds, *Shakspere's Predecessors*, p. 66.

Von Stein[1] goes so far as to say that the formal character of Shakspere's dramatic work is "a fixed mimetic improvisation," — whatever that may mean. Of the fact, however, there is no question. Tom Nash, in his *Lenten Stuffe*,[2] telling of the trouble he had from that "imperfit embrion of my idle houres, the Isle of Dogs," explains this description of his play by saying that having "begun but the induction and first act of it, the other foure acts, without my consent or the least guesse of my drift or scope, by the players were supplied," — a source of mischief for all hands. It was from Italy that the custom came to improvise even tragic speeches; and the passages in the *Spanish Tragedy*,[3] where Hieronymo is preparing his play, show what was expected: —

> It was determined to have been acted
> By gentlemen and scholars too;
> Such as could tell what to speak. . . .
> Here, my lords, are several abstracts drawn,
> For each of you to note your parts,
> And act it, as occasion's offered you.

Italy, to be sure, may have influenced the habit of improvisation in formal drama; but the custom is a survival rather than a growth, and the statement that Sir Thomas More in his youth — the tradition is preserved also in a tragedy which bears More's name as the subject — showed extraordinary power of improvisation in a play, must not be taken[4] as indicating a tendency in Henry VIII's time which came to be a widespread habit under Elizabeth. Such skill of improvisation in plays diminishes as artistic and deliberate drama comes to the fore. So with the mask. At first a dance, with songs and improvised dialogue for the maskers, it

[1] *Vorlesungen über Aesthetik*, pp. 84 f.

[2] Ed. Grosart, V. 200.

[3] Hazlitt-Dodsley, V. 149, 151.

[4] As, for example, Schwab takes it: *Das Schauspiel im Schauspiel*, Wien u. Leipzig, 1896, p. 32.

offered great opportunities for artistic work; Ben Jonson and Milton can tell how the process went on, and with what results.

Improvisation in the drama of comparatively modern times could be followed into remoter places, for example into Persia, where the comedies are mainly in extemporaneous dialogue. Even in Tahiti what passes for drama is improvised;[1] and all evidence makes for this state of things in the primitive play. The earliest form of the drama consists mainly of action and gesture in the dance,[2] so as to repeat a contemporary event of communal interest, — war and the chase, or, with farming folk, and more in reminiscence, the doings of seedtime and harvest; it is clear that the rude songs and shouts that went with step and gesture[3] and mimicry must have been improvised. In late stages of tribal life, certain dances and the songs that go with them become absolutely fixed, a ritual calling for unusual care in the learning of it; such is the American buffalo dance.[4] But in the earliest drama dance, gesture and choral song were the main elements, and the variation from those repeated shouts took, so it would seem, the path of short improvised and individual utterance. Those improvised stanzas, to be sure, which plagued the frustrated Faroe fisher, dancing perforce to his

[1] Bruchmann, *Poetik*, p. 17.

[2] The material has been set forth above in the section on the communal dance; for early dramatic dances of fight, hunting, and the like, see especially pp. 336 ff., and the passage on *lâc*, p. 340.

[3] On gesture as common and universally understood expression, see Darwin, *Descent of Man*, 2d ed., I. 276 f. "Men of all races" have a "mutual comprehension of gesture-language"; they all have "the same expression on their features," and "the same inarticulate cries when excited by the same emotions." See also Tylor, *Early History of Mankind*, chapters on Gesture-Language; and *American Antiquarian*, II. 219, G. Mallery on Indian Sign Language. This universal validity of gesture is highly significant for the beginnings of poetry, for the rude cries which precede language are probably of the same order as the gestures. See Chap. II., Wundt's *Völkerpsychologie*.

[4] Bastian, "Masken und Maskereien," *Zst. f. Völkerpsych.*, XIV. 347.

own shame before the dancing and singing throng, led to a narrative song, a ballad, and so in time might lead to an epos; but in the making of the stanzas, along with mimicry and dance, there is more of the dramatic than of the epic element.[1] The improvised song-duel, of which so much has been said, is incipient drama; and all those songs sung in cadence by groups of workers in the wine-press, at reaping, pulling, even when marching, and rushing into the fight, have the dramatic trait so far as they go with the appropriate action. So, too, the festal recapitulation of labour, with its appropriate songs and movement, would lend itself to dramatic improvisation more easily and hence earlier than to narrative; the art of telling a tale, as may be learned from ethnology as well as from the observation of children's games, is an accomplishment which comes much later than the art of mimicry and rude improvisation at the dance. The improvising singer and dancer detaches himself from the throng to give an isolated part of the action,[2] and may put it into words to suit his gesture and steps; or two persons may dance, gesticulate, and sing alternately in what answers dramatically to the amœbean song, — an actual fight may have found this kind of recapitulation at a very early stage of the poetic art. True, as was noted above, Wallaschek will not allow that this primitive form of drama had anything to do with poetry; it was pantomime, he says, without words, like the mimic dances of the Damaras, the Fans, and other savage tribes. But it is beyond question that rude songs are often sung along with the acting and the mimicry; and every

[1] See Grosse on the two "roots" of the drama, *Anf. d. Kunst*, pp. 254 f. On the mimicry of different tribes in the communal dance, see Bruchmann, *Poetik*, pp. 208 ff.; Wallaschek, *Prim. Music*, Chap. VIII.

[2] The conspicuous performer, — the "entertainer" or soloist, — grows less and less prominent as one gets upon lower levels of culture. The earliest distinction of this sort was probably achieved by the priest, conjurer, medicine-man, shaman, or whatever his special function.

consideration[1] makes it probable that the pantomime pure and simple, with distinct repression of the desire to give vent to the feelings by shout and word and song, is an artistic not to say artificial development[2] of the original drama along the lines of a painful, concentrated imitation, and is almost a professional affair. Then there is the "speaking pantomime," so called.[3] In short, the communal origin of the drama was surely where Wagner declared it to be, in a combination of gesture, dance, and song, the whole man active "from top to toe," and also, one may add, active as a member of a thoroughly and concertedly active throng. Even the animal and bird dances, favourite among savage tribes, and supposed to be pure pantomime, have the imitated cries of the model in time with the dance; and this is a kind of poetry, lingering in refrains like Walther's *tandaradei*. More than this, it is fairly certain that word and gesture[4] went together in the early stages of speech. As Letourneau points out,[5] the word was too uncertain to stand by itself, and needed the bodily movement that went with it;[6] while the sounds instinctively

[1] As Wallaschek recedes from his proposition, the examples have more and more mention of words and song together with the action; for example, pp. 217 ff.

[2] This must always be taken into account. As Wallaschek says of an Australian "corrobberee," however primitive it may seem, "it is a well-prepared and elaborated dance, which it takes both time and practice to excel in."

[3] Wallaschek, pp. 223 f.

[4] From gesture back to facial expression and other signs now unknown because speech has taken their place, is an inviting path, but not to be trodden now. From the *Kansas City Star*, date unfortunately lost, may be quoted an interview with Hagenbeck, the lion-tamer. "We can't see," he said, "the expression of a lion's face, except of rage, but his companions can. . . . Did you ever see one animal fail to understand another? I never saw such an instance. . . . I am inclined to think that what we call mind-reading is mere survival here and there of the lost sixth sense, which was probably common to primitive man, and which animals possess to this day." Mr. Hagenbeck could furnish an interesting supplement to Darwin's book *On the Expression of Emotions*.

[5] Work quoted, p. 28, speaking of Australian song and dance. See also p. 201.

[6] Sign-language of later date, as studied by Mallery among the American Indians, cannot be regarded as primitive in this genetic sense. It comes to be a

uttered in tune to the cadence of labour and play were felt to lend force to the dramatic representation and fill out the mere suggestion of gesture. An artistic series of movements alone,[1] an artistic series of words alone, would be a later triumph; improvisation of new words to the traditional cadence, and to the given, and in a sense obligatory gestures, would mark early progress in the making of this primitive kind of poetry.

Drama, then, in the widest sense, is the "imitation" of life by means of remembered and repeated movements, induced by the feeling of social elation, and made possible by the cadence of social consent in the dance, accompanied by sounds which instinctively follow this cadence of the action and find their stay as well as their suggestion in the regular recurrence of rhythm. It must have followed hard upon the discovery of consent in common step and common cry, which, if one choose, one may call primitive lyric; the other may pass as primitive drama. In perspective they seem almost contemporaneous in origin. The question of priority, debated with so much warmth, thus becomes a question of names, and not a very important question at best. It is a matter of differentiation and growth from a common origin, which may be described as dramatic or lyric, according as one understands the terms, and which certainly had both elements in it. It was rhythmic, and it was an outlet for communal emotion; it was imitated action,

highly developed art and calls for considerable skill in the making as well as acuteness in interpretation.

[1] As in dances of the Greeks, now felt to be a lost art. On this matter of gesture and signs, see an excellent book by Sittl, *Die Gebärden der Griechen und Römer*, Leipzig, 1890; his accounts of the attempt "die Völker durch die Zeichensprache zu verbrüdern," with reference to Leibnitz and others; of orgiastic ecstasies; and, of course, the study of Greek gesture in art and poetry, are all instructive. For primitive relations, Darwin's book *On the Expressions of Emotions*, etc., 1872, is still main authority. Gestures, like sounds, are either instinctive or called out by the will; and any study of progress in the dramatic art must concern itself with these fundamental elements of acting.

with momentary and spontaneous suggestions; and it can be called narrative or epic only by unwarranted stretching of the words, though the slightly reminiscent factor in the case may be called an epic germ. Finally, the differentiation and growth from this communal poetry of a primitive stage of culture must have been mainly the work of improvisation, or individual assertion, acting on the communal elements, and leading to disintegration and new combinations in processes which varied with the conditions of race and environment.[1] One suggestive fact, however, is to be noted. The drama, in a broad sense, is the beginning of poetry; it is also the end and perfection of the art, and this by a communal reaction. There are centripetal as well as centrifugal forces; if the individual is forever breaking away from the throng and carrying poetry into lonely paths of deliberation, sentiment, artistry, the throng, mainly by that subtle suggestion of consent in rhythm, is forever calling the poet back to his communal point of departure. We have seen how slowly the communal beginnings of poetry, — to us like geological periods, because they have sent down to us no records, and only a few hints of their existence, — yielded even to the tentative progress of individual art, and what long ages must have contented themselves with songs of the horde and the iteration of the refrain in a tribal dance; it is equally

[1] It would be useless to attempt a bibliography of this subject. A. W. Schlegel's historical account of the drama and its relations to epic and lyric is still useful. See especially *Vorles.*, I. 124; II. 317, 321, 325. Eugen Wolff's return to the priority of epic, — *Prolegomena*, etc., p. 10; "Vorstudien zur Poetik," *Zst. f. vgl. Litt.*, VI. 425, — fails to satisfy the student of ethnological evidence; like most writers from the æsthetic point of view, Wolff neglects to study the poetry of the throng, the choral, the dance. Barring this same fault, there is considerable truth in the view of Burdach (letter to Scherer, in the latter's *Poetik*, pp. 296 f.), that epic and drama are wrongly taken as extreme antithesis in poetry, whereas lyric and drama are really "die beiden Urphänomene." Little profit for the historical student of poetry is to be found in essays like Veit Valentin's "Poetische Gattungen," in *Zst. f. vgl. Litt.*, N. F., V. 35 ff.

true that the communal instinct still summons poetry back from its hiding-place with the poet in that "ivory tower," and bids it tread the ways of open and crowded life. In the drama poetry may, indeed, find its final form, as Goethe declared, but it is also coming back in some degree to the instincts and habit of its prime; it is recalling its forces from the scattered and lonely paths of individual thought for a distinctly communal reaction. Even the opera, the ballet,[1] though in less marked degree, show this reactionary communal spirit. The communal elements of action, dance, music, scene,[2] all of which Aristotle had reckoned along with drama and epos as a part of poetry, are thus variously restored. Narrative is banished in favour of the plot, which at least seems to be natural action; deliberate lyric effort, the solitary thought, is rejected for what at least seems to be improvised or spontaneous speech of the actors; dancing and festal expression may or may not be present, and so with music, but the rhythm is deputy for the cadence of dancing feet; and finally there is what seems to be the real world of men, the scene. These realistic effects, these chariot-races and locomotives on the stage, whatever one despises most heartily in the degenerate drama of the day, are the reaction from excesses of subjective poetry toward actual life and the tendency toward communal conditions which art always shows when it deals with a public and abandons the confidences of author and reader.[3] It is perhaps too much to assert that the drama was done to death through

[1] See Blankenburg's excellent article on the ballet in his *Zusätze*, I. 154 ff. La Motte, in his ballet of *Europe Galante*, 1697, made the ballet an object in itself and in its own action; here "entspringt Tanz und Gesang aus der eigenen Gemüthsstimmung der handelnden Personen." This is communal revival.

[2] That is, ὄψις.

[3] "Daudet me dit . . . 'Je crois décidément avoir trouvé la formule; le livre c'est pour l'individu, le théâtre c'est pour la foule.'" *Journal des Goncourt*, VIII. (30 Jan., 1890), 129.

excess of that "lyric cry," and by a tendency which developed character at the expense of action; but the counter movement has been toward the mass and rude effects of force. In the eyes of some uncritical folk, the lack of distinct individual characters, the effect of a homogeneous mob of actors, the crude but vigorous course of events, in early histories and miracle plays, would make better claim to the title of drama than the subtile characterization of Shakspere and the humours of Jonson; *arma*, they might maintain, should come before *virum* for the playwright; and if any comfort can be gathered from our deplorable modern drama, it may possibly lurk in this idea of the return to communal art. In any case, it is the price which our age has to pay for the piercingly subjective character of its lyric poetry. Epic, in any objective and vital form, has vanished, and the drama, desperate in its struggle for life, turns to demos as to a long-forgotten friend.

Before one leaves the beginnings of poetry, its earliest disintegration in point of treatment and theme, and goes back to that improvising poet, in order to glance again at the beginnings of artistry and the decline of communal power, one has two elements of the main subject with which it is well to come to terms. Besides the subject-matter of poetry, there is its style, its form; between the style, or figurative element in poetry on one hand, and on the other hand, its material divisions of drama, epos, lyric, is that vast and ill-defined province assigned to myth. Now claimed as metaphor, and offspring of earliest language, now as drama of nature, now as the tale told by primitive fancy in response to primitive curiosity, now as the lyric or hymn which embodied man's first religious impulse, this fugitive and exquisite creature has had as many masters, has been dragged over as many paths, and has kept as unimpaired beauty, as that famous daughter of the soudan of Babylonia, affianced to the king of Garbo. Of all these temporary masters none is so comprehensive in his gallantry as A. W. Schlegel,[1] who hails myth as the source of poetry, of philosophy even, as the soul of primitive language, as "nature in poetic robes," and goes so far as to say that modern physical science could easily be stated in terms of ancient mythology. Myth, indeed, is such a wide word with Schlegel that it covers the romances of Arthur and Charlemagne;[2] and when one reflects that folklore has since claimed its share of mythological territory, while, on the other hand, brutal folk who speak for a new euphemerism call myth an impudent baggage with no religion in her and only a touch or so of poetry, the case is complicated. Over a path so riddled with pitfalls one is not anxious to walk; but to treat the beginnings of poetry without touching myth is out of the question, and a few steps must be made if only to secure a point of view. We shall consider myth in its relation to primitive verse, and shall then turn to the kindred topic of early figurative language and poetical style.

Concerning the source and function and meaning of myths[3] a long battle has been waged, and noise of it is still ringing in our ears; but the fiercer struggle seems just now to have come to a kind of truce, and the warriors, as in that other contest over the origin of language, appear to be lying on their arms. The more one knows of early civilization, it would seem, the less one feels inclined to dogmatize about the source of myths; while with regard to their meanings, that exhilarating and harmless pastime, where scholar after scholar came forward with his solution, where Bacon in older days turned classic myth into the wisdom of the ancients, and where, in later times, Simrock gave a *haec fabula docet* for

[1] *Vorlesungen*, Stuttgart, 1884, I. 329 ff., 342, 344 ff.

[2] *Ibid.*, III. 110.

[3] See the present author's article on "Mythology" in the new edition of Johnson's *Cyclopædia*.

every shred of Germanic fancy and fable;[1] where Uhland, in his beautiful book on the Myth of Thor, blew one of the most exquisite and irridescent bubbles that ever delighted the poetic eye and broke at the touch of common sense; where Max Müller and his friends converted the primitive Aryan now into a fellow of the prettiest and most fanciful habit of mind, with his interest in sunsets, and stars, and vanishing dewdrops, now into a resolute and saner Lear bent on knowing the cause of thunder; a pastime, finally, in which even Jacob Grimm, for all his "combining" powers, refused to join, — this mania for the direct interpreting of myths has had its day and ceased to be. The end came with the establishment of two facts, one negative and one positive. Anthropology, ethnology, a close study of the history of culture, of social institutions, of religion, led to the sound conclusion that whatever else it might be, the mythology of early man was not conterminous with the religion of early man;[2] for religion in those stages is chiefly a matter of ceremony and ritual forms. Suppose a person ignorant of the rites of the Roman church undertaking to get a notion of its ceremonies, and of the heart of its faith, by a study of the *Legenda Aurea*, or any such body of tales! That was the negative fact; the myth is not primitive religion, and is rarely primitive creed. Again, anthropology, notably through its great exponent Professor Tylor, established the positive fact that myths are due to a kind of poetic faculty in primitive man, the habit of animating, or, in modern phrase not quite

[1] A dozen years ago or more, a professor lecturing on this subject in a German university, after giving all the myths about a certain goddess, spoke somewhat as follows: "Gentlemen, this goddess is either a star or the early summer grass, I am not certain which. I am studying the matter carefully, and hope soon to reach a positive conclusion."

[2] Compare Lucretius, dealing now lovingly with the Venus of myth — *alma Venus*, the beloved of Rome's own god — and now, a few lines below, scornfully, passionately, with the cruel rites of the worship of Diana and the sacrifice of Iphigenia at her shrine: "*illa* Religio," he says, with a touch almost of blasphemy.

accurate for early stages of culture, of personifying what went on about him.[1] Mr. Andrew Lang, while following Professor Tylor in principle, has made room for the obscene, the brutal, the silly, which can be found so plentifully in savage myth and sporadically in the myths which we call classical. To these ways of thinking came the sturdy Müllenhoff, and after him, Mannhardt, an avowed student of customs and popular thought; with Mannhardt's later work, myth-guessing, in which he had once been as wild as any,[2] came to an end. It is now conceded that the source as well as the meaning of most myths is veiled in the obscurity of early animistic processes, while their later development belongs to the poet altogether. "I have learned," wrote Mannhardt[3] to Müllenhoff, "to value poetical and literary production as an essential factor in the formation of mythology." Indeed, it is not considering too curiously when Burckhardt[4] declares that the renaissance in Italy so thoroughly revived the gods of old pagan belief, that poets made new myths in the ancient spirit.

It is a great mistake, however, to infer with certain bold followers of Mr. Herbert Spencer — the German Lippert, for example — that myths have nothing to do with primitive religion and belong altogether to the poetic or fantastic instinct. True, myths of the classic kind, barring the names of god and goddess, were pretty well divorced from faith; but Homer and Hesiod told tales unknown to the primitive worshipper of Greece, and he had myths of his own.

[1] See the chapters on animism and mythology in Tylor's *Primitive Culture*. A. W. Schlegel was on this trail, but let himself be befogged by Schelling's philosophy. See the *Vorlesungen*, I. 329, 337.

[2] See his *Germanische Mythen*.

[3] *Mythologische Forschungen* (*Quellen u. Forschungen*, No. 51, Strassburg, 1884), Vorrede, p. xxv; the lesson came from Tylor's book which Müllenhoff had set Mannhardt reading. This letter was written in 1876. See also Müllenhoff's own definition of mythology in his *Deutsche Alterthumskunde*, V. 1, 157.

[4] *Cultur d. Ren. in Ital.*, I. 288.

Schwartz, a valiant guesser, but rational on certain lines, pointed out forty years ago[1] that perspective must be observed, and that the origin of a myth must be held apart from its development; often, indeed, by a hint here and a survival there, one can feel one's way back from the graceful, celestial romance to a rude myth with all the awe of belief upon it. It may be said with confidence that early myth excluded mere tales of nature, drama of the shifting seasons, the flash of sunlight on the waves, and all the romance of blushing dawns and shepherded or wandering stars; these tales of later origin belonged to the poet and his fantasy. Early man did not go about commercing with the skies, nor did any spur of occasion put him upon the telling of a natural process, duly observed, in terms of a human history proportioned and duly recorded. That is a definite poetical or allegorical process, and means that the mind has a clear idea of two separate systems, and can hold apart the world of fancy and the world of fact, welding them together in conscious purpose. It is poetry,[2] not primitive myth, which sees the heavens as the psalmist saw them: *in them hath he set a tabernacle for the sun, which is as a bridegroom coming out of his chamber, and rejoiceth as a strong man to run a race.* Myth, indeed, may now and then lie at the heart of such poetical achievement; but that elementary myth, the work of unconscious animism, is rude and shapeless by comparison with this finer stuff. Primitive myth is a block of marble with more or less resemblance to some creature, a kind of fetish; poets come and carve it into definite shape, individualize, idealize, polish; next is formed the group, the celestial romance, figures as on the frieze of a temple, with the loves and the quarrels of the gods; and then, last stage of all, alle-

[1] *Zeitschrift f. Gymnasialwesen*, Berlin, Nov., 1861, p. 837.

[2] Mr. Tylor lets animism of this sort have too free a play among quite primitive men.

gorical and satirical poets, a Lucian, a singer like him of the Norse *Lokasenna*, make free with those fragments of myth where no awe of belief can linger and hardly even the vital grace of imagination. In all this coil but one stage has interest for us; what can be said of the beginnings of poetry in their relation to the beginnings of myth?

A good test for the primitive stage of myth is first the necessity, not the possibility of it, and secondly, the unconscious character of the animating process. Dawn, starlight, and laughing waters put no stress of questioning upon early man; but the bolt from a stormcloud which laid low the sheltering tree, or struck down members of the horde, a nameless Terror bursting out of the unknown, came in more questionable shape, and must have found expression in those statements which a communal chorus, as was seen in the case of the Botocudos, is fain to make about the fate and doings of the horde itself. Mere ancestor-worship is not enough to explain such a case;[1] every analogy of human action fails in the presence of this flash and roar and destruction; the unknown was there, as with modern phrase — "it" thunders[2] — and the statement, repeated in indefinite chorus, had in it the awe and fear and yearning about the unknown which still go a long way to make up the idea of religion. But it was

[1] Too much stress is laid by some writers on primitive studies of death, and of dreams about the dead, as productive of myth. Modern peasants, like savages, often show a heavy and stupid indifference in the presence of death; and its problem, though it doubtless suggested a cult of spirits, was far less insistent with early man than the problem of life. Before he thus worked out a world of dead spirits, he knew by instinctive, really unconscious inference, a world of living spirits, not of his own breed, but vaster, subtler, in those operations of nature which struck into his actual life, interfered with it, or conspicuously helped it.

[2] "*It* hurts me; *it* makes me cry," says the child, pointing to the seat of affliction; this "it" corresponds with savage and primitive animism. It is not personification, as one is often told. Human beings do not crawl into other human beings and hurt them; not he or she, but "it" hurts. One remembers the remark of J. Grimm, that the neuter gender means not lack of sex, but the undeveloped, initial stage. *Deutsche Grammatik*, III. 315.

unconscious, this process of animism; before one consciously attributes personality to a force of nature, one must have the two distinct ideas before the mind, and for early man such a clear view was out of the question. Moreover, the idea of a definite force, a definite personality, hardly belongs to the primitive stage of myth; one must look at environment[1] and the social organization. It is known that even the sacred bull, and still more the "father" of the spirits, the chief god, reflect nomadic life under a leader; while the leaderless horde is girt about with a horde of spirits, the "they" of primitive worship corresponding to the "we" of the social group.[2] In this stage of culture only the horde itself, the social group, can be in the case; poetic fancy on one side, ordered bands of deities, high and low, with a supreme god over all, on the other side, must be excluded. Earliest myth is simply communal emotion, in choral statement, provoked by some overwhelming act of vague and unseen powers. Early poetry is always "occasional"; what strikes, like this thunderbolt, into the life of the horde,[3] is a theme quite as solicitous as good hunting, or the fight with rival clans, to fill a refrain with repeated statement of fact, and, in time, to tempt the improvising soloist into a phrase of wonder, awe, pity, propitiation. Here, then, is a common ground for the beginnings of poetry and the beginnings of myth,[4] — in communal, choral statement. True, explanation of these doings of nature may be a fertile source of myth in the later period when

[1] Posnett, *Comparative Literature*, pp. 162 ff. The idea, however, is by no means as new as Posnett thinks it to be.

[2] See above, p. 380.

[3] Vignoli, in his *Myth and Science*, notes that a dog growls or bites at a stick thrust toward him, a kind of animism; although as Spencer said, — with quite unwarrantable inference in the denial of nature-myths among primitive men, — a dog takes no notice of ordinary natural doings, swaying boughs, sunrise, and all the rest.

[4] Max Müller's "disease of language" as source of myth is absurd; the myth does not wait for the misunderstanding of a metaphor, but begins with the metaphor and lives with its life, — both being, of course, unconscious at the start.

poetry and science are allied in a search after causes; but it is clear that stating a fact is a process anterior to any explanation of a fact. Is there not for modern man himself a comfort in the lucid statement of things even before the things are explained? The lawyer who states his case clearly has half explained it and has prepared the jury to accept his explanation of the facts. Scherer says that myth is due to some primitive genius who listened to a thunderstorm, wished to explain it, and conjectured that "the gods were fighting,"[1] a theory adopted by the fellow-citizens of this genius, who thus had "founded" a myth. But communal statement, with unconscious animism in the terms of it, — communal, that is, in its expression, and religious in its source, — is the only formula for early myth which will agree with the conditions of primitive life. To the cadence of the dance, in iterated refrain, the horde as a social group took comfort in getting the facts into a coherent statement; to repeat, in a rhythm which made repetition easy and coherence possible, that the "they" in question had done things which the "we" were now recording, was a process not far removed from the iterated statement that "we" had found a good hunt, made a good catch, or what not. From the awful and inevitable, this communal choral statement could pass to less destructive doings; and from the pandemonium, the rout of spirits, step by step with differentiation of the horde, with the rise of tribal leaders, with the coming of an improvising singer, this statement could pass to the pantheon[2] and hierarchy of gods.

That myths of this sort, statements based on the feeling for animated nature in its more obtrusive forms, were as

[1] A child who saw a flash of lightning once said, "God is winking at me"; and the phrase was seized upon as a fine illustration of primitive myth-making. But the child had been presented, by the whole process of human culture and thought, with at least two-thirds of this "myth," — the idea of God, of a distinct, supreme personality, and the reference to God of whatever goes on in the sky.

[2] See E. H. Meyer, *Indogerm. Mythen*, Berlin, 1883, I. 87.

early as the worship of ancestral spirits, is denied by Mr. Herbert Spencer and his school, but without good cause. It is illogical to affirm the beginnings of reason and in the same breath to deny the beginnings of fancy. If ancestor-worship, belief in "them," was one of the earliest inferences of the human mind, if one of the first conclusions which man made outside the round of his daily struggle for food and safety was to animate an unseen world, as early an act, earlier indeed, was to animate the world he saw. Statements about the doings of an animated nature, a horde of echoes, movements, violent activities, girdling the horde of men, were thus in all probability the earliest form of myth. This statement, however, had less of that scientific leaning than Scherer would make one believe; childish fear of harm and childish hope of gain is a more likely attitude of mind in primitive folk than childish curiosity about causes. The choral statement, one may assume, took most easily a reference to human needs and so became a hymn. The hymn is essentially choral, and even under literary conditions implies a congregation; the majesty and power of a real hymn like Luther's is out of all proportion to its merit as a poem. It is the source of the hymn in a communal emotion, and the direction of it to unseen forces, that give it this majesty; and the poorest words gain might from these conditions alone. A rude hymn of the horde to those spirits unseen but felt, was therefore the probable beginning of myth, — not a performance of the shaman before a passive throng, and not a tale of celestial doings invented by some early genius who took it upon him to pry into the mystery of things. Of course there are fetish myths which have come to be brutal and obscene, but were not brutal and obscene when they were first formed;[1] there are also myths

[1] In the reaction from ideas of a golden age one must not go too far, and "call names" which now mean vice, degeneration, rottenness. It is possible that even

invented in a later stage of culture to account for a ritual or a belief [1] come down from early and obscure origins, often with something of the fetish in them, as is probably the case with the myth of Rome and the wolf; and there are crude tales, due to as crude scientific instinct, to account for physical phenomena, popular everywhere and in all times down to the day of Uncle Remus. But all evidence of ethnology, all the facts which have served to trace the line of poetical evolution, go to make probable the social and communal and choral beginnings of the myth which has the awe of belief upon it. As might be expected, fragments of this old choral refrain which bound the myth to the community and to its religious emotion, have come down to us embedded in later and poetical myth; and it has been shown that a refrain of grief [2] for the loss or departure of a god, demigod, hero, has often been made a proper name and the nucleus for a new myth. This choral cry of the horde has great interest for the student of myths; and if the etymology be probable which makes the word "god" mean "one that is called upon," here is more beckoning that way. Heavier stress should be laid upon the choral hymn as expression of emotion from a homogeneous horde of men toward a homogeneous horde of spirits, and upon the dance and symbolic action which went with the song, taking in time now a ritual and now a dramatic guise.[3] In other words, this choral hymn, danced and sung,—if one will,

earliest myth touched here and there a chord of poetry as we now know poetry, and appealed to that constant element which belongs to our humanity and not to our history.

[1] Or, of course, a tradition; so Prometheus and the origin of fire may account for the stealing of fire from some neighbouring tribe. See Gruppe, *Griechische Culte und Mythen*, p. 206.

[2] See above, p. 236.

[3] Comparetti, *Kalewala*, pp. 154 f., in his excellent remarks on popular myth and popular poetry, has left his analysis incomplete by leaving throng-poetry quite out of the account.

danced and sung about some symbol of animated and superhuman but by no means individualized or "personified" powers, and with accompaniment of sacrifice, with festal recapitulation, even, of action inspired by the help of these powers, — was on one hand the source of religious ceremony, which later, in its mutilated and incomprehensible refrains held so stubbornly in festal worship, with the worshipped powers hovering about unseen, and, on the other hand, source of a secular drama, where, as in Greece, only an altar remained as visible hint of sacred origins, and only the intervention of gods and the abiding sense of fate kept alive the old purpose of the hymn. This chorus, dealing with the doings of spirits, like the chorus that dealt with labour and hunt and communal experience at large, was also the beginning of myths which, like the older refrain, fell under the power of improvisation and so passed into poetic control, keeping pace with the tribal development of hero, chieftain, conqueror, king, blending with legend, and at last finding record in the epos.

The impression of natural forces upon man, and the reactionary process which imposes man's imagination upon natural forces, have another side; they make up not only the material of poetry, but also its manner, its style. The second process, when it animated nature with something like human will, human passion, human fate, and while it did this with the awe of belief upon it, has been seen to pass into myth. Roughly speaking, one may say that the early and unconscious process is myth, and the later, conscious process, when directed not to a statement or story but only to a word or phrase, is the figure or trope of personification. The first process, however, where human life is treated in terms of nature, is conveniently known as metaphor, although precision in the use of these terms is not so much observed as desired; and metaphor, too, must be regarded as first an unconscious and then a conscious process.

Myth and personification need no further comment, and we shall now consider the metaphor as mainstay of poetical style; one word, however, may be in place for an early and unconscious form of personification, which deals with language rather than with fact, and so must be sundered from myth — the grammatical gender of words.[1] A bit of myth may lie, of course, in those expressions which hover between the natural and the grammatical gender, and is not always easy to explain from the primitive point of view, however appropriate the choice may seem to a modern mind; why is the sun feminine in all Germanic languages, and the moon masculine? Day is masculine, night is feminine; earth seems always feminine, and "mother" is no new epithet for her. Death, pestilence, sickness, have personifications that are more than gender; Servians think of the plague as a woman in white who steals upon her victims, and to modern Greeks sickness is also a woman, blind and old, who feels her way from house to house.[2] But even now the process may be unconscious, as one observes in languages like English, which have lost their inflections and can give gender only by pronouns; Grimm's elaborate categories for the three genders are sadly baffled by the habit which calls a ship a "man-of-war" and bids the bystander watch "her" sail by.[3] Again, there is transfer to reckon with; the first name for an object, as will be shown presently to be the case with metaphors, yields later to a name more precise; and when a ship, or the like, is in question, motion and seeming life

[1] Grimm's chapter on gender in the third volume of his *Grammar* remains the masterpiece of investigation in this subject; but his theory has been attacked by Brugmann. See, too, President Wheeler, "Origin of Grammatical Gender," *Journal Germanic Philology*, II. 528 ff. Grimm defines gender, III. 346, "eine in der phantasie der menschlichen Sprache entsprungene ausdehnung des natürlichen auf alle und jede gegenstände."

[2] *Ibid.*, III. 354.

[3] Grimm says the Englishman calls "she" whatever is dear to him — the sailor his ship, the miller his mill; III. 546.

could give one vague name, while later and nearer acquaintance found an appellation in technical qualities. On the whole, it will be best if we leave gender to animism, to incipient myth, unconscious metaphor, and whatever other forces went to the making of words, and turn to metaphor itself.

To those who hold with the Abbé Dubos[1] that poetic style is the most important factor in differencing poetry from prose, and demands the greatest genius in the poet, it may seem a hard saying to call the early stage of figurative language unconscious metaphor. The habit of describing primitive poetry in terms of modern verse imposes on these early stages a teleological element quite foreign to the conditions which ethnology and the sense of evolution compel one to assume for the beginnings of such an art. Poetry, says Cardinal Newman, in his little essay,[2] has to adopt metaphorical language as "the only poor means allowed for imparting to others its intense feelings," which refuse "the feebleness of ordinary words"; and with this *raison d'être* for the metaphor, one goes on to inquire how it is made. The transfer from a literal to a figurative or metaphorical expression, one finds, is made on the basis of a comparison and an observed resemblance, so that a metaphor is compressed or abridged simile, and the simile must be the fundamental figure in poetry. So the schools have taught time out of mind.[3] Even Scherer,[4] eager to hit the new note,

[1] *Reflexions Critiques*, ed. 1770, I. 298. La Poësie du style fait la plus grande différence qui soit entre les vers et la prose. . . . Les images et les figures doivent être encore plus fréquentes dans la plupart des genres de la Poësie, que dans les discours oratoires. . . . C'est donc la Poësie du style qui fait le Poëte, plutôt que la rime et la césure. . . . Cette Partie de la Poësie la plus importante." See also p. 312, in § xxxv.

[2] *Essay on Poetry with Reference to Aristotle's Poetics*, ed. Cook, p. 11.

[3] Some representative definitions of this sort are collected and quoted by Dr. Gertrude Buck in an interesting paper, *The Metaphor: a Study on the Psychology of Rhetoric*, being No. 5 of the "Contributions to Rhetorical Theory," edited by Professor Scott, Ann Arbor, — no date, but about 1899, — p. 40.

[4] *Poetik*, p. 87 f. See also p. 83. On p. 262 he opens, however, a dangerous door for the interests of this theory.

and fixing his gaze on primitive conditions, is sure that poetical figures spring from the innate love of comparison; even Dr. R. M. Meyer,[1] studying old Germanic poetry, finds that its metaphors prove the fundamental character of the simile from which they spring.[2] A little reflection, however, ought to convince candid minds that in the chronological, if not in the logical, order of development, the metaphor comes first and the simile is an expanded metaphor; this is proved not only by the psychological argument, but by the facts in the case. Those similes from Polynesian poetry given by Letourneau[3] represent no primitive stage, and to the long comparisons of Homer[4] no wise man will now appeal as examples of the artless and natural in poetic style. Savages, like Mr. Shandy, may dearly love a comparison; but it is a logical process, a kind of incipient science, in any case subsequent to the unconscious stage of metaphors. For, as a matter of fact, wherever one finds verse which all tests of value show to have the primitive quality, similes and the comparative impulse in general conspicuously fail; this is the case with ballads,[5] with choral and refrain of communal origins everywhere, and with the ruder stages of our old Germanic poetry.[6] Anglo-Saxon poetry, though all its artistic and literary influences urged it to comparison, simile, allegory, — the latter a peculiarly Chris-

[1] *Altgermanische Poesie*, p. 20.

[2] Modern writers on æsthetics make the same error: so Biese, "Das Metaphorische in der dichterischen Phantasie," *Zst. f. vgl. Lit.*, N. F. II. 320, makes the primitive process from simile to metaphor.

[3] On pp. 90 ff.

[4] St. Evremond thinks them distracting; in any case he will banish such things from drama. *Œuvres Meslées*, London, Tonson, 1709, III. 72 f., in an essay, "Sur les poëmes des Anciens."

[5] See above, p. 190.

[6] It is the case with later reaches of poetry. Chaucer, for example, offers very few figures or metaphors as compared with later poets; "no other author in our tongue," says Professor Lounsbury, *Stud.*, III. 441, "has clung so persistently to the language of common life."

tian invention,—is absolutely hostile to the simile except in passages copied almost slavishly from a literary source; and this consideration led the present writer[1] twenty years ago to find ground for opposing the traditional doctrine of metaphors as founded in the first instance upon an observed likeness. Everybody grants that early metaphor differs from late; a child calls the bird's nest a house, not because it compares the nest with a house, but because it has the idea of house and has not the specific idea of nest; and so it would and does call the horse's stable, the rabbit's burrow, what not, a house, until wider knowledge and specific information give a distinct name for each. Then, and not until then, with two separate ideas before the mind, is the metaphor based upon a definite comparison, and the transfer a conscious process. In other words, the metaphor was not a metaphor at the start, save in the unconscious force of it; so with the early myth, where there was no thought of comparing a force of nature and a human act, but simply an effort to express the force along the only possible path, the path of animism. This, moreover, is at first nothing but direct statement. In all primitive verse, including its survival, the ballad, it is simple statement, and not metaphor in any modern shape, that constitutes the style. One cannot express the literal by the figurative until one has got a conception of literal and figurative as discrete things; the first stage of metaphor, then, is unconscious, a confusion, if one will, or, better, a flexibility in application of the small stock of words. In a little article[2] on metaphor and poetry, the

[1] *The Anglo-Saxon Metaphor*, Halle, 1881. The theory of the metaphor there advanced was due to the study of poetical material alone, and had no help from psychology. The latter, however, is quite favourable to the theory of poetic evolution as stated in the text. See the quotations from Taine and others in the essay of Dr. Buck. The false conclusions of Heinzel in regard to simile and metaphor are of little moment compared with the general value of the essay which contains them: *Ueber den Stil der altgermanischen Poesie*, Strassburg, Q. F., 1875, a stimulating piece of work.

[2] *Modern Language Notes*, I. 83.

writer proposed this sequence of development in poetical figures: metaphor pure and simple, what has just been called the unconscious metaphor, stands first;[1] then comes metaphor with the literal peeping through, that is, where literal and figurative are joined, but in a separable fashion, the literal statement involving but not expressing contradiction in its terms; lastly the quite conscious metaphor, where both terms are expressed, and where the mind is fully alive to the gap between reality and trope, a metaphor which may be either the implied simile ("he is a lion") or the stated simile ("he is *like* a lion"). Evidently now, there comes a stage in poetic expression where that need for freshness and force sends the poet back over this path; the logical expression of resemblance is too literal, and he turns to the metaphor again, and so justifies the standing definition of it as a compressed or abridged simile. That, however, is not the history of its evolutionary growth.[2]

Turning to the nearer subject, we may now ask how the differentiation came about in poetic speech, and where it belongs in the beginnings of poetry. It is more than probable that earliest language was social in a sense now hard to understand; so tremendous was this step from brute forms of intercourse to human speech that it must have taken place under a social pressure infinitely removed from

[1] Logically Gerber is right, *Die Sprache als Kunst*, I. 256, in putting interjections at one end of the linguistic process and metaphor at the other; but chronologically, historically, genetically, the assumption fails to hold.

[2] The subject is too wide for further treatment, and can be regarded here only in its relations to the beginnings of poetry. See, however, for the early stages of a metaphor, J. Grimm's essay on "Die Fünf Sinne," *Kleinere Schriften*, VII. 193 ff.; and F. Bechtel, *Ueber die Bezeichnungen der sinnlichen Wahrnehmungen in den indogerm Sprachen*, Weimar, 1879, where he shows how the idea of "bright" underlies so many of our words, — "glad," for instance, which even in Anglo-Saxon meant "gleaming." See, too, in this book the confusion, or flexibility, of words for the "bright" and the "loud," seeing and hearing; also J. Grimm, "Die Wörter des Leuchtens und Brennens," *Kl. Schr.*, VIII. 263 ff.

conditions of what now passes for "conversation." As with the earth itself, these psychical changes were volcanic. The refrain of concerted labour, upon which Bücher has wisely laid such stress, the refrain of festal emotion over a victorious fight, the cadenced sounds in concert with consent of individual energies alert for a common cause, — it was under such vast and unusual social pressure that the greatest of social triumphs came about. Hence it may well seem absurd to talk of earliest song in words as a "heightened" or emotional speech, speech raised above the level of ordinary conversation; for what needs could have produced ordinary conversation before the wholly imperative and extraordinary occasions which called out the greatest resources of social effort? It is to be denied, therefore, that "poetic" expression was lifted out of ordinary and conversational expression; and it may well have been that choral hymns with earliest statement of myth,[1] choral song with earliest statement and gestured imitation of communal achievement, and choral refrains of labour, formed the beginnings of speech, which was mainly a recapitulation of action, and therefore mainly a matter of verbs. It is conceded that verbs came before substantives, for action, as in labour, is easily paired with gesture and sound; names for things, the substantives, the singular forms of the pronoun, are a different affair, and lend themselves more readily to the individual and to improvisation. A statement of action, subjective or objective, contemporary or reminiscent, is easily made by a chorus, whether of primitive men, or of modern children with their "Now we go round the mulberry-bush"; and the statement as naturally repeats itself as refrain to the dancing or whatever cadenced motion is in the case. This

[1] Allegory, now a huge projection of metaphor from the style into the subject-matter, is a consistent series of personifications not unlike the later stages of myth; in fact, late myth is allegory.

is the communal or centripetal impulse. The centrifugal, individual impulse lays hold of an unvaried repetition of rhythm,[1] and evolves couplet and stanza, with variations of rime, assonance, and the like; laying hold of the expression itself, and by a parallel process applied to style instead of to form, this impulse leads to variation in expression,[2] to something in one verse very like the corresponding part of the preceding verse, yet different. Step by step, with the aid of the "Apollinian" instinct, metaphor becomes conscious of itself and of its own effort; it works out a poetic dialect, which, contrary to the common notion, is an increasing and not a decreasing factor in poetry. It begins with flexibility of application, unconscious of a difference, for there is no difference; sees at last a gap between itself and the literal, which has been formed by the rise of a conversational and "ordinary" language; avoids this literal, and shuns this ordinary, until in absurd excess it reaches the scaldic kenning, or finds a pedant[3] making dictionaries of metaphors proper for the poet to use in this or that case. Finally, it returns upon itself, seeking simplicity, if it can find it, with a Wordsworth, but still refusing to join hands with the talk of everyday life.[4] Be all this as it may be, the metaphor of the verb is both older and more communal than the metaphor of the substantive, which better fits the inventor's case and may well

[1] On the tendency of rhythm and music to suggest images and stir the powers of language, see the wild but interesting words of Nietzsche, *Geburt d. Tragödie*, p. 48.

[2] See above, p. 211.

[3] Josua Poole, *English Parnassus*, London, 1677, like Italians just before him, and like Vinesauf and others of earlier time, has an array of kennings whence the poet may pick and choose. Abel, for example (pp. 221 ff.), you may call "death's first fruit," or "death's handsel." Then there are "forms of invocating Muses" (p. 630), followed, alas, by "forms of concluding letters"—in prose.

[4] "The language of the age," wrote Gray to West, April, 1742, "is never the language of poetry."

have been the origin of the riddle,[1] conceded to be a very ancient form of literature. As in the beginning, so even now. The more individual, artistic, and subjective poetry becomes, the more it tends to deal in intricate metaphor, the less it has of the simplicity due to statement of action in simple because communal phrase; and whenever reactions set in toward that communal state of things, action comes to the front, intricate figure vanishes, verbs have more to do, substantives less, and adjectives almost nothing.[2] A reactionary movement of this sort lies before us in the verse of Mr. Kipling.

[1] Kennings often read like riddles: so in Finnish, "contents of Wainamoinen's milk-bowl," — the sunshine. See, moreover, Scherer, *Geschichte d. deutsch. Lit.*, pp. 7, 15; and R. M. Meyer, *Altgerm. Poesie*, p. 160.

[2] In this sketch of differentiation in poetic style only outlines are essayed. The subject is uncommonly attractive, and a book on the history of metaphor would be welcomed by all students of style. Nothing has been said here of symbolic metaphor from animals and the like. See Brinkmann's study of "Thierbilder in der Sprache," *Die Metaphern*, Bd. I. Bonn, 1878. His researches in German, English, French, Spanish, Italian, Latin, Greek, should be extended to half civilized and savage conditions, and should take a historical and genetic range. Of course, the æsthetic side of this whole subject is treated in Gerber's well known book, quoted several times on preceding pages, *Die Sprache als Kunst.*

CHAPTER VIII

THE TRIUMPH OF THE ARTIST

FROM this brief raid upon the territory of poetic style, we return to the fortunes of improvisation and its defeat at the hands of a more deliberate art.[1] Among the countless passages in which the poet has talked of his profession, not the least notable is that *impromptu* of De Musset in which he says: —

> Faire un travail exquis, plein de crainte et de charme,
> Faire une perle d'une larme,
> Du poëte ici-bas voila la passion, —

that is, of the poet whom one takes seriously, the artist, the solitary maker of things beautiful. Quite different is the idea of the poet implied in a pleasant little jest that passed between De Musset and Sainte-Beuve. The critic had declared that in the majority of men there is a poet who dies young while the man himself survives; whereupon De Musset pointed out that Sainte-Beuve had unwittingly put his thought into a good Alexandrine, and thus had helped to prove that the poet in the case was not dead but asleep. Between this poet who dies young or slumbers in each of us, and the artist in verse who makes pearls out of tears, there is now only a fantastic and fugitive connection; in mediæval times, in rude agricultural communities, and under primitive conditions,

[1] It is noteworthy that Aristotle excludes improvisation from poetry; and in modern times Gerber (*Die Sprache als Kunst*) finds this rude kind of verse so opposed to his definition of poetry ("die Kunst des Gedankens," *ibid.*, I. 50; "enthusiasm plus deliberation," I. 77), that he too rules it out, and says it belongs simply to "the art of language." It is not well to drag such a ball-and-chain by way of definition when one is dealing with primitive poetry.

this slumbering poet was awake and active, and the step from his ranks to that of artistry was of the easiest and shortest kind. The story of the poet is simple. Detaching himself from the throng in short improvisations, he comes at last to independence, and turns his active fellows into a mute audience; dignity and mystery hedge him about, his art is touched with the divine, and like his brother, the priest, he mediates between men and an imaginative, spiritual world, living, too, like the priest, at the charges of the community. This was the upward path; another path led the minstrel into ways of disrepute, where dignity and mystery were unknown, where the songsmith was made a sturdy beggar and an outlaw by act of parliament, and where there was little comfort even in being the singing-man at Windsor. With the upward path there is no space here to deal; the poet by divine right, moreover, has had chroniclers enough and to spare, and it only remains to note the later stages through which his communal brother passed on the way to what seems an everlasting silence.

As the chosen singer stands out single from the throng and the throng lapses passive into the background, so the poem which this singer makes becomes a traditional and remembered affair, with epic movement and an interest which causes art and substance of the song to outweigh any mere expression of contemporary emotion. This, indeed, lingers in the chorus or refrain of a ballad; but even the choral impulse passes away as the story and the style of the poem increase in importance, and it disappears behind the rhapsode,[1] who chants or recites his verses to a listening

[1] See above, p. 215. There is a lively if exaggerated account of the rhapsode in Blackwell's *Enquiry into the Life and Writings of Homer*, pp. 104 ff. Limits already transgressed forbid the author to add any material on the minstrel in his relations to the making of poetry. See a brief account, with a few references, in *Old English Ballads*, pp. 310 ff. Further, see Piper, *Spielmannsdichtung* (Vol. 2 of the *Deutsche National-Litteratur*); Scherer, *Gesch. d. deutsch. Dichtung im*

crowd. With permanent record, with the making of manuscript,[1] poetic art at its best ceases to be a matter of voice and ear; two silent men, the poet and his reader, communicate by means of the written or the printed page, itself the result of solitary thought, and subject, at the other end of the process, to the same deliberation and inference in the appreciation of it as the poet employed in the making.[2] But the obvious advantages of immediate contact, of living voice, gesture, personal emotion, in the poet, and palpable interest, whether active or passive, on the part of the audience, made the disintegration and decay of this primitive group a very slow affair. It survives even yet in the popular "reading," and, with higher pretensions, on the stage; but a far more interesting survival, and more complete, is found among that people of strong poetic impulses who gave the *improvvisatore* his place of honour down to quite recent times. The art was so common that it got the compliment of parody; Pulci imitates the *improvvisatori* in his *Morgante*,[3] and worse yet, the luckless bards who made extemporaneous verses at the table of Leo X were whipped if these verses were not of the smoothest. But this is only the shady side of the art. Quadrio[4] thinks that if the human mind anywhere puts forth its noblest powers, it is in that craft called *canto all' improv-*

11 u. 12 Jhrh. (*Quellen. u. Forschungen*, XII.); Wilmanns, *Walther v. d. Vogelweide*, especially pp. 39 ff.; the general account in Axel Olrik's *Middelalderens Vandrende Spillemaend* (*Opuscula Philologica*), Copenhagen, 1887; Freymond, *Jongleurs und Menestrels*, Halle, 1883 (for the Romance side of the question); and portions of many other works, such as Jusserand, *Théatre en Angleterre*, p. 23, note; F. Vogt, *Salman und Morolf*, pp. cxxiii f.; notes here and there on Widsith and Déor, the earliest types of English minstrel; and so on.

[1] There were pedants before paper, however, in the days of great mnemonic feats. See Max Müller, in the *Nineteenth Century*, November, 1899, pp. 798 ff.

[2] This evolution of the solitary and deliberate poet has been outlined in Chap. IV.

[3] Burckhardt, *Ren.*, I. 172. See also p. 250.

[4] *Della Storia e della Ragione d'ogni Poesia*, Vol. I., Bologna, 1739, pp. 155 ff.

viso;[1] this, he says, was the beginning of poetry, and is still one of its best achievements; and he goes on to give some hints for the ambitious. Every one knows the romantic figure of Corinne; but a better example for the present purpose is Perfetti, an actual *improvvisatore* whose feats drew attention abroad as well as at home. He is mentioned in Spence's *Anecdotes;* and a few facts about him[2] may be given here in order to show how the fatal breach between poetry of mere entertainment, now in full process of degeneration at the hands of the minstrel and balladmonger, and poetry of creative and imaginative art, now veiled in mystery and seen of none but consecrated eyes, was thought to be healed by the rapt strains of these improvising poets of Italy. What grace, they argued, could be lacking to one that was crowned at the Capitol, and stood in the stead of Petrarch? Son of a cavalier and a noble lady, Perfetti began very early his office as a bard; his Latin biographer, with vast gravity, says the child made "what in our tongue is called rime" at eleven months; small wonder that he became famous when still a youth, and was welcomed at parties of every sort, weddings, social discussions, what not, where he exercised his gift of extempo-

[1] "Tutta volta bisogna ancor confessare, che questo fu il primo genere di Poesia, che fosse al Mondo." There is a long account of improvisation in Crescimbeni, *L'Istoria della Volgar Poesia,* Venice, 1731 (written in 1697), pp. 219 ff. An old and very interesting *gradus ad Parnassum* is Ruscelli, *Del Modo di Comporre in Versi nella Lingua Italiana,* Venice, 1582 (a new edition), "nel quale va compreso un pieno ordinatissimo Rimario," and there are directions for using the voice both for prose and for verse. The seventh chapter is on the "stanze d'ottava Rima," and treats of improvisation, mentioning even an infant phenomenon in this art ("essendo ancor fanciullo . . . non arrivava ai sedici anni"), who made verses off-hand on any subject which was given to him.

[2] From two books, one Italian, *Saggi di Poesie parte dette all' improvviso e parte scritte dal Cavaliere Perfetti patrizio Sanese ed insigne Poeta estemporaneo coronato di laurea in Campidoglio* . . . dal Dottor Domenico Cianfogni, 2 vols., Florence, 1748 (Vol. II. has the account of the crowning); and a Latin pamphlet of 56 pp., *Josephi Mariani Parthenii S. J. de Vita et Studiis Bernadini Perfetti Senensis Poetae Laureati,* Rome, 1771. They are interesting in many ways.

raneous song. Of a summer night[1] he would improvise songs in praise of some family, singing under their windows, an amiable fancy. Cianfogni heard him on these occasions, and says that the poems were often taken down in writing by persons concealed from the poet's view; but he rarely wrote verses of his own, finding that sort of composition by no means to his taste. He refused to undertake an epic, though the pope urged him thus to rival Tasso and Ariosto. *Ottava rima* was his favourite verse, and he was fond of a musical accompaniment. His memory, too, was prodigious; in brief, Cianfogni hopes that this Moses will lead poetry back from its exile in a land of paper and print to its old glories of the living voice and the hearing of the ear. The Latin pamphlet, which has some interesting remarks on related matters in poetry, says that Perfetti learned his art at Sienna from one Bindius "poeta extemporalis," who excelled in that sort of verse which Berni composed, and which was called from its founder Bernesque. Come to his full powers, Perfetti shunned no kind of poem, and excelled in every branch of the art. His songs were repeated on all sides and passed current among the people; while, for the rest, he could sing *majora* too, winning applause from the pope himself, and getting crowned at the Capitol in a function of unusual splendour. Physically, his poetic ardour was formidable and "almost passed belief," eyes aflame, brow contracted, panting bosom, and a flow of words so vehement and swift that his harp-player was often left far in the rear; the song done, Perfetti could hardly stand for exhaustion, and slept but little on the ensuing night.[2] So strenuous a life told on his health, one must think; at any rate, he died of paralysis in July, 1747.

[1] Latin, xix.

[2] The pious father tells elsewhere of mitigating contrivances: "Frigida inter canendum uti solebat, ad fauces nimirum recreandas et ad nimium fervorem, quo incendebatur, restringuendum!"

This account of Perfetti is amusing, but much may be learned from it. Significant is the fact that he always sang his verses as he composed them, kept to one fixed rhythm, and had a harp to accompany him, — music once more in her original function as muse. Significant, too, is his aversion from pen and paper, his sensible refusal to try epic and poems of great length. That physical excitement and that reaction, too, are in line with the old communal elation, and are at no great remove from similar states of the body in medicine men, magicians, priests of the oracle, and even the rapt poet of a traditional prime. Significant, finally, is the feeling on the part of his friends that with him poetry was going back to first principles, and could thus bathe in the fountain of youth. But it was not to be. The communal fashion of poetry was already a lost cause. *Soli cantare periti Arcades;* the "poet in every man" is passive and not active; and the gift of improvisation comes now in vain, for the conditions which once gave it sole validity are vanished beyond recall. Shakspere's kindred three, the lunatic, the lover, and the poet, once frankly accepted as public and privileged characters, sacred even, must now play the fool nowhere but in their own houses.

Whatever it gained by the process, poetry has been forced to give up its immediate power over men, and to console itself with what Herder called a "paper eternity." This triumphant artist, who now holds its destinies in trust, stands at such a remove from its beginnings, his very art seems so opposed to rude songs of the prime, and the public making of verse[1] has

[1] Along with Perfetti's moribund art of individual improvisation dies as well the improvised flyting, even in its more complicated and artistic phases. Through sundry references made above (pp. 208, note, 325, 416 f.) in regard to the inter-

become so deject and wretched, that one must face again, and this time in conclusion of the whole matter, a question of identity. Is it all one and the same art? Has all this pother about refrain and rhythm concerned the beginnings of actual poetry, or only hints and forewarnings as alien to poetry itself as the brute beast is alien to civilized man? Three answers may be made to this question. With Aristotle, or rather with what one takes to be the meaning of Aristotle, one may sunder as into two distinct arts the improvisation of primitive throngs and the deliberate poetry of maker and seer. Here, of course, is a denial of identity. Again, with Scherer,[1] one may ignore improvisation by throngs, recognize only the difference between oral and written record, and assume for earliest poetry conditions analogous to those of modern times, — the need for entertainment on the part of a "public," and the answering performance of an "entertainer" who languishes or thrives according to the state of the literary market. Here is identity outright, but far too much of it. Whatever the merits of his *Poetik*, and it has great merits, Scherer was doomed to failure from the first, because, as Bücher[2] rightly objected, no one

laced stanzas of ballad and song, I have come into a bit of unintentional and quite explicable confusion. These *serranas* were called artificial, and yet were cited in the proof of communal origins. Artistic and even artificial these *serranas* undoubtedly become; and yet so does the refrain. They are very common; as Professor Lang points out in his *Liederbuch des Königs Denis von Portugal*, Halle, 1894, pp. xlvii, lxiii, they make "die Norm des altportugiesischen Kunstgedichtes," and are found alike in songs of love and in the various kinds of flyting. Here, in the public song-duel, one crosses into communal territory; and the *serranas* go back to that rivalry of variation based upon a refrain or a repeated traditional verse.

[1] See above, p. 349.

[2] I regret that all references to Bücher's *Arbeit und Rhythmus* have been made from the first edition, and not from the second, which came to my hands after the foregoing chapters were printed. In bulk the book has more than doubled, increase lying mainly in new songs and refrains of labour, particularly of *Bittarbeit* and *Frohnarbeit*. Neither this new edition, however, nor the new edition of

can arrive at the spirit of primitive art by setting out from the categories of modern art. Moreover, Scherer flies in the face of facts, while the facts which go with that Aristotelian theory are surprisingly accurate. Not a syllable in Aristotle's brief account of poetic origins has been assailed by all the evidence gathered for modern ethnology, and by all the historical and comparative work undertaken on the basis of this new material. Nevertheless, one hesitates before the Aristotelian theory of absolute difference, just as one hesitates before the notion of absolute identity. True, one must sunder the epoch of instinct, of throngs, and of improvisation, from the epoch of deliberate and solitary art; but this does not warrant one in granting to the second epoch alone the name and fact of poetry. There is a third answer to the question, reasonable in every way, which would neither transfer modern conditions to the remote past, nor yet blot out one of the two periods of poetry, but would see in all manifestations of the art, early and late, the presence and play of two forces, one overwhelmingly conspicuous at the beginning, the other overwhelmingly conspicuous now; forces which, in their different adjustments, have conditioned the progress of song and verse at every stage.

For it is clear that two forces[1] have been always active

Bücher's *Entstehung der Volkswirthschaft* (see my note above, p. 107) changes materially his theory as quoted in defence of communal poetry. Not so much the priority of play is conceded as the early lack of a definite boundary between play and work. Again, references have been made above to Yrjö Hirn's book, *Förstudier till en Konstfilosofi;* this material, and much more of the sort, are now to be found in the same author's *Origins of Art*, London and New York, 1900. Possibly some modification, due to the chapter on "Erotic Art," should be made in the statements of ethnologists with regard to the lack of this motive in savage poetry.

[1] The science of poetry has had its share of wild theories meant to establish "laws" of progress. See Tarde, *Les Lois Sociales*, pp. 24 ff. But the play of collective and individual forces is too evident, too reasonable, to be classed with Vico's *Ricorsi* and with Plato's or Bacon's cycles.

not only in letters but in human life, and that these forces answer to the communal influence dominant in early poetry and the centrifugal, individual tendency in modern verse. One phase of this dualism in poetry has been discussed above;[1] it is now in order to look at it not with separation and analysis in view, but rather with an eye to the higher synthesis. No one questions the antithesis between man solitary and man social; and few will question the relative dominance of this or that type for any given age of the world. There are times so stamped by the individual impulse that all kinds of covenant, system, institution, are attacked, and nowhere more fiercely than in affairs of religion and of state. Seventeenth-century England is a case of this kind; individuals rush off to the wilderness to think and dream, and then rush back again to found a new sect. On the large stage the state is Cromwell, and on the small stage Quakerism is George Fox. Again, and for the other view, seventeenth-century France[2] is a place of order, tradition, and collective peace. True, names are also current along with creed and rule, Bossuet, Boileau, and the great Louis himself; but it is dogma and order, not disintegration, that they proclaim. Consent is supreme here, as dissent is supreme across the Channel. In any line of human effort, and at any given time, one of these forces is dominant. But after all, it is only of a relative dominance that one can speak, and these labels that the historian puts upon his entire epoch are good until another historian, with another phase of it in mind, takes up the brush. There is constant play of those opposing forces, and if the collective spirit brought order, tradition, cohesion, to the late seventeenth and the early eighteenth century, the individual spirit even

[1] In Chapters III and VII.

[2] See the brilliant description of this epoch in the opening chapter of Pellissier's *Mouvement Littéraire au XIXe Siècle*, 5th ed., Paris, 1898.

then fostered, as never before, the idea of a great man as mainspring in social progress. So, too, if disintegration ruled in seventeenth-century England, there was no lack of the collective and communal force; witness the social organization and religious democracy of the Quakers themselves. It was a time of sects and schisms; it was also a time of commonwealths spiritual, political, and social.

With this constant play and change of the two forces in mind, one may return to poetry itself and attempt a summary of the whole case, noting the alternation of communal and individual impulses, and seeking, by a study of their manifestations, to bring the beginning of the art into line with its present condition. It has been shown how easily confusion besets a discussion of that savage culture which is now declared communal in every way, and now painted as individual to the extreme of brute selfishness. So, too, when one says that early poetry was overwhelmingly choral and communal, that modern poetry is overwhelmingly individual, one has full warrant of facts; but it is well to remember just what these facts are, and so avoid ill-considered criticism. Poetry was a social creation and essentially communal at the start; although some of the most careful investigations in the early history of man [1] are now putting stress upon the fact that for perhaps thousands of years humanity was hovering on the far border of communal organization, and led a mainly selfish and unsocial life. Man of this period did not have to unite with his fellows for purposes of mutual help and for defence against a common foe; like many wild animals, he could have roved about in smallest groups, each member of which got its own food for itself, often, as in favoured climates, with a minimum of exertion. Hence, too, for long stretches of time, no need of organized labour, of any eco-

[1] Notably Bücher, *Entstehung der Volkswirthschaft*,[2] Tübingen, 1898, "Der Urzustand."

nomic system. But these needs all came at last;[1] and when primitive man confronted them, he began his social history, and communal life was a fact. Here, too, in these rude communal beginnings, consent and rhythm played their parts. Now it is no argument whatever against the assumption that earliest poetry was strongly communal to say that earliest social man himself was only feebly and tentatively communal; the point is that where he was communal it was to a degree rendered utterly impossible for the present, and almost incredible for the past, by reason of the very social progress in which that communism, that consent, formed the first step. So, too, when it is said that the individual element in primitive poetic art was at a minimum, there is nothing counter to this assertion in the fact that early man was close to the absolutely individual and centrifugal state; whenever the individual made himself felt in poetry, it was as an individual bound by the new social tie, and his individual expression was a part of the communal expression. But, as was just said, the new communal element, so far as it went, was communal to an almost exclusive degree; not until after long ages of alternating collective and individual forces, working within the social union, was the individual socially free to make himself master in a wholly social art. It is a fact full of significance that the nearer social groups, like the Veddahs and the Botocudos, stand to the brutish, unstable, isolated, and wandering life of earliest man, so much the closer and more emphatic is their tentative expression of social consent in the dance, which is almost a continuous ring of humanity, with just two prominent characteristics: the tightest possible clasp of individual to individual, and the most exact consent of rhythm in the limbs that are free to move. Yet when the dance is past, and the ring is broken,

[1] See Professor Keasbey, *International Monthly*, April, 1900: "The Institution of Society."

its individual members go back to a life marked by hardly any social traits. As to labour, Bücher[1] puts stress on the priority of women in gregarious songs of toil; while men were stalking game, the women combined in movements and chorals of work,[2] and a certain antithesis is not far to seek which would give women the primacy in early stages of poetry, while men lord it almost exclusively in these latter days. No woman, with the doubtful exception of Sappho, has crossed the bounds of what is known as minor poetry; no woman, though women sing and have most need of song from the cradle to the death-bed, has been a great composer; no woman, not even George Eliot or any of her clever cousins in New England, has yet laid hold of that quality which goes with triumphs of the individual poet, the quality of humour. Why women were so prominent in the communal poetry of the beginnings, is easily answered and is a question to be asked; why women fail as individuals to reach the higher peaks of Parnassus, is a question perhaps not to be asked, although the answer might well seem a distinct recognition of woman's great services to the art. At certain stages of poetry women have been nursing mothers without whose love and zeal for song poetry would have fallen into evil ways indeed. In any case, woman looms larger than man in that shadowy world of beginnings; her life was more consistently social, and her quicker emotional nature, whatever it may seem to modern eyes, gave her an advantage over the more stolid and more solitary male.

How is one to bind these beginnings to the present condition of poetry? With that alternation of social, choral impulses and impulses of the individual, poetry is not simply

[1] *Arbeit u. Rhythmus*, 2d ed., p. 340.

[2] In dances, of course, as well. To references scattered through the preceding pages, add Mommsen on the Camenae, *Hist. Rome*, trans. Dickson, 2d ed. London, 1864, I. 240.

swinging back and forth between two positions, but makes a steady advance. As in social progress, at each fresh occasion on which the individual isolates himself from society, he takes with him the accumulated force that society, by its main function, has stored up from traditions of the past, and as whenever he returns to society, he brings back as his own contribution a fresh strength derived from more or less unfettered thinking over vital problems, so it is with communal and artistic forces in poetry. For the mere case of poetry as a body of literature, on one hand, and the poet as an individual on the other hand, this relation is plain enough, and speaks for itself. Poetry does even more for the poet than the poet does for poetry. But when one passes from materials to conditions and elements, asking for what is social or communal in the modern poetry of art at its best, few answers, if any, are to be heard. Some answer, however, is demanded, and it must try to rise to the height of so great an argument. Where, then, is the trace of direct communal elements in great poetry?

The modern artist in poetry triumphs mainly by the music of his verse and by the imaginative power which is realized in his language, often merely by the suggestion in his language; for poetry, as Sainte-Beuve prettily remarked, lies not in telling the story but in making one dream it. For present purposes, then, it will be enough to look at the formal quality of rhythm and the more creative quality of imagination. Assuming that the second chapter of this book proved what it set out to prove, one must see in rhythm, or regularity of recurrence due to the consenting cadence of a throng, the main representative of communal forces; although repetition in its other forms goes back to the very condition of choral poetry itself. Because the critics take rhythm and verbal repetition largely for granted in the work of any great poet, and look rather to his excellent differences in thought and in variation of style, one must not ignore the immense significance of those communal forces in the poetry of art. It is not the mere rhythm, grateful, exquisite, and powerful as that may be, but it is what lies behind the rhythm, that gives it such a place in poetry; it appeals through the measures to the cadent feet, and so through the cadent feet to that consent of sympathy which is perhaps the noblest thing in all human life. The triumphs of modern prose are great, but they fail one and all to take the place of rhythmic utterance; they fail even to do at their best what poetry often does in its mediocrity. The short story commands pathos to an almost intolerable degree; Balzac's heartless daughters bring old Père Goriot close to the plight of Lear, so far as this pathos is concerned; and when Ibsen wishes to touch the quick of things in a play, he does well, from his point of view, to discard jingling verses and to use the prose of common conversation, thus bringing one face to face with the pathos of bare and actual life, — very actual and very bare. Pathos, indeed, all these prose triumphs show, and pathological is the word for them. They belong to surgery. Poetry, recoiling from bare and actual life, has a very different function. Significant is the popular use of this word, poetry; when one says that the poetry has gone out of one's life, one means that something very like Ibsen has come in, that one can no longer idealize life and can see in it only its flatness and bareness. The cadence of those feet has ceased, and with it the hint of consent and sympathy. For when the Veddahs leave their solitary and often desperate search for food, come together, cling each to each as close as may be in that arrow-dance of theirs, and sing for hours their monotonous chorus, it is certainly not done in order that they may see bare and actual life, but rather that they may escape it and forget it. It is not surgery they seek, but medicine, and this either tonic or opiate; indeed, the twofold function of poetry could be ranged under such a head. Tonic were the cheery chorals of actual labour, old as social man, songs of battle and the march, festal recapitulation of hunt and work and fight. They idealized life; they appealed to sympathy, and heartened the solitary by a sense of brotherhood. So, in these latter days, tonic are the passages which stir the heart of a young man who reads wisely his Goethe, and tonic too — why not? — all those jingling platitudes beloved and quoted of the youth who make valedictory speeches in the village school; tonic, in fine, whatever *gedenke zu leben* rings out from poets of the virile and the sane. And from the beginning to the end, this tonic poetry falls naturally into the rhythm of a march. On the other hand, poetry is an opiate; the solitary man ran to a choral throng not only that he might find brotherhood and sympathy, but also that he might forget himself, — a task which the wild chorus of Dionysos could accomplish no less surely and thoroughly than the very grapes and vintage of the god. Like these, poetry helped man to forget his troubles; like these, the whirl and motion of cadenced dancing brought about a kind of intoxication; and the graceful words with which Sir William Temple concludes his essay on poetry have gained a deeper and yet a more literal meaning through the researches of ethnology and the proof which now lies before us of the extent to which primitive man has found in dance and song a refuge from the bare hideousness of life. For this early art, for this soothing and flattering function of it, the main force lay in rhythm; and if one wishes to call rhythm the conventional part of poetry, one degrades it not a whit by the name. Early poetry was exactly that, — a conventional affair, an idealized view of life, now tonic and now opiate in its aim. But whether to hearten or to soothe, stimulant or sedative, poetry found its initial source of energy in rhythm; most intimate of all the arts, and nearest to the heart of man, poetry will part with this pulse of rhythm only when the sea shall part with its tides.

Rhythm, then, binds in a single bond both the beginning and the end. But its formula is one which any rimer can use with more or less skill, and modern verse makes far wider and deeper claims, claims which no one has thought to carry back to the beginnings of poetry. Where, in those early days, was that rare quality of imagination to which the critic now appeals when he sets off a masterpiece of poetry from its rivals? To answer this question, one cannot cite mere history; chorus and refrain and shards of rustic rime must be left aside; and one must even beg a little help from æsthetics itself: *so muss denn doch die Hexe dran.*

Described in its simplest form, the quality of modern poetic imagination seems to be a power, by suggestive use of musical and figurative human speech, to put the solitary reader into the mood which would arise naturally in him under the pressure of certain actual events or of a certain actual scene. To repeat the phrase of Sainte-Beuve, "la poésie ne consiste pas à tout dire, mais à tout faire rêver." Even primitive poetry was an idealization, an abstraction, a narcotic, a kind of waking dream; modern poetry is also a dream, but with deeper and wider issues, and with a purpose far more clearly defined. Now the great passages of poetry, such as those which Matthew Arnold used as tests for excellence, easily fall into one of the two categories; they revive, even create, the mood felt either in the pressure of actual events or in the presence of an actual scene. That beautiful line which Arnold quotes from Dante is simply the imaginative and conventionalized sense of beatific worship such as all men have felt in varying degree; while for the thousand cases where nature is treated, there can be no doubt whatever of the tie which binds even the most imaginative and solitary poet to the old singing throng. Nature is nothing without man to interpret it; and neither man nor nature could stand in this mutual relation had not social consent and social processes created these abstract ideas, this very "man," this very "nature," by the reciprocal working of communal and individual forces. It was thus a social process which brought man to read his condition and fates in terms of nature, or else to read nature in terms of his own condition and fates. His own condition and fates were ideas that came to him through a kind of social reflection; and nature grew "poetic" only by reason of man's social organization, which sprang from consciousness of kind, took shape in consent, and has begotten first the communal idea and then the idea of humanity. Only the eye "which hath kept watch o'er man's mortality" can see the "poetic" side of nature; and even man's mortality is a fact which came home to him in this poetic sense only when social organization had put the notion of humanity before his mind. So much is said of being "alone with nature" as a necessary condition for the enjoyment of its poetic side, and for sympathy with it, that one forgets what sympathy means. The social foundation is now forgotten; without it, however, there would be no poet's solitary rapture at all. Sympathy of the poet at its highest is only rising to a new pitch in the sense of kind; and although the prayer of St. Francis[1] has been quoted nigh unto death, one may be allowed to revive it, not merely because of its wide sympathy, embracing "my brother, the sun," and all created things, but also because this sympathy is the poetic expression of an idea which St. Francis put into actual working on earth, in that community of brothers in the bonds of divine and human love.

Nature, however, and the fates of man are not always so stupendous or so abstract in their relations. There is a

[1] See above, p. 155.

close, familiar tie, now cheery in its kind, and now sad, in the coming and going of the seasons. How much of modern poetry is bound up with this simple and obvious motive; and how easily one finds here the connection between new song and old! In a preceding chapter it was the difference we sought; here it is the identity, not merely of rhythm, but of imaginative force. Much has been said of that lyric appeal to the season and to the scene with which rude songs of the dance, and, later, actual ballads, were wont to begin: *Sumer ys ycumen in*, and *Lenten is comen with Love to toune*, are fossil bits of English verse in this kind. So, too, as the coming season was welcomed, the parting season had its lyric regret. What more is done by the most imaginative poem of our day, than to revive in the solitary reader that immediate delight or sorrow of the singing and dancing throng? When one says that the poet ennobles this actual scene, and adds something which was not present in sunshine and woods and waters and green earth, not even in the song of the birds, what else does one mean but that the poet has brought these things under the spell of human emotion, precisely as the human emotion of the dancers mingled with the scene of their festivity? Nothing is more common in folk-song than lament for wintry desolation, for the silence and absence of the birds. Walther von der Vogelweide touches the old motive and the old cadence with slight but graceful art; and it is "I" instead of "we," although the communal emotion is not far away. Then comes the full power of imagination in a certain sonnet, and in a certain line of it:—

> Bare, ruin'd choirs where late the sweet birds sang.

Take away the "ruin'd choirs," and of course one takes away Shakspere; but there is another alternative. Take away the older festal throngs of summer, the sorrowing throngs at its close; take away that cadence of consenting feet which echoes in the verse; take away the human sympathy which was so fostered by this consent, — and those "ruin'd choirs" are left as purposeless and idle as the void of space.

So, too, with other forms of imagination in poetry. Nature apart, and on themes as abstract as one will, great artistic poetry is still powerless to sever its connection with this communal imagination of sympathy and consent. Some of the strong passages in later poetry derive their energy from despair. "Man's one crime," says the Spaniard, "is to have been born;" while between Fitzgerald and the tentmaker lies the credit for that verse which bids God take as well as give pardon for the wickedness of mankind. This is called sublime. When the savage beats and breaks his gods, or reviles them in reiterated verse, he is called silly; but perhaps his disillusions, put into choral statement, may bring him something of that grim comfort which civilized man finds in a rhythmic defiance not absolutely different in kind. Nor, again, was the passing of a god, or of a system of gods, the same thing for communal chorus with those mounting races in the prime, as with these belated and stunted hordes. Defiance, however, apart, on the positive religious side choral praise is still a fact; and choral comment on the ways of God with man, that enthusiasm for which imagination is only a substitute, that *sursum corda* of congregational singing, that lapse of the individual and that triumph of the community, are enough to check one's impulse to think of early communal singing in terms of a Gilbert and Sullivan opera. It is hard, indeed, to pass back from conditions of solitary and artistic imagination to conditions of communal imagination; but the process is not impossible. If one will simply open a Shakspere and read aloud the passage where Ophelia tells her father how Hamlet came to her closet and bade her that silent farewell; the praise of friendship chanted so finely by Hamlet to Horatio; the parting at dawn of Romeo and

Juliet; the declaration of Portia;[1] the last speech of Othello; Macbeth arming for the final fight; Prospero at the end of the mask: familiar as these all are, the mere series of impressions will give one a new sense of the varied creative power to be found in a single field of poetry. Then, with all this ringing in one's ears, let one read aloud the shorter version of *Sir Patrick Spens*, and compare its imaginative range with the imaginative range of Shakspere. Neither simplicity alone, nor the change from drama to ballad, will cover this difference.[2] The strongest differencing element is the antithesis of individual artistic imagination in widest range, and of sympathy concentrated upon a small, but compact group. It is a step from the great world to a little canton, from humanity to a clan; spaces have shrunk, and sympathy almost lies in that actual touch of hand and hand, which once did for primitive poetry what imagination now does for the poet. At the heart of them both, however, drama and ballad, is this sympathy and consent of kind. True, the ballad is late and has its share of art; but the line drawn to it from the drama is a curve to be projected into prehistoric conditions, and able to connect the crude sympathy of kind expressed in choral repetition with noblest imaginative achievements of the perfected art.

To create the communal elements, poetry had to pass through ages of preparation. Dreary ages they seem now, and rudest preparation, in contrast with present verse; but it may be said that the poetry was not insipid for its makers and hearers, and the art was not crude for the primitive artists. One must ignore with equal mind the romantic notion of a paradise of poetry at the prime, as well as a too fondly cherished idea of ethnology that belated if not degraded

[1] You see me, Lord Bassanio, where I stand . . .
—*Merch. Ven.* III. 2.

[2] See above, pp. 140, 155.

wanderers on the bypaths of human culture are to stand as models for the earliest makers of song. Let one think of that poetry of the beginnings as rude to a degree, but nobly rude, seeing that it was big with promise of future achievement, and not a thing born of mere stagnation. Circling in the common dance, moving and singing in the consent of common labour, the makers of earliest poetry put into it those elements without which it cannot thrive now. They put into it, for the formal side, the consent of rhythm, outward sign of the social sense; and, for the nobler mood, they gave it that power by which it will always make the last appeal to man, the power of human sympathy, whether in love or in hate, in joy or in sorrow, the power that links this group of sensations, passions, hopes, fears, which one calls self, to all the host of kindred selves dead, living, or to be born. No poetry worthy of the name has failed to owe its most diverse triumphs to that abiding power. It is in such a sense that prehistoric art must have been one and the same with modern art. Conditions of production as well as of record have changed; the solitary poet has taken the place of a choral throng, and solitary readers represent the listening group; but the fact of poetry itself reaches below all these mutations, and is founded on human sympathy as on a rock. More than this. It is clear from the study of poetic beginnings that poetry in its larger sense is not a natural impulse of man simply as man. His rhythmic and kindred instincts, latent in the solitary state, found free play only under communal conditions, and as powerful factors in the making of society.

INDEX

A

Accent, 39.
Addison, 136.
Adonis, 236.
Æschylus, 369.
Æsthetics, 119, 468.
Afghans, songs of the, 395.
Africa, songs of, 200, 204, 249 f., 252, 270 f., 289, 329, 394, 397 f.
Albania, poetry of, 217, 228.
Algeria, songs of, 203.
Allegory, 145, 307.
Allen, F. D., 85, 260.
Alliteration, 68 f., 75, 86 ff., 256, 267.
Amœbean, 123, 144, 200, 400 f., 408 ff., 458 f.
Animals, songs of, 8, 100.
Anthology, 32.
Arabic verse, 79.
Arabs, 395.
Arcadia, the, 61.
Aretino, 144.
Aristotle, 1, 42 ff., 113, 132, 136, 369 f., 433, 453, 459 f.
Armenia, songs of, 203.
Arnold, M., 410, 421, 468.
Arval hymn, 69, 260 f., 297 f., 334.
Aryan verse, 85 ff.
Ass, feast of the, 301.
Assyria, poetry of, 261.
Attila, 264; funeral of, 223 f.
Aubrey, 225, 289, 302, 304.
Augustine, St., 222.
Ausonius, 287 f.
Australia, songs of, 171, 330; *vocero* in, 248.

B

Babylon (ballad), 195 f.
Bacon, 33 f., 45, 435, 460.
Bagehot, 36, 169.
Bain, 57, 365.
Baldwin, J. M., 9, 16, 364, 384.
Ballad, 27 f., 64, 70, 72 f., 116, 130, 134, 156, 164 ff., 168 f., 172, 175, 314, 316 ff., 321, 327, 342, 415, 422, 454, 472; epithets in the, 193 ff.; making of the, 184; material of the, 179; passing of the, 164 ff., 177, 211, 271 f., 292 f., 303.
Ballade, 257.
Ballads, not indecent, 169 ff.; omissions in, 197 f.; rank in, 177; recited, 189, 326; style of, 189 ff.
Ballati, 231.
Ballet, 433.
Ball-playing, 97, 337.
Balzac, 466.
Barbour, 265.
Baring-Gould, 168, 342.
Barnes, Dr. Thomas, 50.
Barth, 360.
Bartsch, 242.
Basques, the, 234, 395.
Bastian, 330, 361, 385, 428.
Batteux, 108.
Baudelaire, 32, 59.
Baumgarten, 38.
Beattie, 35.
Beaurepaire, 293.
Bechtel, 449.
Bell, 307.
Béowulf, 193, 222 ff., 331.
Béranger, 140.
Berger, A. E., 136, 164.
Bergk, 85.
Bernheim, 362.
Berni, 457.
Bertrand, 32, 59.
Bible, 48, 56 ff., 124 f., 186 f., 226 f., 261 ff., 271, 361, 423.
Biedermann, 75 f., 256.
Biology, 13, 363 f.
Bion, elegy of, 237.
Bistrom, 188, 198, 211.
Blacksmith, songs of the, 276 f.
Blackwell, 131, 454.
Bladé, 203, 218, 233, 234 ff., 279, 341.
Blank verse, preaching in, 80.
Blankenburg, 433.
Blémont, 170, 382.
Boas, 96.
Boat-songs, 98, 265, 272 ff., 289 f.
Böckel, 70, 72, 110, 168, 185, 270 ff., 307.
Böhme, 182, 281, 283, 308, 328, 343, 415.
Bolte, 426.
Borrow, George, 234.

Borrowing in literature, 351 ff.
Bosanquet, 56.
Botocudos, 94 f., 189, 209, 312, 330, 374, 390 f., 421, 439, 463.
Bourdeau, 362.
Boynton, J. H., 317 f.
Brandl, 413.
Brand's *Antiquities*, 218, 276, 294, 296 f., 303 f., 306 f., 343
Branle, The, 341.
Brazilians, songs of the, 246 ff.
Breath-lengths, 94, 100 f.
Brenner, 406.
Breton ballads, 183.
Bright, J. W., 148.
Brinkmann, 452.
Brinton, D. G., 190, 253, 313 f.
Broadwood and Maitland, 294 f., 302.
Brown, Baldwin, 251, 367 f.
Brown, Dr. John, 96.
Brown, T. E., 410.
Browning, R., 30, 347.
Bruchmann, 64, 70, 171, 428 f.
Brücke, 81.
Brugmann, 445.
Brugsch, 236.
Brunetière, 6, 26 f., 377, 389.
Bücher, 10, 63, 107 ff., 270 ff., 345, 369, 373, 386, 459 f., 462, 464.
Buck, Dr. Gertrude, 446, 448.
Buckle, 127, 175.
Budde, 62, 186, 218, 226 f., 262.
Bugge, 180.
Bujeaud, 166, 258.
Burckhardt, 141, 144, 158, 160, 425, 455.
Burdach, 432.
Burden, 275, 316 ff.
Burette, 346.
Burns, 170, 209, 308, 410.
Bushmen, 90.

C

Cædmon, 403.
Calmet, 124 f.
Campbell, J. F., 72, 179, 192, 400.
Cante-fable, 71 f., 97.
Caracolu, 231.
Carlyle, 51, 59.
Carmen, 68.
Carmina Burana, 207 f., 323.
Carole, the, 341.
Carstanjen, 359.
Carver, 249, 333.
Casaubon, I., 44 f.
Castrén, 200.
Catullus, 207, 217, 220, 258, 382.
Cell, the, 357 f.
Celts, *vocero* of the, 239 ff.
Chambers, 323.
Chant, 80, 82 ff.
Chappell, 294, 305 f., 316, 319, 411.
Charles of Orleans, 150.
Charms, 205, 245, 283 f., 300.
Châteaubriand, 60.
Chaucer, 64, 146, 222, 229, 239, 447.
Child, Professor, 70, 164, 181, 307, 317, 319, 413 f.
Children, 9 ff., 102 ff.; games of, 209, 297, 322 ff., 335 f., 344, 429; songs of, 284.
China, drama in, 72; songs in, 282.
Chorus, 27, 67, 70, 83, 86, 91 ff., 100, 105, 186, 219, 221, 236 f., 238, 249, 257, 260, 262 f., 270 f., 295, 308 f., 315, 332, 420 f., 422, 425, 440, 442 ff., 450, 454, 467, 471; cereal, 255, 310; Greek, 72, 186, 257, 261, 369, 372.
Church, the mediæval, 153.
Cnut, song of, 275.
Coleridge, 35, 51, 421.
Colour in ballads, 213 f.
Commedia dell' Arte, 425.
Communal poetry, 116 ff., 122, 125, 129 ff., 158, 163 ff.; elements of, 172.
Comparative literature, 352 ff.; method, 31, 40.
Comparetti, 64, 177, 352, 355, 402, 443.
Comte, 152, 360, 378.
Condorcet, 10.
Consent, communal, 91, 101, 105, 107, 220 f., 255, 332, 348, 364, 376, 383, 386, 440, 461 f., 466.
Cook, voyages of, 331 f.
Coplas, 401, 405, 425.
Corsica, *vocero* in, 231 ff.
Counting-out rimes, 201, 203 f.
Courthope, Professor, 181.
Coussemaker, 226, 280, 302 f., 324.
Crane, 325.
Crescimbeni, 229, 341 f., 456.
Criticism, 6, 31, 216.
Cumulative songs, 98, 200 ff., 278.

D

Dance, 84 f., 105, 106, 147, 174, 184, 188, 202, 209, 217, 222 f., 231, 246, 248, 250, 260 f., 275, 291, 299, 301, 305, 311 ff., 318 ff., 322 ff., 327 ff., 354 f., 367, 370, 409, 412 f., 415, 428 ff., 431, 441, 443, 463 f., 466 f.; in churches, 335; by pairs, 321, 340 f.; and rhythm, 69, 78.
Dances, panic, 338; of the savage, 18 f., 90 ff., 95 f., 328 ff.

D'Annunzio, 60 f., 206, 230 f.
Dante, 45, 122 f., 142 f., 145, 341 f., 361, 468.
Darmesteter, 259, 395.
Darwin, 8, 24, 88, 357 f., 428, 431.
Daudet, 433.
Declamation, 82, 86 f., 99.
Degeneration, 16, 18.
Dekker, 47.
Déor, song of, 147, 266.
De Quincey, Thomas, 58.
Dialect, 190.
Dickens, 276 f.
Dilthey, 141.
Dithyramb, 66, 370.
Dixon, J. H., 294 f.
Donovan, 104 ff., 186, 345, 365, 368 f., 386, 392.
Don Quixote, 425.
Döring, 370, 420.
Douglas, Sir George, 167 f., 173.
Drack, M., 424.
Drama, 39, 66, 83, 106, 117, 189, 338, 424 ff., 434.
Drayton, 303.
Dryden, 59, 295.
Dualism, 116 ff., 136 ff.
Dubos, 35, 446.
Dunbar, 146, 151, 161.
Dunger, 406.
Düntzer, 68.

E

Earle, Professor, 197.
Ebert, 258, 306.
Egger, 215.
Egypt, poetry of, 271, 285; *vocero* in, 237 f.
Ehrenreich, 94 f.
Elements, The Four, 322 f.
Elliott, Ebenezer, 52.
Eloquence, 53.
Elyot, Sir T., 345 f.
Emerson, 35.
Emotion, 13, 83, 100, 105, 151 f., 155, 266, 364 f., 374 f., 386.
England, ballads of, 168, 183, 187, 326 f.
Enthusiasm, 126 f.
Epic, 39, 66, 117, 174, 179, 189, 324, 420, 422 ff., 434.
Erotic dances, 336, 367; songs, 8, 20, 88 f., 239, 401 f., 407, 420, 460.
Eskimo, 96 f.; songs of the, 243, 311, 313, 391, 400.
Esthonians, 272.
Ethnology, 14 ff., 92 ff., 375; evidences of, 19 ff., 22.
Ethology, 6.
Euphuism, 61.
Evolution, curves of, 26 ff., 84, 163, 172, 178, 422, 472.

F

Fabyan's Chronicle, 265.
Fame, 141 f.
Faroe Islands, songs of, 318 f., 337, 399 f., 428 f.
Fauriel, 217, 227, 415.
Fell, Dr., 80.
Festal origin of speech, 104 ff.
Finns, poetry of the, 166, 198, 213, 252, 270, 355, 402, 452.
Firmenich, 204, 219, 287 f., 292, 302, 308, 324, 408 ff.
Flanders, ballads in, 226, 294, 303, 324.
Fletcher, Alice C., 254; Rev. Mr., 308.
Flyting, 144, 200, 212, 227, 279, 287 f., 306 ff., 321, 391, 399 ff., 429, 458 f.
Folksong (see Ballad), 106.
Fontenelle, 117.
Foresinger, 315, 318 f., 327.
France, songs of, 139, 320, 325.
France, Anatole, 9, 139.
Francke, K., 152, 182.
Freericks, 259.
Freytag, 360.
Fuegians, 253.
Funeral, songs of the, see *Vocero*.

G

Gab, 331.
Gaelic ballads, 192.
Garnett, 425.
Gascoigne, 45.
Gascony, ballads and songs of, 203, 233, 235 f., 247, 279 f.
Gautier, 33, 359.
Gayley and Scott, 6, 54.
Geijer, 327.
Gender, 445 f.
Genius, 126.
Gerber, 370, 449, 452 f.
Germanic epic, 191, 198, 209, 447 f.; poetry, 64; verse, 86 ff.
Germany, ballads of, 168, 182 f., 190, 216.
Gesture, 330, 428, 431.
Giddings, F. H., 360, 372, 385.
Gnomic poetry, 95, 421.
Goethe, 2, 49, 73, 116 f., 118, 315, 410, 433.
Goldsmith, 36.
Goncourt, Journal des, 359, 433.
Gorgias, 66.
Gottsched, 10, 13, 64, 124.

Grasserie, R. de la, 76 ff.
Gray, T., 162, 197, 451.
Greek communal poetry, 266, 271, 284 f.; poetry, modern, 192, 217, 227, 273, 415.
Greenes Funeralls, 206.
Grimm, J., 65, 133 f., 136 f., 182, 256, 283, 300, 341, 350, 436, 439, 445, 449.
Groos, 102, 337, 365.
Grosse, 14, 18, 22, 90, 178, 239, 336, 345, 378 f., 381, 383, 385.
Grube, 299, 315.
Grundtvig, 167, 176, 275, 317.
Gruppe, 14, 443.
Guest, 316, 318.
Guilds, 142, 149, 153, 160, 165 f.
Gumplowicz, 15, 359, 378.
Gurney, Edmund, 55, 89, 256.
Guyau, 3, 40, 121, 348, 387.

H

Haeckel, 9.
Hahn, J. G., 217, 228.
Halliwell, 284.
Hamann, 125.
Hampson, 276, 301.
Hardy, Thomas, 25, 114, 292, 344.
Harmony, 92, 109.
Harrison, Frederic, 56.
Hartmann, von, 361.
Harvest, Highland, 289 f.
Harvest-home, 178, 280 f., 286, 291, 294 f., 309.
Harvey, Gabriel, 207.
Haym, 152, 382.
Hazlitt, 36.
Hebrew prophets, 262 f.
Hebrews, dance of, 336, 346.
Heckewelder, 309 f.
Hegel, 33, 53 f., 423.
Heine, 161, 410.
Heinzel, 159, 177, 209, 448.
Henderson, 181.
Hennequin, 6, 359, 378, 388.
Herder, 119, 122, 125 f., 131 f., 171, 346, 458.
Hero and Leander, 179, 196.
Herodotus, 238, 374.
Herrick, 305.
Hesiod, 216, 437.
Higginson, Colonel, 97 f.
Hildebrand Lay, 212.
Hirn, Y., 260, 328, 336, 460.
Historical school, 122 ff.
History, 53.
Hoffmann, 94; von Fallersleben, 269.
Hogg, James, 173.
Homer, 44, 49, 175, 221, 285, 333 f., 337, 361, 370, 382, 423, 437, 447.
Homogeneous community, 167 f., 176 ff., 244 f., 357, 374 ff., 443.
Hook, Theodore, 396.
Horace, 107, 142, 186, 404, 411.
Hudson, 366.
Hugo, Victor, 49, 121, 142 ff., 362.
Humboldt, W. von, 41, 133, 357, 382.
Humour, 159 ff., 464.
Hungary, poetry of, 64.
Hyde, Douglas, 404 f.
Hylas, 238.
Hymn, 153 f., 442 f.

I

"I," in children, 9.
"I," the, in ballads, 182 ff., 187 f.
"I," the, in the Psalms, 186 f.
Ibsen, 466.
Iceland, songs of, 318 f., 337, 400 f.
Imagination, 35, 37, 136, 391, 468 ff.
Imitation, 352, 362, 369, 375, 386 f.
Improvisation, 92, 95, 97, 113, 180, 199, 212 f., 222, 227, 234, 240, 273, 275, 287 ff., 292, 311, 355, 369 f., 394 ff., 396 ff., 401 ff., 404, 415 ff., 418 f., 421, 424 ff., 428 f., 432, 441, 455 ff.; two kinds of, 396.
Inarticulate sounds, 30, 253, 260.
Indians, American, 93, 189, 245 ff., 253 ff., 273, 309 ff., 313 f., 333 f., 394.
Individual, 139, 141 ff., 151, 153, 155, 183, 212, 371 ff., 377 ff., 381, 382 ff., 389, 391 ff., 393 f., 407, 421, 429, 432, 452, 464; and society, 110 f., 116, 126, 147.
Infant, 12 ff., 100.
Instinct, 355 f., 363 ff., 383.
Invention, 349 ff., 361, 386 f.
Iranian verse, 85.
Isis, *vocero* of, 237 f.
Italy, improvisation in, 424 ff., 455 ff.

J

Jacobowski, 11 ff., 254, 345.
Jacobs, Joseph, 71, 164.
Jacobsthal, 69, 93.
Japan, poetry of, 64; songs of, 282.
Jeanroy, 174, 179, 207, 258, 308, 320 f., 341 f., 401, 405.
Jeremiah, 230.
Jessopp, 286, 291.
Jews, poem of the, 205.
Jigs, 342, 426.
Job, 58, 261.
Johnson, Dr., 37, 289 f., 347.

Jonson, Ben, 34, 169, 316.
Junod, 105.

K

Kalevala (see Comparetti), 64.
Kawczynski, 349 ff.
Keane, A. H., 378.
Keasbey, L. M., 463.
Keats, 157.
Keening, 240 f.
Kenning, 191, 209, 452.
Khorovod, 327.
Kîna, the, 226 f.
Kind, sense of, 115, 348, 385 f., 472.
Kingsley, Miss, 254.
Kipling, 388, 452.
Kirn (see Harvest-home), 290 f.
Kleinpaul, 176.
Koester, 221.
Kögel, 74, 189, 218, 220, 261, 298 f., 340, 417.
Kollo, the, 339.
Krejči, 373 f.
Krohn, 166.

L

Labour, songs of, 70, 78, 91, 107 ff., 202 f., 269 ff., 317, 369, 402, 419, 450.
Lâc, 340.
Lafitau, 248, 252, 311.
La Motte, 433.
Lamprecht, 360.
Landstad, 166, 414, 418.
Lang, Andrew, 436.
Lang, H. R., 459.
Language, origin of, 392, 450.
Lapps, the, 92, 129.
Largess-shilling, the, 297.
Latin communal poetry, 271, 273, 283, 285, 404 f., 424.
Layamon, 265.
Le Bon, 6, 360, 377 f., 382.
Lefebvre, 2.
Legend, 189.
Lery, 246 ff., 252, 312 f.
Lescarbot, 247, 252, 333.
Lessing, 84.
Letourneau, 7, 11, 42, 308, 430, 447.
Leyser, 46.
Like Wil to Like, 342.
Limburg Chronicle, 182.
Linos, 236 f., 285.
Lippert, 437.
Literary evolution, 23.
Lithuania, songs of,
Lityerses, 238, 285.
Livy, 424.
Longinus, 53, 58, 79.
Loquin, 167.
Lost arts, 17.
Lotze, 365.
Lounsbury, T. R., 447.
Lowth, 47 f., 262, 346.
Lucian, 219, 222, 324, 336.
Lucretius, 299, 436.
Lundell, 418.
Lyke-wake, 239 f.
Lyngbye, 194, 232, 399.
Lyric, 39, 117, 147, 173, 420 ff., 431, 434; origin of, 8, 12.

M

McLennan, J. F., 22.
Maeterlinck, 60 f., 206.
Magic, 67, 283.
Mahomet, 1.
Maine, Sir H., 379.
Mallery, 428, 430.
Malmesbury, William of, 301.
Malory, 56.
Maneros, 238, 285.
Manley, J. M., 337.
Mannhardt, 238, 283, 294, 310, 343, 437.
Mansöngvar, 401.
Marcaggi, 229, 231 ff.
Marching-songs, 204, 269.
Masing, 119 f., 256.
Masson, 57.
Matriarchate, 10.
May songs, 281, 305 f.
Meier, John, 164.
Mendelssohn, Moses, 119.
Meredith, 114.
Mérimée, 231.
Metaphor, 161 f., 190 ff., 444 f.
Metre, 180.
Metres, origin of, 110.
Meumann, 81 ff., 88, 99.
Mexico, songs of, 334.
Meyer, E. H., 166 f., 216, 272, 279, 283, 300, 306, 417.
Meyer, Gustav, 172, 181, 405, 407 ff.
Meyer, R. M., 176, 188, 209, 256 f., 259 f., 267, 447, 452.
Michel, F., 183, 234, 395.
Milieu, the, 358.
Mill, J. S., 51 f.
Milton, 49, 207.
Minstrel, the, 181, 215 f., 272, 315, 322, 403, 454.
Mitchill, Senator, 19 ff.
Möller, 86 ff., 267.
Mommsen, 464.

Monboddo, 50, 354, 357.
Montaigne, 6, 129 f.
Montanus, 296.
More, Sir T., 427.
Morgan, Lloyd, 121, 363, 365, 387.
Morhof, 124.
Mucke, 378.
Müllenhoff, 154, 218, 222, 267 f., 284, 336 f., 388, 437.
Müller, D. H., 262.
Müller, K. O., 265.
Müller, Max, 136, 436, 440, 455.
Müller, W., 301.
Muse, 106.
Music, as muse, 106; in poetry (see Rhythm), 55.
Musset, A. de, 453.
Myth, 284, 293, 434 ff.

N

Nash, Tom, 61, 280, 427.
Nature, 25, 126, 468 ff.; and art, 118 ff., 133, 135, 137, 165; in ballads, 188, 192 f., 321, 413.
Nauze, M. de la, 124.
Negro slaves, 97 f.
Neidhart, 323.
Neniae, 221, 244.
Neocorus, 218, 318 f., 321, 340 f.
Nerthus, 299 f., 339.
Newell, W. W., 179, 284.
Newman, Cardinal, 446.
Newton, 2.
Nietzsche, 24, 59, 371 ff.
Nigra, Count, 180, 185, 405.
Nisard, 169.
Noiré, 365, 392.
Norden, 65 ff., 74, 87, 145, 403.
Northall, 160, 276, 278, 284.
Northbrooke, 305.

O

Objective, 139 f., 158.
Ontogenesis, 9 ff.
Opera, 424, 431.
Oratory, 79 f.
Ortoli, 231 f., 279.
Overbury, 277, 291.

P

Pellissier, 461.
Pantomime, 336, 429 ff.
Parallelism, 62, 214.
Paris, Gaston, 150, 174, 185, 334, 341, 352.
Park, Mungo, 397 f., 422.
Pastourelle, 326.
Pater, Walter, 55, 61, 258.
Patten, 147.
Paul, 81, 360.
Peacock, T. L., 1, 10.
Pearson, 8, 10, 216.
Peele, George, 281.
Pennant, 239, 270.
Pennillion, 403.
People, mind of the, 360 f.
Percy, Bishop, 181.
Perfetti, 456 ff.
Persia, Comedy in, 428.
Pervigilium Veneris, 258.
Petrarch, 2, 45, 145.
Pfannenschmid, 238, 283, 286, 292 f., 343.
Phillips, 118.
Phœnician *vocero*, 236 f.
Phylogenesis, 9 ff.
Planch, 229.
Plato, 1, 33 f., 460.
Play, 365 ff., 369.
Play-excitement, 368.
Plutarch, 66, 270, 395.
Poe, 51.
Poet, the, 347, 388, 390 ff., 406, 433, 453 f., 465, 470.
Poetic sentence, 33, 53.
Poetics, 7.
Poetry, art of, 3; attacks on, 1 ff.; beginnings of, 4, 123, 464 ff.; biological basis of, 8; communal elements of, 433; defence of, 1 ff.; definition of, 4, 30, 51, 118, 158; earliest form of, 210 f., 314; elements of, 29, 163, 172; historical treatment of, 5; Latin, 141; laws in, 74 f.; meaning of, 4; reading of, 63; and science, 2; singing of, 64, 72, 75 f., 139, 173, 180, 272.
Poland, songs of, 270.
Pope, 47.
Porthan, 198 ff., 269 f.
Portugal, songs of, 208, 320 f.
Posnett, 7, 142, 257, 260, 265, 336, 381 f., 440.
Praefica, 225, 229, 248.
Praetorius, 242.
Prickard, A. O., 43.
Processions, communal, 224, 298 ff., 304.
Prose, artistic, 65 ff.; periodic, 69; poems in, 32, 38, 41, 59 ff.; priority of, 63 ff., 75 ff.; rhythmical, 67 ff.; and verse, line between, 62.
Psalms, the, 36, 153, 186 f., 209, 261 f., 420, 438.

Psychology, 364 ff., 374 f., 8 ff., 81.
Pulci, 455.
Pulszky, 26, 383.

Q

Quadrio, 43, 455.
Quatrains (see *Schnaderhüpfl*), 213, 418.

R

Radloff, 71, 211 ff.
Rain-song, the, 300.
Ralston, 166.
Ranke, 360.
Recitative, 91 f., 104, 310.
Réclus, 378.
Refrain, 92, 97, 129, 174, 183, 190, 209, 225, 230, 232, 253 f., 256 ff., 287, 291, 308 f., 313 ff., 354, 415 f., 430, 443, 450; in Germanic poetry, 267; in Greek, 266; nature of, 314 ff.
Refrains, agricultural, 279 ff.
Reifferscheid, 288.
Relativity, 14, 16.
Religious rites, 204, 220, 238, 260 f., 282 ff., 292, 300 f., 305, 313, 333 ff., 338 f., 392, 436, 444.
Renan, 2.
Repetition, 76, 193 ff., 205 ff., 231 f., 236, 245, 251, 255 f., 313, 416, 451; classes of, 206; incremental, 194 ff., 198 f., 208 f., 213 f., 252, 254 f., 319, 325 f., 423.
Rhythm, 246, 332, 345, 348 ff., 356, 383, 386, 390, 421, 432, 463, 465 ff.; and music, 79; nature of, 99 ff., 109; derived from prose, 63 ff.; as a social factor, 93.
Ribot, 100, 104, 140, 151, 364 f., 369, 384.
Riddles, 212, 452.
Rime, 56, 68 f., 75.
Rimed prose, 61.
Ritson, 307.
Robin Hood, ballads of, 327.
Romance, 179 f.
Romanes, 364, 398.
Romans, dance of the (see Arval hymn), 334, 345.
Ronsard, 45, 63, 122, 146, 150.
Rose, Romance of the, 362.
Rosières, 258 f., 266.
Rosenberg, 275, 317, 353 f.
Roumania, ballads of, 72.
Round, the, 341 f.
Rousseau, 127, 151, 157, 389.
Rückert, 315.
Rudimentary growths in literature, 17.
Rundâs, 406.
Ruodlieb, 341.
Ruscelli, 456.
Russia, ballads of, 166, 188, 198, 327.

S

Sachs, Hans, 281.
Sainte-Beuve, 6, 148 f., 388, 453, 465, 468.
St. Evremond, 447.
St. Francis, prayer of, 155, 469.
St. Victor, 231, 233 f.
Saintsbury, Professor, 55.
Sandys, 303.
Sappho, 464.
Sarcasm, songs of, 288 f.
Satire, 404 f.
Satura Menippea, 73.
Saturnian verse, 68.
Savages, 9, 11, 13 ff., 19 ff., 65, 82, 90 ff., 95 f., 127, 374 ff.; character of, 111; poetry of, 252 ff., 308 ff., 370.
Scaliger, J. C., 3, 34, 43 f., 122 f.
Scandinavia, songs of, 188, 191, 270, 353 f.
Scéaf, 284 f.
Scherer, 8, 88 f., 133 f., 178, 336, 349, 381, 441, 446 f., 452, 454, 459 f.
Schiller, 49, 113, 119, 375.
Schipper, 315.
Schlegel, A. W., 9, 40 ff., 48, 101, 108, 119, 122, 132 ff., 254, 327, 346, 369 f., 396, 415, 423, 432, 435, 437.
Schlegel, F., 5, 38.
Schleicher, 398.
Schleiermacher, 39, 117, 420.
Schmeller, J. A., 405 f.
Schnaderhüpfl, 144, 200, 297, 299, 403, 405 ff.
Schoolcraft, 245, 248 f., 308 ff.
Schopenhauer, 371.
Schröder, 68.
Schuchardt, 403.
Schultze, 9, 374 f., 383.
Schwab, 427.
Schwartz, W., 438.
Science, 126.
Scotland, ballads of, 173, 183, 327; songs of, 265, 273.
Scott, Sir W., 156, 168 f., 173, 181, 414.
Seasons, poetry of the, 470.
Selden, 2, 80.
Sentiment, 25 f., 147 f., 156, 159, 421, 432.
Sermons in verse, 80.
Serranas, 459.
Servia, songs of, 299 f.
Seville, dance in cathedral of, 335.
Shaftesbury, 46, 126.
Shakspere, 113 f., 316, 426 f., 470 ff.
Shaman, 221, 244, 338, 379, 392 f., 429, 442 f.

Shelley, Mary, 253.
Shelley, Percy Bysshe, 10, 336.
Siberia, songs of, 211 ff., 243.
Sidney, 34 f., 122, 130.
Siebs, 74.
Sievers, 62, 86 ff., 267.
Silius Italicus, 336.
Simile, 446 f.
Simonides, 220.
Simplicity, 190.
Simrock, 435.
Sittl, 221, 431.
Skeat, 291.
Skolion, 395, 403.
Smend, 186.
Smith, Adam, 14, 23, 50, 96, 256, 336, 354.
Smythe, H. W., 217, 258, 266, 285.
Society, 220, 368, 449 f., 462 f., 473; and poetry, 1, 7, 52, 89 f., 101, 120.
Sonnet, 145.
Souriau, 55, 350.
Southey's *Doctor*, 278.
Spanish Tragedy, the, 427.
Spencer, H., 18, 89 f., 243, 328, 350, 365, 372, 377 ff., 383, 385, 391, 398, 437, 442.
Spencer, Dr. John, 346.
Spens, Sir Patrick, 172, 472.
Spenser, E., 118, 122, 206, 241.
Spinning-songs, 277 ff.
"Spirituals," 98.
Spontaneity, 65, 350 f., 355 ff., 369, 373.
Stedman, E. C., 120.
Steenstrup, 187, 190, 327, 343.
Stein, von, 427.
Steinthal, 352, 361.
Stev, 401, 418 f.
Stevenson, R. L., 314.
Storm, G., 355.
Stornelli, 401, 405.
Strabo, 64, 66.
Strambotti, 401, 404 f., 418.
Street-songs, 166, 169.
Style of poetry, 35, 54, 161 f., 189 ff., 434, 444 ff.
Sublime, the, 53.
Sully, 365.
Summer and winter, songs of, 306 f.
Swift, 61, 375.
Sword-dance, 268, 336 f.
Symonds, J. A., 426.
Sympathy, 115, 471 ff.
Syria, poetry of, 218, 227, 236.

T

Tacitus, 86, 205, 299, 336 f., 392.
Taine, 6, 359, 388.
Talvj, 167, 182, 395.
Tammuz, 237.
Tarde, 137, 348, 351, 356 ff., 362 f., 374, 376 f., 380, 423, 460.
Tartars, songs of the, 71.
Télémaque, 38, 46, 60.
Temple, Sir William, 46, 467.
Ten Brink, 176, 213, 306, 326, 361, 403, 424.
Tennyson, 82, 156, 190, 220, 388.
Texte, 359, 389.
Theocritus, 405, 418.
Thought, 83, 113, 139, 152, 374 f., 383, 420 f.
Thucydides, 17.
Tibullus, 277, 299.
Ticknor, 425.
Tille, 276.
Tirade, 211.
Tobler, 188, 194.
Tragedy, Greek, 257, 338, 369 f., 371 ff., 424, 444.
Translations in prose, 49, 55, 57 ff.
Trapp, 46.
Turgot, 15, 59, 126.
Tusser, 297.
Twining, 1, 43.
Tylor, E. B., 18, 24, 204, 238, 283, 379, 428, 436 ff.

U

Ubi Sunt, 148 ff.
Uhland, 220, 281, 298, 306, 338, 343, 415, 436.
Usener, 69, 84, 213, 350, 421, 423.

V

Valentin, 319.
Variation, 194, 209 ff., 213 f., 236, 256, 408 f., 423, 451.
Varro, 66.
Veddahs, the, 330, 390 f., 463, 466.
Veisa, 355.
Verbs, 450 ff.
Vergil, 58, 73, 207, 298, 306, 334, 404 f., 418.
Verse, oldest European, 85.
Verse (see Rhythm), 54.
Vico, 10, 128, 460.
Vigfusson and Powell, 257.
Vignoli, 440.
Vigny, De, 154, 373.
Villemarqué, 183 f.
Villon, 148 ff., 161.
Vinesauf, 229.
Vocero, 100, 168, 219 ff., 321, 419; literary form of, 228 f.; of savages, 243 ff.
Vogüé, E. M., de, 115, 144.
Vossius, G. J., 44, 123.
Vossius, I., 46.

W

Wackernagel, W., 320.
Wagner, R., 103, 120 f., 171, 327 f., 430.
Waitz, 327, 329, 379 f.
Wakes, 303.
Wales, songs of, 288 f.
Wallace, A. R., 365, 403.
Wallaschek, 13, 91 ff., 99 ff., 260, 328 f., 366, 381.
Walther von der Vogelweide, 430, 470.
War, songs of, 86, 268 f., 311, 388.
War-dance, 311, 331 f.
Wasf, the, 219.
Warton, Joseph, 47.
Watts, Theodore, 57.
Webster, John, 59.
Wedding, songs of, 202 f., 216 f., 324.
Weismann, 4, 363.
Werner, R. M., 420.
Westphal, 84.
Whately, 42, 48, 51 f.
Wheeler, B. I., 445.
Williams, Talcott, 16.
Wilmanns, 85, 87.
Witchell, 364.
Wold, 293.
Wolf, F., 71, 167, 176, 257 f., 280, 315, 327, 340.
Wolff, Eugen, 164, 432.
Women, songs of, 199 f., 222, 226, 228, 240 f., 250, 263 f., 269 f., 329, 339, 341, 397 f., 419, 464.
Woodberry, G. E., 162.
Wordsworth, 150, 155, 162, 451.
Wright, Thomas, 303, 307.
Writing, invention of, 252.
Wundt, 360, 363, 366, 428.

X

Xenophon, 34, 337.

Z

Zell, 198, 260, 271, 283, 404.